W9-ABQ-499

The Psychology of Gender

The Psychology of Gender

SECOND EDITION

Edited by

ALICE H. EAGLY
ANNE E. BEALL
ROBERT J. STERNBERG

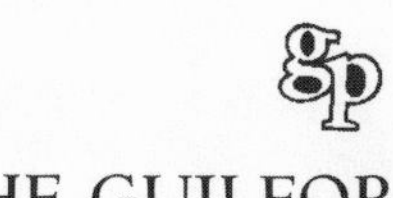

THE GUILFORD PRESS
NEW YORK LONDON

A Division of Guilford Publications, Inc.
72 Spring Street, New York, NY 10012
www.guilford.com

Printed in the United States of America

This book is printed on acid-free paper.

Last digit is print number: 9 8 7 6 5 4 3 2 1

Library of Congress Cataloging-in-Publication Data

The psychology of gender / edited by Alice H. Eagly, Anne E. Beall, Robert J. Sternberg.— 2nd ed.
p. cm.
Includes bibliographical references and indexes.
ISBN 1-57230-983-0 (hardcover : alk. paper)
1. Sex differences (Psychology)—Textbooks. I. Eagly, Alice Hendrickson. II. Beall, Anne E. III. Sternberg, Robert J.
BF692.2.P764 2004
155.3′3—dc22

2003023603

About the Editors

Alice H. Eagly is Professor of Psychology and faculty fellow in the Institute for Policy Research at Northwestern University. She received PhD and MA degrees from the University of Michigan and a BA from Radcliffe College of Harvard University. Dr. Eagly is particularly known for her research on the psychology of gender and the psychology of attitudes. She received the Distinguished Scientist Award from the Society of Experimental Social Psychology and the Donald Campbell Award for Distinguished Contribution to Social Psychology from the Society for Social and Personality Psychology.

Anne E. Beall is President of Beall Research and Training, a firm that applies principles and findings from psychology to the business world. She received MS, MPhil, and PhD degrees in social psychology from Yale University and a BA from the University of Delaware. Dr. Beall conducts training seminars on gender, nonverbal communications, persuasion, sales, and detecting deception. She also conducts marketing research on a variety of strategic business issues. She has held positions at The Boston Consulting Group and National Analysts and has written book chapters and articles about emotional expressions, consumer psychology, and marketing.

Robert J. Sternberg is IBM Professor of Psychology and Education at Yale University. He received a PhD from Stanford University and a BA from Yale. Dr. Sternberg has published over 950 books, articles, and book chapters and was the 2003 President of the American Psychological Association.

Contributors

Albert Bandura, PhD, Department of Psychology, Stanford University, Stanford, California

Anne E. Beall, PhD, Beall Research and Training, Chicago, Illinois

Leslie C. Bell, MA, MSW, Department of Sociology, University of California–Berkeley, Berkeley, California

Deborah L. Best, PhD, Department of Psychology, Wake Forest University, Winston-Salem, North Carolina

Chris Bourg, PhD, Department of Sociology, Stanford University, Stanford, California

Victoria Brescoll, MS, Department of Psychology, Yale University, New Haven, Connecticut

Kay Bussey, PhD, Department of Psychology, Macquarie University, Sydney, Australia

Mary Crawford, PhD, Department of Psychology, University of Connecticut, Storrs, Connecticut

Alice H. Eagly, PhD, Department of Psychology, Northwestern University, Evanston, Illinois

Shira Gabriel, PhD, Department of Psychology, State University of New York at Buffalo, Buffalo, New York

Wendi L. Gardner, PhD, Department of Psychology, Northwestern University, Evanston, Illinois

Elizabeth Hampson, PhD, Department of Psychology and Graduate Program in Neuroscience, University of Western Ontario, London, Ontario, Canada

Melissa Hines, PhD, Department of Psychology, City University, London, United Kingdom

Mary C. Johannesen-Schmidt, PhD, Department of Behavioral and Social Sciences, Oakton Community College, Des Plaines, Illinois

Douglas T. Kenrick, PhD, Department of Psychology, Arizona State University, Tempe, Arizona

Marianne LaFrance, PhD, Department of Psychology, Yale University, New Haven, Connecticut

Jeanne Marecek, PhD, Department of Psychology, Swarthmore College, Swarthmore, Pennsylvania

Scott D. Moffat, PhD, Department of Psychology and Institute of Gerontology, Wayne State University, Detroit, Michigan

Florrie Fei-Yin Ng, MA, Department of Psychology, University of Illinois, Urbana–Champaign, Illinois

Elizabeth Levy Paluck, MS, Department of Psychology, Yale University, New Haven, Connecticut

Eva M. Pomerantz, PhD, Department of Psychology, University of Illinois, Urbana–Champaign, Illinois

Danielle Popp, MA, Department of Psychology, University of Connecticut, Storrs, Connecticut

Felicia Pratto, PhD, Department of Psychology, University of Connecticut, Storrs, Connecticut

Cecilia L. Ridgeway, PhD, Department of Sociology, Stanford University, Stanford, California

Robert J. Sternberg, PhD, Department of Psychology, Yale University, New Haven, Connecticut

Jill M. Sundie, PhD, Department of Marketing, University of Houston, Houston, Texas

Jennifer J. Thomas, MA, Department of Psychology, Wake Forest University, Winston–Salem, North Carolina

Melanie R. Trost, PhD, Department of Communication Studies, University of Montana, Missoula, Montana

Angela Walker, MA, Department of Psychology, Quinnipiac University, Hamden, Connecticut

Qian Wang, MA, Department of Psychology, University of Illinois, Urbana–Champaign, Illinois

Wendy Wood, PhD, Department of Psychology, Texas A & M University, College Station, Texas

Contents

1

Introduction

ANNE E. BEALL
ALICE H. EAGLY
ROBERT J. STERNBERG

> Class, race, sexuality, gender—and all other categories by which we categorize and dismiss each other—need to be excavated from the inside.
>
> —ALLISON (1994, pp. 35–36)

Dorothy Allison, novelist and feminist, and many other authors and scientists have written about how consequential social categories such as gender are to life experiences. Gender functions as a social label that is applied to people instantly and generally automatically, without deliberation. And much of the power of gender emerges from the universality of this categorization. Although scholars have pointed to the wisdom of considering that humanity comprises more than two sexes and is in fact a continuum of people between the dimorphic ideals of man and woman (e.g., Fausto-Sterling, 2000), dividing the world into men and women is fundamental to all cultures. For all but a small proportion of individuals who are born intersexed, sex-typed bodies place individuals in the social category of female or male. Although there are multiple ways to construe gender personally, being born into one of these categories and not the other has a profound impact on how individuals are treated, what they expect of themselves, and how they lead their lives.

That gender has considerable impact on people's lives is obvious when viewed from the perspective of aggregate global statistics. Consider the following findings (United Nations Development Programme, 2002):

- Women constitute 64% of all illiterate adults.
- Women's income is 75% that of men for comparable hours of paid employment.
- The proportion of men in national parliaments is 86%.
- Every year, approximately 500,000 women die in childbirth.

These statistics underscore the different lives that women and men lead. Gender permeates most aspects of human life and often manifests itself in terms of female disadvantage. As editors of this volume, which addresses the question of why gender is so important, we believe that the discipline of psychology provides a major part of the answer. Because research and theory on the psychology of gender provide powerful insights into the differences and similarities in the lives of women and men, we decided to edit a second edition of *The Psychology of Gender* to share the advances that have occurred within this field in the past decade. These advances are impressive.

In this edition, as in the earlier one, we faced the problem of our inability to include all topics that fall under the rubric of the psychology of gender. Therefore, we decided to produce a book whose main focus is on sex differences and similarities in cognition, personality, and behavioral tendencies. This question of difference and similarity has been the core gender issue for psychologists in psychology departments for many decades and is crucial for answering the question of why women and men so often lead different lives. If men and women were the same except for genitalia and some details of secondary sex characteristics, women would not end up being positioned differently in society, generally with less access to resources than men. By focusing on similarity and difference, we are leaving out other, very important research areas within which psychologists have studied the particulars of the lives and experiences of women and men—for example, research on sex discrimination, sexual harassment, and mental health. Thus, we realize that this book does not (and, practically speaking, could not) cover all that is important to understanding gender, although we have adopted the inclusive title, *The Psychology of Gender.*

DIFFERING PERSPECTIVES ON THE PSYCHOLOGY OF GENDER

Since the first edition of this book was published in 1993, much has changed in the study of the psychology of gender. Far more research is executed by a larger and more intellectually diverse group. Many authors of these chapters would not have been recognized as gender researchers 10 years ago, and some of their chapters present either entirely new perspectives on gender or substantially revamped versions of older perspectives. Even perspectives that were well known 10 years ago have matured and spawned new work. Although the authors of these chapters are at various career stages, all are currently active investigators of the psychology of gender. Their perspectives are developing and producing new research. Because these authors represent many different theoretical perspectives about gender, readers of this book should get a sense of the challenge and excitement of intermingling theories that emanate from very different assumptions and research traditions.

In sharpening our mission of presenting the best work on similarity and difference, we planned a book that fosters exchange between psychologists who represent different subareas—especially psychobiology and developmental, social, and cross-cultural psychology. Given this breadth, contributors' chapters vary in the particular approaches and specific questions they pose. By studying diverse perspectives within a single book, scholars and students should be stimulated to think about gender in ways that bridge these perspectives. Although some of these perspectives may appear to compete with one another, we regard the different viewpoints in this volume as a collection of perspectives with one overarching set of questions: Why, how, and when does gender have an impact on life?

We hope that the notable range of our book fosters healthy and open exchange between researchers in biological and sociocultural camps. In the past, researchers representing one of these emphases have often remained isolated from and suspicious of those representing other emphases. It is obvious to us that both the biology with which people are born and the society into which they are born must be understood in their interactive impact on the lives of both sexes. Given the synergies between biology and life experience in society, a one-sided emphasis on one set of variables brings even less than a partial understanding. Therefore, we have designed this book to be wide-ranging, in the hope that biologically inclined psychologists and students of psychology will contemplate the sociocultural chapters, and that socioculturally inclined psychologists will contemplate the biological chapters. And we hope that persons in both camps will give particular attention to the chapters that attempt to integrate aspects of biological and sociocultural causation. The future of the psychology of gender will emerge from these biosocial interactions.

NEW COMFORT WITH THE QUESTION OF SIMILARITY AND DIFFERENCE

Although readers of this volume will not encounter harmonious interrelations among all of the chapters, they will find that all authors appear to be comfortable addressing the question of similarity and difference. When the first edition was published, many psychologists were profoundly uncomfortable with this question, especially from a feminist perspective. Their fear was that, in our unequal world of female disadvantage, difference would imply deficiencies of women, whose interests would be better served by psychologists either claiming that similarity prevails or looking elsewhere for their research questions (Eagly, 1995). The greater comfort with the similarity versus difference question, at least among many gender psychologists in the United States, may reflect the remarkable upward shift in the status of women in the last decades. Perhaps as a result of this shift, contemporary discussions of gender in the media in recent years have begun to feature as many stories of female advantage and male disadvantage as of female disadvantage and male advantage. For example, the author of *Business Week's* cover story, "New Gender Gap: From Kindergarten to Grad School, Boys Are Becoming the Second Sex," despaired about growing male disadvantage and maintained that "men could become losers in a global economy that values mental power over might" (Conlin, 2003, p. 78). With less fear that the study of sex differences would harm women, scientists have been freed to take a close look at the causes and consequences of similarity and difference.

Stimulated by the sophisticated quantification of the meta-analysis (Lipsey & Wilson, 2001), research psychologists now think of the similarities and differences of women and men as a continuum, not as a dichotomous arrangement whereby the groups are either similar or different. That dichotomous way of thinking reflected an older philosophy about statistics, whereby a comparison between the sexes was judged by its statistical significance, with a verdict of significance indicating a difference, and one of nonsignificance indicating no difference. With the acceptance of the idea that effect sizes provide a far more meaningful metric than significance tests for understanding difference and similarity, the question is not whether men and women are psychologically different or the same. Instead, the question has become the extent to which the distributions of men and women are overlapping. Sometimes researchers find no difference between the sexes and completely overlapping distributions; other times, they find small but not necessarily unimportant differences and largely overlapping distributions; and still other times, they find larger differences and less overlapping distributions. Given this continuum understanding of similarity and difference, the debate about whether sex differences "exist" is now dead among research psychologists. Much debate remains, however, about whether small differences are important or unimportant.

THE GROWTH OF THEORY

One of the notable developments in the psychology of gender is that researchers are posing increasingly subtle questions about the contextual patterning of difference and similarity. Under what conditions are differences smaller or larger, and under what conditions does similarity or near-similarity prevail? It is impossible to make progress on this question without good theory about how sex and gender interact with other variables. As the chapters of this book illustrate, theory has been improving, allowing psychologists to understand the variability of sex difference and similarity across person and situational variation.

Especially important in terms of relatively new theoretical developments is the focus of some psychologists on the question of the ultimate origins of sex differences—that is, the distal causes in addition to the proximal causes that lie in one's personal history of socialization and current environment of physiological regulation, self-regulation, and reactions to social pressures. In the past, psychologists dealt primarily with such relatively proximal causes of sex differences and similarities, thereby giving only partial answers to causal questions. For example, social psychologists often emphasized the effects of stereotypes and social expectations but did not consider why those expectations have certain content. If they did identify the source of the expectations, generally in social roles and other aspects of social arrangements, they did not address in any depth the question of why those social arrangements exist.

Explaining the origins of sex differences and similarities challenges psychologists and other scientists, because theories of origins involve multiple levels of causation in which proximal causes are embedded within more distal causes (Wood & Eagly, 2002). Use of knowledge from these differing levels of causality requires intellectual breadth on the part of investigators and interdisciplinary investigations that do not rely solely on constructs within one subdiscipline of psychology, or even within psychology itself. With the growth of evolutionary psychology, some definite answers have been provided to the question of the ultimate origins of sex differences (e.g., Kenrick, Trost, & Sundie, Chapter 4, this volume; Mealey, 2000). These answers have stimulated other psychologists to provide alternative answers—for example, Eagly, Wood, and Johannesen-Schmidt's (Chapter 12, this volume) alternative biosocial origin theory is included in this book. The biologically oriented authors whose work is also featured in this book help build understanding of the ultimate origins of psychological sex differences (Hines, Chapter 2, this volume; Hampson & Moffat, Chapter 3, this volume).

INTRODUCTION TO THE CHAPTERS

In the first two chapters that follow our introduction, the authors discuss biological influences on the behavior of women and men. Chapter 2, by Melissa Hines, emphasizes the organizational effects of gonadal hormones. She explores the extent to which the prenatal environment and exposure to estrogen and androgen influence human brain development and, therefore, gender identity, personality, sexual orientation, and social behavior. In Chapter 3, Elizabeth Hampson and Scott D. Moffat consider the activational effects of hormones that circulate in the bodies of women and men. These hormones affect the expression of various behavioral and cognitive functions. Understanding the organizational and activational effects of hormones is a rapidly developing area of psychobiology, in which progress is speeded in part by advances in technology that allow more precise measurements of physiological states and processes.

In Chapter 4, Douglas T. Kenrick, Melanie R. Trost, and Jill M. Sundie take the evolutionary psychology approach to gender. They assert that evolutionary processes account for many current sex differences in behavior and, drawing heavily on sexual selection theory (Trivers, 1972), argue that modern male and female behavior has its roots in the differential parental investment of men and women.

The book then features researchers who have explicitly considered developmental issues. In Chapter 5, Kay Bussey and Albert Bandura discuss the various processes by which children are socialized to become men and women. Important in their approach is the principle that children do not passively absorb gender roles from society but are important actors who cognitively construct the categories of gender and the man or woman they will become. In Chapter 6, Eva M. Pomerantz, Florrie Fei-Yin Ng, and Qian Wang explicate the implications of the clear-cut behavioral sex differences that appear in early childhood. They argue that although parents socialize children, the sex-typed attributes of children are important influences on the effects of socialization pressures.

In Chapter 7, Leslie C. Bell reviews the remarkable growth of the psychoanalytic perspective in successive waves of scholarship by feminist psychoanalytic theorists. She examines how unconscious and unresolved conflicts within childhood influence personalities, producing not only certain universal features but also endless variety in the specific manifestations of gender.

In Chapter 8, Wendi L. Gardner and Shira Gabriel introduce the concepts of relational and collective interdependence and argue that men and women emphasize different forms of interdependence, with women oriented relationally and men, collectively. These different ways of being "social" influence how men and women view themselves and behave with others.

In Chapter 9, Jeanne Maracek, Mary Crawford, and Danielle Popp discuss the social constructionist view of gender. This perspective presents the multiple ways in which our understanding of gender is a social product. Thus, individuals favor differing versions of gender, each of which is the result of language, cultural beliefs, and discourse among people. The social constructionists challenge our understandings of gender and maintain that both gender and sexuality are more fluid and complex than the representations provided by most other theories.

Relative to issues of gender and power, in Chapter 10, Cecilia L. Ridgeway and Chris Bourg discuss expectation states theory, a social psychological theory with important implications not only for explicating gender but also for understanding other social cleavages, such as race and social class. These authors contend that gender, like certain other human attributes, is inextricably linked with status through consensual stereotypes. When status beliefs are salient in goal-oriented contexts, they lead to hierarchy by which gender inequalities develop in assertiveness, power, influence, and esteem. Chapter 11, by Felicia Pratto and Angela Walker, also addresses the issue of men's greater social power. As they point out, in no known society do women wield more overall power than men, and they describe four bases of power and contend that all of these are disproportionately held by men.

In Chapter 12, Alice H. Eagly, Wendy Wood, and Mary C. Johannesen-Schmidt present and illustrate the social role theory of sex differences and similarities by explaining its implications for mate selection. These authors argue that, in general, sex differences in social behavior arise from the distribution of men and women into social roles within a society. The different positions of men and women in the social structure yield sex-differentiated behavior through a variety of proximal, mediating processes that include socialization and the formation of gender roles. Therefore, as men and women become more similarly positioned in social roles in postindustrial societies, sex differences in mate selection preferences erode.

In Chapter 13, Deborah L. Best and Jennifer J. Thomas provide an overview of the cross-cultural approach to understanding gender. Their review of cross-cultural studies indicates that male and female stereotypes exist in all societies, as does a gender division of labor. Yet their research on gender stereotypes across cultures reveals both the rigidity and malleability of gender.

Finally, Marianne LaFrance, Elizabeth Levy Paluck, and Victoria Brescoll, in Chapter 14, present commentary on the totality of the chapters. They provide a critical perspective that recognizes progress in the psychology of gender but urges attention to issues that have been insufficiently addressed. This stimulating chapter should help to bring gender researchers forward to new issues and richer understandings in the coming decades.

As the chapters of this book reveal, numerous valuable perspectives on gender are insufficiently integrated into broader theories. A complete account of the psychology of gender will ultimately incorporate insights from all of these perspectives. There is much more to know—more questions to ask and many more answers needed. Therefore, we hope that readers are stimulated and challenged by these chapters, and that many readers will personally contribute to the psychology of gender in the coming years.

REFERENCES

Allison, D. (1994). *Skin: Talking about sex, class and literature.* Ithaca, NY: Firebrand Books.

Conlin, M. (2003, May 26). The new gender gap: From kindergarten to grad school, boys are becoming the second sex. *Business Week*, p. 78f. Retrieved July 3, 2002, from *http://www.businessweek.com/@Suqvqiyql4La*w8a/magazine/content/03_21/b3834001_mz001.htm*

Eagly, A. H. (1995). The science and politics of comparing women and men. *American Psychologist, 50,* 145–158.

Fausto-Sterling, A. (2000). The five sexes, revisited. *Sciences, 40*(4), 18–23.

Lipsey, M. W., & Wilson, D. B. (2001). *Practical meta-analysis.* Thousand Oaks, CA: Sage.

Mealey, L. (2000). *Sex differences: Developmental and evolutionary strategies.* San Diego: Academic Press.

Trivers, R. (1972). Parental investment and sexual selection. In B. Campbell (Ed.), *Sexual selection and the descent of man: 1871–1971* (pp. 136–179). Chicago: Aldine.

Wood, W., & Eagly, A. H. (2002). A cross-cultural analysis of the behavior of women and men: Implications for the origins of sex differences. *Psychological Bulletin, 128, 699–727.*

United Nations Development Programme. (2002). *UNDP human development report: Deepening democracy in a fragmented world.* New York: Oxford University Press.

2

Androgen, Estrogen, and Gender

Contributions of the Early Hormone Environment to Gender-Related Behavior

MELISSA HINES

The amniocentesis had revealed a Y chromosome and no chromosomal errors, so Samantha and Richard were expecting to take a healthy baby boy home from the hospital. His name—William, after Samantha's father—had been chosen, the nursery was decorated with trains, and blue clothes filled the bureau drawers. However, when the baby was born, the pediatrician congratulated the new parents on their beautiful baby girl. What had happened?

Samantha and Richard's baby had an extremely rare genetic condition called complete androgen insensitivity syndrome (CAIS). People with CAIS have male (XY) chromosomes but lack receptors for androgens, the major masculinizing hormones. Because androgens from the male gonads (the testes) direct development of the external genitalia, people with CAIS look like girls at birth, despite their Y chromosome. Most babies with CAIS are not suspected of having any disorder at birth and are raised as girls. The syndrome is usually detected at puberty, when menstruation fails to occur and a physical examination reveals undescended testes instead of ovaries. A genetic analysis then also reveals the previously unsuspected Y chromosome.

Samantha and Richard were told that, despite the Y chromosome, their baby should be raised as a girl. They decided to name her Janice, after Samantha's mother, and redecorate the nursery with fairy princesses. The blue clothes were replaced with pink dresses. But how successful could they expect Janice to be as a girl? And would her Y chromosome, the absence of ovaries, or her lack of androgen receptors have psychological consequences?

To answer these questions, we need to review what is known about sexual differentiation, or development as a male versus a female. Because of space limitations, this review is brief; interested readers can find more detailed information and additional primary references for many of the topics covered in this chapter in Hines (2002, 2004).

GONADAL HORMONES AND SEXUAL DIFFERENTIATION

Although sexual differentiation begins with the sex chromosomes (XX or XY), these chromosomes do not exert most of their influences directly. Instead, their main job is to direct the gonads to develop as either testes or ovaries. After that, hormones from the gonads, particularly androgens from the testes, provide the major biological influences on sexual differentiation. The influences of hormones on sexual differentiation begin early in gestation, and involve the internal and external genitalia, as well as the brain and behavior. They have been studied extensively in nonhuman mammals, ranging from rodents to primates, and appear to apply, at least to some extent, to human development as well. These hormonal influences do not mean that the social environment is unimportant for gender development. However, infants enter the world with some predispositions to "masculinity" and "femininity," and these predispositions appear to result largely from hormones to which they were exposed before birth.

The gonads are originally identical in both XY (male) and XX (female) embryos. However, in XY individuals, genetic information on the Y chromosome causes the gonads to become testes, and by week 8 of human gestation, they are producing hormones (particularly the primary androgen, testosterone). If the gonads do not become testes, they become ovaries, which do not appear to produce appreciable amounts of hormones prenatally. Consequently, XY fetuses have higher levels of testosterone than XX fetuses, particularly between weeks 8 and 24 of gestation. After that, and until birth, gonadal hormone levels are low in both sexes. However, with a surge of testicular hormones after birth, testosterone is again higher in boys than in girls from about the 1st to the 6th month of infancy.

Other mammals show similar hormonal differences during early life, and the times when testicular hormones are elevated in males correspond to critical periods for sex-related development (Goy & McEwen, 1980). For instance, male rats have elevated testosterone during late prenatal and early neonatal life, and treating female rats with a single injection of testosterone on the day of birth causes them to show increased male-typical and decreased female-typical sexual behavior as adults. Similar hormone treatment later in life, after the critical period, will not have the same effect. Early treatment with testosterone also promotes male-typical development of other behaviors that differ for male and female rats, including play and aggressive behaviors (Collaer & Hines, 1995). Although these hormonal influences have been studied most extensively in rodents, similar effects have been seen in nonhuman primates. For example, treating pregnant rhesus monkeys with testosterone masculinizes sexual and play behaviors in female offspring.

Hormones appear to exert these permanent influences on behaviors that demonstrate sex differences by influencing brain regions that show sex differences. One example is the sexually dimorphic nucleus of the preoptic area (SDN-POA), located in the anterior hypothalamic preoptic area (AHPOA). Although the specific function of the SDN-POA is not known, the larger AHPOA within which it lies is involved in sexual and maternal behavior, and regulation of gonadal hormone release (Allen, Hines, Shryne, & Gorski, 1989). The SDN-POA is several times larger in male than in female rats, and early treatment with testosterone increases SDN-POA size in females. Similar neural sex differences and hormone effects have been observed in other species and in other brain regions (De Vries & Simerly, 2002). Sometimes hormone-sensitive brain regions that show sex differences are larger or more complex in males; other times, they are larger or more complex in females. Regardless, early exposure to testicular hormones consistently sculpts a more male-typical brain.

A few more points aid discussion of the role of hormones in human development. First, one implication of evidence that female-typical development occurs in the absence of testicular hormones is that hormones from the female gonads, the ovaries, are not needed for feminization. In fact, in rodents, and perhaps in primates as well, androgen is converted to estrogen within the brain, before it exerts some of its effects. Consequently, treating females with estrogen during early development can produce the same effects as treating them with testosterone (Collaer & Hines, 1995; Goy & McEwen, 1980). Although ovarian hormones occasionally have feminizing behavioral effects, these effects are far more limited than the masculinizing effects of androgen or estrogen produced from it. In addition, when feminizing effects of estrogen are seen, they appear to occur relatively late in development (Fitch & Denenberg, 1998). Thus, although estrogen has feminizing influences at puberty (e.g., promoting breast development), its primary impact during early development appears to be the promotion of male-typical neural and behavioral characteristics. A second important point is that hormonal influences are graded. For XX animals, the larger the dose, the greater the effect. For XY animals, adding hormone rarely, if ever, enhances male-typical characteristics. However, partial reduction in hormones can partially reduce male-typical behavior. Thus, hormonal differences during development could contribute to behavioral differences within each sex, as well as to differences between the sexes. Finally, different behaviors that demonstrate sex differences are influenced by hormones via somewhat different mechanisms (Hines, 2002) that can involve the specific hormone responsible (e.g., testosterone vs. estrogen produced from it), the times when hormones are influential, or the dosage of hormone required for an effect. This diversity provides mechanisms whereby different individuals can develop different mixtures of male- and female-typical traits. For instance, a hormonal abnormality during a short span of early life could alter one behavior linked to gender, without influencing others.

GONADAL HORMONES AND HUMAN BEHAVIORAL DEVELOPMENT

Hormones clearly influence the human genitalia. Baby Janice is one example. She has a Y chromosome and normal levels of androgen. However, because her cells cannot respond to androgen, her external genitalia look feminine. Similarly, girls exposed to elevated androgen prenatally, because of genetic conditions, or because their mothers took androgenic hormones during pregnancy, tend to be born with ambiguous genitalia (in between those of males and females), a situation that is sometimes called an *intersex condition.*

Hormonal influences on human behavior are harder to establish than are influences on the genitalia, partly because behavioral sex differences are subtler than genital sex differences, and because behavior is subject to social (and other) influences after birth. In addition, because it is generally unethical to manipulate hormones experimentally in humans during early life, research such as that conducted in other species is largely impossible. However, some information has come from situations in which hormones have been perturbed for other reasons, and from studies relating normal variability in hormones during early development to subsequent behavior. These investigations have focused on childhood play behavior; sexual orientation; core gender identity (or the sense of self as male or female); personality characteristics, such as aggression and nurturing; and cognitive abilities, including spatial, mathematical, and verbal abilities. These characteristics have been studied because they show sex differences, and animal research suggests that influences of gonadal hormones are limited to behaviors that show sex differences. Some researchers also have attempted to evaluate hormonal influences on the developing human brain by looking at behavioral manifestations of neural asymmetry (language lateralization and hand preferences), or by looking directly at brain structure and function. The remainder of this chapter summarizes findings from these investigations, outlines areas of current research activity, and evaluates baby Janice's prospects given her diagnosis with CAIS.

Childhood Play Behavior

The strongest evidence that prenatal hormones influence human behavior comes from studies of childhood play. One syndrome that has been studied extensively, congenital adrenal hyperplasia (CAH), is a genetic disorder that results in the production of high androgen levels by the adrenal gland, beginning prenatally. Girls with CAH are usually diagnosed near the time of birth, because they typically have partially masculinized genitalia, caused by their prenatal androgen excess. They are then treated postnatally to normalize hormones, sex-assigned and reared as girls, and surgically femininized. Boys with CAH are born with normal male genitalia and do not appear to have dramatically or consistently elevated androgen levels prenatally, perhaps because their testes are able to reduce androgen production to compensate for the excess hormone from the adrenal gland.

Behaviorally, girls with CAH show increased preferences for toys usually preferred by boys, such as cars and other vehicles, and reduced preferences for toys usually chosen by girls, such as dolls (for review, see Hines, 2002, 2004). These findings have been reported by researchers in several different countries, using interviews and questionnaires, as well as direct observation of children's toy choices. The differences also are seen in comparison to various control groups, including unaffected sisters of girls with CAH and girls matched for demographic background. Girls with CAH also show altered playmate preferences. About 50% of their favorite playmates are girls, and 50% are boys, whereas, for their unaffected relatives, 80–90% of favorite playmates are children of their own sex (Hines & Kaufman, 1994).

Figure 2.1 illustrates the scores of girls and boys with CAH and of unaffected male and female relatives on a standardized measure of childhood gender role behavior, the Pre-School Activities Inventory (PSAI; Golombok & Rust, 1993). The PSAI assesses a broad range of sex-typed interests, such as playing with dolls or trains, playing with girls, dressing up in girlish clothing, and enjoying rough-and-tumble play. On the PSAI, as well as on measures of toy and playmate preferences, the behavior of girls with CAH is more male-typical than that of unaffected girls, but not as male-typical as that of unaffected boys. The difference between the behavior of girls with CAH and control boys could reflect the influences of postnatal factors, such as socialization, because girls with CAH are reared as girls. Alternatively, although girls with CAH appear to have prenatal androgen levels as high as those of boys, other aspects of their androgen exposure (e.g., its timing) may differ.

So it is clear that girls with the genetic disorder CAH show altered play behavior, but what does this imply for normal development? Girls with CAH typically are born with ambiguous genitalia, and despite surgical feminization, knowledge of this ambiguity could alter their self-perceptions or the ways in which their parents treat them, and this could

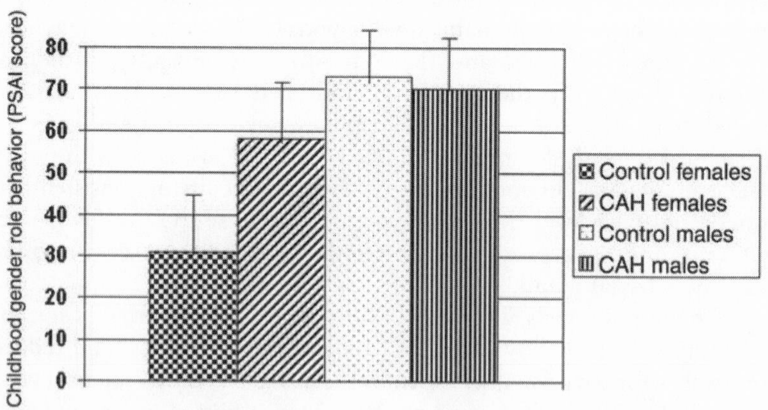

FIGURE 2.1. Mean scores on the PSAI (a standardized measure of sex-typed toy, playmate, and activity preferences) in males and females with CAH compared to unaffected controls. Females with CAH differ significantly from both control females and control males. Males with and without CAH do not differ. Adapted from Hines (2004). Copyright 2004 by Melissa Hines.

change their behavior. However, parents of girls with CAH are told to raise their daughters as they would any other girl, and they report that they do so (Berenbaum & Hines, 1992; Ehrhardt & Baker, 1974).

In addition, normal variability in prenatal androgen appears to influence sex-typical play, without causing genital ambiguity. Testosterone levels during pregnancy have been found to be higher in mothers of healthy girls with extremely male-typical toy, playmate, and activity preferences than in mothers of girls with extremely female-typical behavior (Hines, Golombok, et al., 2002). Similarly, high levels of available testosterone in the maternal circulation during pregnancy, along with the daughters' own levels of testosterone in adulthood, have been found to predict male-typical gender role behavior in daughters at 27–30 years (Udry, Morris, & Kovenock, 1995). Causes of individual variability in testosterone during pregnancy could be genetic. In addition, in other mammals, drugs (e.g., alcohol and cocaine) and stress have been found to influence testosterone levels during pregnancy. However, prenatal stress does not appear to have an appreciable impact on gender-related behavior in humans (Hines, Johnston, et al., 2002), and the influences of drug use on testosterone levels during human pregnancy remain largely unexplored.

Baby Janice's disorder, CAIS, usually is not diagnosed until girls fail to menstruate, allowing only retrospective assessment of childhood behavior. However, females with CAIS recall typically feminine toy, playmate, and activity preferences (Hines, Ahmed, & Hughes, 2003). This finding suggests that Janice's complete lack of androgen receptors, coupled with her female upbringing, will result in female-typical childhood play behavior.

Core Gender Identity

Most boys and men have a male gender identity and most girls and women have a female gender identity. This is probably the most dramatic psychological sex difference in humans. However, even here, there is diversity. Some individuals have gender identity disorder (GID), meaning a strong and persistent cross-gender identification or desire to be the other sex, and persistent discomfort with the assigned sex and its gender role (Green & Blanchard, 1995; American Psychiatric Association, 2000). Adults with GID are often treated with sex reassignment, including hormones to promote development of secondary sexual characteristics, and genital surgery. The strong, persistent desire to change sex, and the willingness to undergo surgery and hormone treatment despite formidable obstacles, including, in some cases, social stigmatization and job loss, may suggest a biological imperative. Efforts to identify genetic or hormonal abnormalities in adults with GID have been largely unsuccessful. However, the hormone environment during prenatal development may influence gender identity.

Given the influences of hormones on brain development and behavior, prenatal hormones might seem the most likely source of any such biological imperative. However, most individuals with prenatal hormone abnormalities develop a gender identity consistent with their sex of rearing, regardless of its direction. For instance, Money and Daléry (1976) compared 7 XX individuals with CAH, 3 reared as boys and 4 as girls. All were successful in the assigned gender, whether male or female. Currently, almost all XX individuals with CAH are reared as girls (with surgical feminization if thought necessary), and this is usually successful. However, in one study of 53 XX individuals with CAH, 1 individual had been diagnosed with GID and was now living as a man, despite assignment and rearing as a girl. The authors estimated that GID occurs in about 1 in 30,400 women in the general population, and calculated the odds that 1 in 53 women with CAH would have GID by chance as 608 to 1 (Zucker et al., 1996). Another study found 4 XX individuals in the New York area with CAH who were living as men, despite having been reared as girls (Meyer-Bahlburg et al., 1996). These authors estimated that GID occurs in 1 in 30,000–100,000 women, and that CAH occurs in about 1 in 14,000 live births. Based on these estimates, they calculated the probability that the two conditions would occur together by chance is 1 in more than 420 million.

Women with CAH also appear to experience somewhat reduced satisfaction with the female sex of assignment, without having GID. One study found that 5 of 16 women with CAH indicated that they sometimes wished they were a person of the other sex, whereas all of the control women said they never, or almost never, had this wish (Hines, Brook, & Conway, in press). The CAH women also scored higher on a quantitative measure of gender dissatisfaction, although none of them were dissatisfied enough to be diagnosed with GID.

Girls with CAH also may experience reduced satisfaction with being female, without having GID or wishing to change sex. In one study, fewer girls with CAH than control girls said they were content to be, or preferred to be, a girl (Ehrhardt, Epstein, & Money, 1968). In another study, girls with CAH were more likely than unaffected sisters to say they might have chosen to be a boy, or might be undecided as to whether to be a boy or a girl, if given the choice (Ehrhardt & Baker, 1974). Nevertheless, severe unhappiness with being a girl was found to be rare or nonexistent in both studies. In contrast, in a third study (Slijper, Drop, Molenaar, & de Muinck Keizer-Schrama, 1998), 2 of 18 girls with CAH met the diagnostic criteria for GID, as did 5 of 29 other children reared as girls but exposed to high levels of androgen prenatally, caused by other intersex conditions. GID also has been reported in women with other intersex disorders involving elevated prenatal androgen (Zucker, 1999).

XY individuals with CAIS appear content to be women (Hines et al., 2003; Masica, Money, & Ehrhardt, 1971; Wisniewski et al., 2002). Their inability to respond to androgen, combined with being reared as girls, appears to produce a female gender identity, even in the absence of a second X chromosome or ovaries. Thus, Janice's parents can expect her gender identity to be unambiguously female.

Information about hormonal influences on gender identity also has come from studies of individuals with deficiencies in enzymes needed to produce the full range of testicular androgens. These enzymatic deficiencies usually cause the genitalia to appear ambiguous or feminine at birth. However, high levels of androgen at puberty masculinize the external genitalia and produce male-typical patterns of hair and muscle development. In some instances, these individuals then change to live as men, despite having been reared as girls. In other individuals, particularly in Europe and North America, the gonads are removed before puberty to avoid physical virilization, and the individuals continue into adulthood as females (Wilson, 2001; Zucker, 1999). Different outcomes for different individuals may reflect cultural factors; it is more common to change to a male identity in societies in which the status of men is markedly higher than that of women. However, this cultural factor is confounded with hormonal and physical virilization at puberty, because the testes are unlikely to be removed prior to puberty in the same cultures in which the social status of men and women differs dramatically. Thus, cultural factors, physical appearance, or hormonal changes at puberty may play a role in the ability of these individuals to change gender.

A final source of evidence regarding hormonal influences on core gender identity comes from XY individuals who have a normal male hormone environment prenatally but have been surgically feminized in infancy and reared as girls (e.g., because of limited penile development or the complete absence of a penis). One source suggests that these individuals experience problems with core identity (Reiner, Gearhart, & Jeffs, 1999), although others do not (Schober, Carmichael, Hines, & Ransley, 2002). Perhaps the most dramatic evidence has come from studies of boys whose penises were damaged so severely in infancy that they were surgically feminized and their sex assignment was changed to female. One widely publicized case involved an identical twin whose penis was accidentally cauterized at the age of 8 months during a surgical procedure. Reassignment to the female sex was reported as successful during childhood (Money & Ehrhardt, 1972), but by adulthood, this individual was living as a man and recalled being unhappy as a female for many years (Diamond & Sigmundson, 1997). This outcome could suggest that early exposure to androgen irreversibly masculinized his gender identity. However, for at least the first 8 months of life, he was socialized as a boy, and it is unknown how quickly or successfully his parents, or others in his social environment, were able to change to treating him as a girl. In a second case, in which reassignment from male to female occurred earlier, following penile damage at the age of 2 months, the outcome was different. At 16 and 26 years, this individual had a female gender identity, with no evidence of gender dysphoria (Bradley, Oliver, Chernick, & Zucker, 1998).

Thus, it seems that hormones influence core gender identity, but other factors are also important. In fact, the ability of some individuals to change sex following physical virilization at puberty, and of some infants to be reassigned to the female sex, despite a Y chromosome and early exposure to testicular hormones, suggests that this basic aspect of human identity is surprisingly flexible.

Sexual Orientation

The two male infants who were surgically feminized and reassigned as girls following penile damage also illuminate the role of hormones in sexual orientation. In both cases, sexual orientation was pushed in the masculine direction. The infant reassigned after the age of 8 months was erotically interested only in women as an adult (Diamond & Sigmundson, 1997), and the child reassigned after the age of 2 months was interested in both men and women (Bradley et al., 1998).

Women with CAH also are less likely than other women to be strongly heterosexual. In one study, more women with CAH than women with other clinical syndromes said they were bisexual or homosexual (Money, Schwartz, & Lewis, 1984). Other studies also suggest increased homosexual or bisexual orientation in women with CAH, and perhaps reduced sexual interest in general compared to unaffected female relatives (Dittman, Kappes, & Kappes, 1992; Hines, Brook, & Conway, in press; Zucker et al., 1996). It is not clear, however, that this shift in sexual orientation can be attributed to a direct influence of androgen on the developing brain. Women with CAH experience genital surgery, and the outcome of this surgery is often less than ideal (Schober, 1998). Their knowledge of exposure to masculinizing hormones and of physical virilization at birth also might influence their sexual behavior. Data on women with prenatal exposure to the synthetic estrogen diethylstilbestrol (DES) address these issues. DES masculinizes brain development and behavior in other species but does not masculinize the genitalia. Therefore, women exposed prenatally to DES might show changes in sexual orientation, although their genitalia are not masculinized. In fact, this outcome has been reported for three samples comprising 90 DES-exposed women and various controls (Meyer-Bahlburg et al., 1995). In these studies, about 40% of DES-exposed women versus 5% of their unexposed sisters were found to be bisexual or lesbian. For DES-exposed women and matched controls, the figures were about 25% and 6%, respectively.

What about XY individuals? Does exposure to reduced androgen or to differing levels of estrogen influence sexual orientation? XY women with CAIS are almost always heterosexual (Hines et al., 2003; Wisniewski et al., 2002) and are just as likely as other women to form long-term heterosexual relations or to marry (Hines et al., 2003). Thus, baby Janice should be as likely to grow up to be heterosexual and to marry as are women in general. This may result from her inability to respond to androgen, but her feminine physical appearance and socialization could also be important.

Little is known about sexual orientation in XY individuals with enzymatic deficiencies that impair androgen production. Some live as men and may have a wife or female partner, but others live as women and may have a husband or male partner. However, their erotic interests have not been studied systematically. Men exposed to estrogens, such as DES, do not show altered sexual orientation (Kester, Green, Finch, & Williams, 1980; Meyer-Bahlburg, Ehrhardt, Whitehead, & Vann, 1987). This finding is not unexpected, because estrogen typically does not promote female-typical development or interfere with male-typical development in other species.

Thus, sexual orientation, like core gender identity, appears to be influenced by the early hormone environment. In fact, hormonal influences on sexual orientation appear to be more dramatic than influences on core gender identity. However, again, hormones are clearly not the only important factor, because outcomes can vary for individuals with the same hormonal history.

Personality

There are some sex differences in personality. For instance, questionnaire and interview assessments suggest that males are more aggressive than females, whereas females are more nurturing than males (for reviews, see Hines, 2002, 2004). Hormones could contribute to these differences.

Aggression and Dominance

One study reported that girls and boys whose mothers took androgenic hormones during pregnancy were more likely than their unexposed siblings to say they would respond to provocation (e.g., another child pushing ahead of them in line) with physical aggression (Reinisch, 1981). A role for genital virilization in this outcome was unlikely, because all the children were born with normal-appearing external genitalia.

Aggressive response tendencies also have been examined in individuals with CAH. Two studies that focused on involvement in fights found no differences between girls with and without CAH (Ehrhardt & Baker, 1974; Ehrhardt et al. 1968). Studies using questionnaires to assess aggression and related personality characteristics have produced inconsistent results. In one study, females with CAH reported more indirect aggression and detachment than matched controls, but did not differ on six other personality dimensions (somatic anxiety, muscular tension, psychic anxiety, guilt, monotony avoidance, and suspicion), which also showed sex differences, or on seven personality dimensions that did not, including irritability and verbal aggression (Helleday, Edman, Ritzen, & Siwers, 1993). Another study compared three samples of individuals with CAH to unaffected relatives (Berenbaum & Resnick, 1997). One sample of female adolescents and adults with CAH showed enhanced tendencies toward physical aggression, but a second sample did not. This corresponded to the pattern of sex differences; controls in the first sample, but not the second, showed a sex difference on the measure used. In the third sample, which involved younger children, boys showed higher propensities toward physical aggression than either girls with CAH or unaffected girls, but girls with CAH and unaffected girls did not differ. A final study with a larger sample than the others found a sex difference among unaffected adolescents and adults in propensities to physical aggression, and that females with CAH resembled males in this respect (Mathews, Fane, Conway, Brook, & Hines, 2003). This study also assessed dominance/assertiveness using Cattell's 16 Personality Factor Inventory (16PF; Cattell, Eber, & Tatsuoka, 1970) but found no difference between females with and without CAH, despite observation of the expected sex difference favoring males in controls.

In contrast to males exposed to androgenic progestins prenatally, males with CAH have been found to show either no alterations in propensities to physical aggression (Berenbaum & Resnick, 1997) or reductions both in this area and in dominance/assertiveness (Mathews et al., 2003).

Thus, although androgen may promote aggressive response tendencies in females, this is not always the case. Among boys, results are even less consistent; prenatal exposure to androgenic hormones has been associated with increased, reduced, or unaltered tendencies toward aggression, depending on the study.

Nurturing and Interest in Infants

The reduced interest in dolls among girls with CAH could reflect reduced nurturing interests. In addition, three studies, based on interviews, suggest that girls with CAH show reduced interest in babysitting or other aspects of child care, including plans to have children (for reviews, see Hines, 2002, 2004). Two studies using questionnaires also suggest that girls with CAH, but not boys, show reduced interest in infants compared to unaffected relatives of the same sex (Leveroni & Berenbaum, 1998; Mathews et al., 2003). Mathews et al. (2003) also used Cattell's 16 PF to assess nurturing/tender-mindedness. As in prior studies, control females indicated more nurturing than males. In addition, females with CAH indicated less nurturing than unaffected female relatives. Males with CAH reported more nurturing than unaffected males.

One study has measured dominance/assertiveness and nurturing/tender-mindedness in individuals like Janice, who have CAIS. No differences were found in either characteristic for women with CAIS compared to female controls, although, as expected, male controls scored higher than female controls on dominance/assertiveness, and female controls scored higher than male controls on nurturing/tender-mindedness (Hines et al., 2003). This suggests that Janice will resemble other women in regard to these particular personality characteristics.

Cognition

Early reports on individuals with CAH, and those exposed to androgenic progestins prenatally, concluded that they had enhanced IQ (Money & Lewis, 1966). In retrospect, it is easy to question the conclusion that gonadal hormones enhance IQ, because there is no sex difference in IQ. Selection factors could explain the apparent IQ enhancement in the hormone-exposed groups (Collaer & Hines, 1995). People who received hormone treatment during pregnancy, or who participated in university-based research, probably had higher IQs than the general public. Subsequent studies have found no differences in IQ or other measures of general intelligence in individuals exposed to elevated hormone levels prenatally compared to their unexposed relatives (Hines, 2002, 2004). To guard against selection biases, most studies now use unexposed relatives of similar age as controls, or try to match controls carefully for demographic background.

Although general intelligence does not show a sex difference, some specific cognitive abilities do. Males tend to excel on certain measures of spatial and mathematical abilities, whereas females tend to excel on measures of verbal fluency and perceptual speed. The magnitude of behavioral sex differences can be described with use of the effect size index, *d,* where a value of 1.0 equals one standard deviation. In general, *d* values of 0.8 or more are considered large; those of 0.5, medium; those of 0.2, small; and those less than 0.2, negligible (Cohen, 1988). The size of cognitive sex differences varies greatly for different tasks (reviewed by Collaer & Hines, 1995; Hines, 2004). There is a large sex difference (d = 0.9) for three-dimensional (3-D) mental rotations (the ability to rotate stimuli, e.g., shapes, in the mind rapidly and accurately), although two-dimensional (2-D) mental rotation tasks generally show smaller sex differences (d = 0.3). Sex differences on measures of spatial perception (the ability to position stimuli, such as lines, accurately despite distracting information, such as a tilted frame) are moderate (d = 0.5), as are sex differences in perceptual speed (the ability to identify or compare stimuli, such as numbers or letters, rapidly and accurately). Sex differences in verbal fluency (the ability to produce words with certain characteristics rapidly) are even smaller (d = 0.3). For mathematics, measures of problem solving show small sex differences (d = 0.3), although some standardized tests, such as the Scholastic Aptitude Test and the Graduate Record Examination, show moderate-to-large sex differences (d = 0.5 and 0.7, respectively). To place these sex differences in context (Figure 2.2), the largest of them, that in 3-D mental rotations, is less than one half the size of the sex difference in height (Tanner, Whitehouse, & Takaishi, 1966) and less than one third the size of the sex difference in childhood play behavior (Hines, Golombok, et al., 2002). Most other verbal, spatial, and mathematical tests, including measures of vocabulary, reading comprehension, general verbal ability, spatial disembedding, computational ability, and understanding of mathematical concepts, show negligible-to-small sex differences (d = 0.0–0.2)

The prenatal hormone environment has been suggested to be an important determinant of cognitive sex differences, particularly of male advantages in spatial and mathematical abilities (Benbow, 1988; Kimura, 1999). However, empirical evidence provides little support for these suggestions. For instance, although some studies of females with CAH suggest enhanced spatial abilities, others suggest no alteration, or even impairment (Hines, 2004; Hines, Fane, et al., 2003). Similarly, studies of math ability in individuals with CAH generally suggest impairment rather than the assumed androgen-related enhancement (reviewed in Hines, 2002, 2004).

Studies of individuals exposed prenatally to the synthetic estrogen

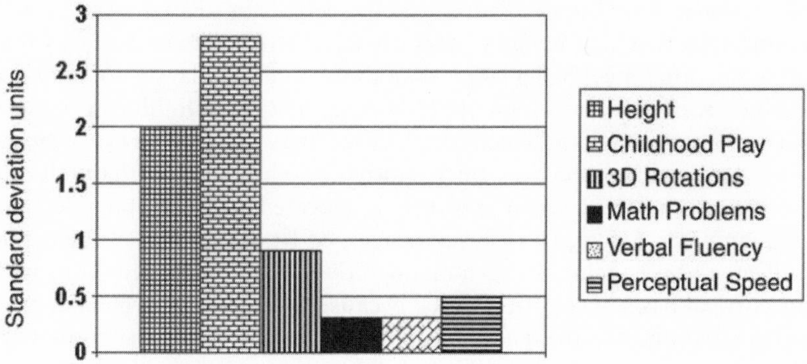

FIGURE 2.2. The sizes of sex differences in psychological characteristics compared to the size of sex difference in human height. Childhood play behavior (assessed using the PSAI) shows a larger sex difference than that in height. Sex differences in cognitive abilities, including 3-D mental rotations, mathematical problem solving, verbal fluency, and perceptual speed, are substantially smaller than the sex difference in height. Adapted from Hines (2004). Copyright 2004 by Melissa Hines.

DES also do not support influence of hormones on spatial abilities. Women exposed to DES do not show alterations in 2- or 3-D mental rotations, or in spatial perception or other spatial abilities (Hines & Sandberg, 1996; Hines & Shipley, 1984). Other cognitive abilities that favor males or females also are unchanged in both males and females following prenatal DES exposure (Wilcox, Maxey, & Herbst, 1992). These studies used relatively large samples, and one (Wilcox et al., 1992) included over 300 DES-exposed males and females, and a similar number of placebo-treated controls who were offspring of pregnant women who had taken part in a study of the efficacy of DES in preventing miscarriage. One study of 10 DES-exposed males compared to 10 unexposed brothers reported reduced spatial performance (Reinisch & Sanders, 1992), but the tasks showed negligible sex differences, suggesting that the result may have been an anomalous finding.

Cognitive outcomes also have been studied in other syndromes involving early hormonal abnormalities, including CAIS, Turner syndrome (a condition that involves a missing or abnormal X chromosome, ovarian regression, and a resultant lack of ovarian hormones), and idiopathic hypogonadotropic hypogonadism (IHH; a disorder that causes reduced androgen). Both XY individuals with CAIS and those with IHH have been found to show deficits on some spatial tasks (see Hines, 2002, 2004, for reviews), but the deficits do not correspond to patterns of sex differences, suggesting that nonhormonal aspects of the disorders might be responsible. Females with Turner syndrome show deficits on spatial tasks, as well as on tasks at which females generally excel, with deficits on tasks that show sex differences being larger than those on tasks that do not (Collaer, Geffner, Kaufman, Buckingham, & Hines, 2002). The finding of reduced performance on tasks at which females excel may suggest that estrogen has some feminizing influences on cognitive development, perhaps during early postnatal life, when estrogen is elevated in developing females (Bidlingmaier, Strom, Dörr, Eisenmenger, & Knorr, 1987). A feminizing influence of postnatal estrogen on cognitive development would fit with the cortical basis of cognitive tasks, because cortical development continues postnatally, and the feminizing effects of estrogen in other species appear to occur relatively late (Fitch & Denenberg, 1998). However, girls with Turner syndrome have many abnormalities in addition to their hormonal deficit, and these could contribute to cognitive outcomes.

Studies relating hormone levels during normal development to subsequent cognitive abilities also do not support the assumption that androgen enhances spatial or mathematical abilities. Although one study reported that testosterone in prenatal amniotic fluid related *positively* to the speed of mental rotations performance, the predicted relationship to accuracy on the task was not seen (Grimshaw, Sitarenios, & Finegan, 1995). In addition, a prior report on the same children at a younger age found an opposite result of that predicted; prenatal androgen related *negatively* to measures of mathematical and spatial abilities in girls (Finegan, Niccols, & Sitarenios, 1992). A separate report on hormones in amniotic fluid also produced a result in the direction opposite that predicted, with testosterone relating *negatively* to spatial ability in girls (Jacklin, Wilcox, & Maccoby, 1988). No relations between hormones and cognition were seen in boys.

The great majority of studies of both abnormal hormone levels and normal hormonal variability have found no relationships to abilities at which females excel, such as verbal fluency and perceptual speed, for either prenatal androgen or estrogen (Hines, 2002, 2004). One problem in studying hormonal influences on cognitive sex differences at which females excel, as well as those at which males excel, is that sex differences in these areas are not as large as those found in childhood play, sexual orientation, or gender identity. Therefore, large samples would be needed to provide adequate power to evaluate hypotheses. To date, very few studies of cognition have included more than 20 participants per group, and it is not unusual for groups to include 10 or fewer individuals. Firm conclusions regarding hormonal contributions to human cognition await studies of larger samples, although it is probably safe to say that factors other than prenatal hormones are the major determinants of these abilities.

What does this suggest about baby Janice? In theory, Janice should not experience any cognitive alterations owing to CAIS. Most aspects of cognitive performance do not show sex differences and are therefore unlikely to be influenced by her inability to respond to androgen. In addition, there is no convincing evidence that prenatal hormones influence those abilities that do show sex differences. However, one study of 10 people with CAIS reported reduced performance on some spatial measures, despite no change in overall IQ (Imperato-McGinley, Pichardo, Gautier, Voyer, & Bryden, 1991). The spatial impairments did not correspond to patterns of sex differences normally seen on the tasks, suggesting that they may have been anomalous or related to nonhormonal aspects of CAIS. If the latter is true, Janice might show some reductions in these particular spatial abilities, without alteration in overall intelligence.

Language Lateralization and Hand Preferences

Most individuals are right-handed for writing and other skilled manual tasks. However, this is not always the case, and men are somewhat more likely than women to be left-handed. Similarly, most people rely largely on their left hemisphere for language, although men show more reliance than women on the left hemisphere (Hines & Gorski, 1985). Several studies have examined the role of hormones in hand preferences and language lateralization.

Four studies of handedness in individuals with CAH have produced somewhat different outcomes. Increased left-handedness has been reported in females, but not males, with CAH (Nass et al., 1987), in males, but not females, with CAH (Mathews et al., in press), and in both males and females with CAH (Kelso, Nicholls, Warne, & Zacharin, 2000). The fourth study, which involved only females with CAH, found no differences in hand preferences (Helleday, Siwers, Ritzen, & Hugdahl, 1994). In contrast, three studies of women exposed to DES prenatally suggest increased left-handedness (Schachter, 1994; Scheirs & Vingerhoets, 1995), with exposure by week 9 of gestation being particularly effective (Smith & Hines, 2000). The sex difference in hand preferences is not large, and the studies of DES-exposed women had larger samples than the studies of individuals with CAH, perhaps explaining the more consistent findings.

Regarding language lateralization, one study suggested an enhanced male-typical pattern in DES-exposed women (Hines & Shipley, 1984), but a second did not (Smith & Hines, 2000). Language lateralization also appears to be unaltered in women with CAH (Helleday et al., 1994; Mathews et al., in press). Females with Turner syndrome show reduced left-hemisphere language lateralization, perhaps suggesting that early estrogen deficiency produces extremely female-typical lateralization (Hines

& Gorski, 1985), although, as noted before, the many other consequences of Turner syndrome might be responsible. One difficulty in studying hormonal influences on language lateralization is that the sex difference is negligible (d = 0.1; Voyer, 1996). Thus, extremely large samples might be needed to detect hormone effects. Given the small sex difference in language lateralization, the research focus on hormonal determininants might seem surprising. This focus probably resulted from the popularity of a theory that appeared before the size of the sex difference was known, speculating that testosterone contributed to learning disabilities and other cognitive problems via an androgen-induced delay in development of the left posterior cerebral hemisphere, and a consequent reduction in left-hemisphere language dominance (Geschwind & Galaburda, 1985).

SEX DIFFERENCES AND THE HUMAN BRAIN

Intelligence and Brain Size

There is a sex difference in brain size: Male brains, like male bodies, are larger and heavier than female brains. Some methods for statistically adjusting for body size suggest that the sex difference in brain size remains, but others do not (Hines, 2002, 2004). The sex difference in brain size also is substantially smaller than the sex difference in height (Figure 2.3). Nevertheless, suggestions that the larger male brain produces greater male intelligence have persisted for over a century (e.g., see Gould, 1981, for a historical review). Currently, intelligence tests are designed to show negligible sex differences, although sex differences on intelligence tests tended to be trivial even before this sex equality was designed into them (Loehlin, 2000). Within each sex, intelligence correlates positively with brain size (r = .20–.35; Vernon, Wickett, Bazana, & Stelmack, 2000), but the relevance of these correlations to sex differences is questionable given the lack of a sex difference in intelligence. In addition, female brains appear to be packed more densely than male brains, as indicated by a higher percentage of gray matter, greater cortical volume, and increased glucose metabolism, thought to reflect increased functional activity (reviewed in Hines, 2004). All of these lines of evidence suggest that understanding sex differences in intellectual functioning requires more than comparisons of overall brain size.

Sexual Orientation, Gender Identity, and the Brain

One sex difference in a specific subregion of the human brain appears to correspond to a hormonally determined sex difference in other species.

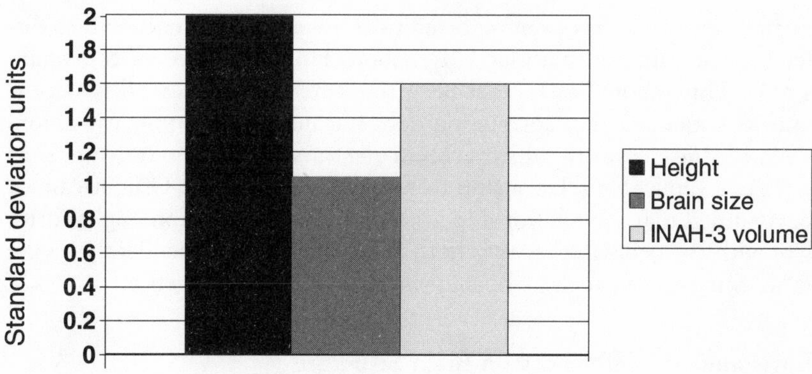

FIGURE 2.3. The sizes of the sex difference in human brain size and in volume of INAH-3 compared to the size of the sex difference in height. The sex difference in brain size is about half the size of the sex difference in height.

The best documented sex difference is in the third interstitial nucleus of the anterior hypothalamus (INAH-3), which appears to correspond to the SDN-POA, originally found to show a sex difference in rats. Three studies have found that the volume of INAH-3 is greater in men than in women (Allen et al., 1989; Byne et al., 2001; LeVay, 1991). The sex difference in INAH-3 is larger than the sex difference in overall brain size (Figure 2.3) and remains significant when brain size is controlled statistically (Allen et al., 1989). INAH-3 resembles the rodent SDN-POA in both its location and the types of neurons it contains. Although the function of INAH-3, like that of the SDN-POA is unknown, two studies have found that its volume is smaller (i.e., more female-typical) in homosexual men than in presumed heterosexual men (Byne et al., 2001; LeVay, 1991). However, Byne et al. (2001) also counted the number of neurons in INAH-3 and found no difference for heterosexual versus homosexual men, rendering the functional significance of the volumetric difference unclear.

Other regions that have been reported to differ in heterosexual versus homosexual men include the anterior commissure (a fiber tract connecting anterior regions of the two cerebral hemispheres) (Allen & Gorski, 1992) and the suprachiasmatic nucleus (SCN; a region intrinsic to the "biological clock") (Swaab & Hofman, 1990). However, a second study failed to replicate the finding for the anterior commissure (Lasco, Jordan, Edgar, Petito, & Byne, 2002), and the SCN does not show a sex difference corresponding to the difference reported in heterosexual versus homosexual men. A portion of the bed nucleus of the stria terminalis (a region connected anatomically to the AHPOA and involved in sex-related functions) has been reported to show a sex difference and to differ in men with and without GID (Zhou, Hofman, Gooren, & Swaab, 1995). This report has not yet been replicated. Regardless, it is important to remember that correlation does not necessarily imply causation. Even in those cases in which a brain region shows a sex difference, as well as a replicable relationship to sexual orientation or GID, it cannot be assumed that the relationship is causal. The brain region might correlate with the behavior because both are influenced independently by the same third factor, such as hormones or postnatal experience.

Environmental Influences on Brain Structure

A second brain region that has been investigated for sex differences is the corpus callosum, the main fiber tract connecting the cerebral hemispheres. The shape of the corpus callosum has been reported to differ in men and women, with posterior regions (the splenium and isthmus) being somewhat larger, particularly relative to brain size, in women, and anterior regions perhaps somewhat larger in men (de Lacoste-Utamsing & Holloway, 1982; Witelson, 1989; see also Hines, 2004, for discussion of controversy about sex differences in the corpus callosum). For the isthmus, the sex difference is seen only in men and women who are consistently right-handed. Variation in the corpus callosum has been related to language lateralization and to cognitive functions that show sex differences. One study linked a larger corpus callosum to greater right-hemisphere language dominance (O'Kusky et al., 1988). A second linked larger posterior callosal regions to reduced left-hemisphere language dominance and enhanced verbal fluency, suggesting that a more female-typical corpus callosum is associated with more female-typical cognitive function (Hines, Chiu, McAdams, Bentler, & Lipcamon, 1992). Subregions of the rat corpus callosum do not show sex differences in size. However, there are sex differences in the types of fibers in posterior callosal regions in rats, and these sex differences can be changed by rearing animals in enriched versus impoverished environments. Sex differences in some regions of the cerebral cortex of rodents also can be enhanced, reduced, or even reversed by altering rearing conditions (Juraska, 1991). This adds a new dimension to understanding the causes of sex differences in brain structure, suggesting that they might be altered by postnatal experience.

Sex Differences in Brain Function

Techniques such as magnetic resonance imaging (MRI) and positron emission tomography (PET) allow investigation of sex differences in both brain function and structure. Although male and female brains function similarly in most respects, there appear to be some differences. Many of these differences involve the extent to which both cerebral hemispheres are activated during language tasks, with men sometimes, but not always, showing more left-hemisphere activation than women (Rossell, Bullmore, Williams, & David, 2002; Shaywitz et al., 1995; but see also Gur et al., 2002). Identification of sex differences in brain function is more complex than it might at first appear. Many factors influence results and might explain different outcomes across studies, including age and hand preferences of participants, whether or not they are completing a task, the specific task being completed, its difficulty level, their skill or experience with the task, the means by which they respond, the imaging technique being used, and the statistical procedures for quantifying functional activity. Thus, although these techniques promise great advances in understanding human sex differences, they have thus far produced mainly tantalizing glimpses of what may be to come.

GONADAL HORMONES AND HUMAN BRAIN DEVELOPMENT

There is almost no information on changes in human brain structure following variation in the early hormone environment. One approach would be to examine sex-related brain regions, such as INAH-3, in individuals with unusual hormonal histories. However, this has not been done, perhaps because INAH-3 cannot be visualized in the living brain with techniques such as MRI, only in brains obtained at autopsy. Another approach involves studying the brains of individuals with unusual hormone histories, without focusing on regions known to show sex differences. One such study found that individuals with CAH showed increased signal intensity in white matter, but that this increase did not relate to cognitive or affective outcomes (Sinforiani et al., 1994). Another study found that both individuals with CAH and their unaffected relatives showed more structural abnormalities, as well as more learning disabilities, than matched controls (Plante, Boliek, Binkiewicz, & Erly, 1996). It is not clear that this last finding relates to androgen, because only individuals with CAH, not their unaffected relatives, would have been exposed to excess androgen. Like early reports of increased IQ in individuals with CAH, the finding could relate to selection biases. Females with Turner syndrome may show ventricular enlargement and alterations in the cerebral cortex, particularly in parietal and occipital regions, (see Collaer et al., 2002, for a review), although, as already noted, findings in Turner syndrome are hard to attribute to hormonal factors, because the syndrome has so many consequences. Nevertheless, research on neural alterations in individuals with atypical hormone histories, like the imaging of sex differences in brain function, is in its infancy and offers great promise for future understanding of the neural mechanisms underlying sex differences in human behavior.

RESEARCH DIRECTIONS

Research to date suggests that the prenatal hormone environment contributes to the development of some human behaviors that show sex differences, including childhood toy, activity, and playmate preferences, and to a lesser extent, sexual orientation and gender identity. For other behaviors, including personality characteristics such as aggression, cognitive abilities such as spatial abilities and verbal fluency, and neural asymmetries such as hand preferences and language lateralization, relationships to hormones have not been studied extensively or documented consistently. Firm conclusions in these areas await more powerful studies, for example, those using larger samples.

In addition to specifying the range of human behaviors influenced by the early hormone environment, areas of current research activity include identifying the neural mechanisms underlying any such influences and specifying how hormones augment or interact with other types of factors (e.g., postnatal socialization) to mold gender development. For instance, the gender-related behaviors linked most closely to the early hormone environment, those in childhood play, also relate to postnatal social cognitive processes. Children model others of the same sex (Perry & Bussey, 1979) and, if told that certain objects or activities are for children of their own sex, come to prefer these (Masters, Ford, Arend, Grotevant, & Clark, 1979). It is easy to imagine how modeling and responses to gender labels could produce sex differences in toy, playmate, and activity preferences. What might be surprising is that hormones influence these behaviors too. One question of current interest in my laboratory is whether girls exposed prenatally to androgen respond to models of the same sex and to gender labels in the same way that other girls do. If not, the effects of the early hormone environment on behavior could be mediated by changes in responses to same-sex models or to gender labels. Such mediation could provide a mechanism for children to acquire gender-related behavior, even if conceptions of what is "masculine" or "feminine" change, for example, from one time period or culture to another. High levels of androgen prenatally would lead to preferences for objects and activities modeled by males or labeled as being for males, regardless of what these were, whereas low levels would have the opposite effect. In contrast, if modeling and labeling were unaltered in girls exposed to androgen prenatally, hormonal influences on childhood play might seem to operate independently from modeling and labeling, suggesting that convergent influences, both biological and social cognitive, push children toward gender-related behaviors.

Information regarding hormonal influences on gender development has both clinical implications and implications for the scientific understanding of gender. Most notably, this information should aid the treatment of individuals like baby Janice, whose sex chromosomes, hormone levels, or genital appearance are not consistently male or female. In many cases, these individuals are assigned and reared as females, often because reducing genital ambiguity is considered important, and surgical feminization is generally more successful than surgical masculinization. In Janice's case, female assignment will almost certainly be successful. Not only are her external genitalia feminine, but her inability to respond to androgen, along with her unambiguous socialization as a girl, makes her just as likely as any other girl to develop a successful female identity. One issue that she will face is an inability to become pregnant, because she lacks ovaries, as well as internal female reproductive organs (a testicular hormone that does not act through androgen receptors has caused the structures that would normally form the uterus and fallopian tubes to regress). Women with CAIS can and do adopt children and in our brave new technological world might also have children through other means (e.g., surrogacy). In other respects, however, Janice's life should be typical of women in general, which again testifies to the supremacy among biological factors of testicular hormones (or the lack thereof) in gender development. Neither a second X chromosome nor ovaries are needed for psychological success as a female. Unlike CAIS, most intersex conditions are not associated with uniformally successful psychosexual development. As I discussed earlier, assignment and rearing as a female is usually, but not always, successful. Increased understanding of the role of gonadal hormones in human gender development may help reduce, or even eliminate, these unhappy outcomes.

ACKNOWLEDGMENTS

My thanks to Richard Green, as well as the editors, for comments on a prior version of this chapter, and to the United States Public Health Service (Grant No. HD24542) and the Wellcome Trust for their support of my research. I am grateful to Stacey Sorrentino, Paul Williams, and Greta Mathews for help with the preparation of the manuscript and figures.

REFERENCES

Allen, L. S., & Gorski, R. A. (1992). Sexual orientation and the size of the anterior commissure in the human brain. *Proceedings of the National Academy of Sciences USA, 89,* 7199–7202.

Allen, L. S., Hines, M., Shryne, J. E., & Gorski, R. A. (1989). Two sexually dimorphic cell groups in the human brain. *Journal of Neuroscience, 9,* 497–506.

American Psychiatric Association. (2000). *Diagnostic and Statistical Manual of Mental Disorders* (4th ed., text rev.). Washington, DC: Author.

Benbow, C. P. (1988). Sex differences in mathematical reasoning ability in intellectually talented preadolescents: Their nature, effects and possible causes. *Behavioral and Brain Sciences, 11,* 169–232.

Berenbaum, S. A., & Hines, M. (1992). Early androgens are related to childhood sex-typed toy preferences. *Psychological Science, 3,* 203–206.

Berenbaum, S. A., & Resnick, S. M. (1997). Early androgen effects on aggression in children and adults with congenital adrenal hyperplasia. *Psychoneuroendocrinology, 22,* 505–515.

Bidlingmaier, F., Strom, T. M., Dörr, G., Eisenmenger, W., & Knorr, D. (1987). Estrone and estradiol concentrations in human ovaries, testes, and adrenals during the first two years of life. *Journal of Clinical Endocrinology and Metabolism, 65,* 862–867.

Bradley, S. J., Oliver, G. D., Chernick, A. B., & Zucker, K. J. (1998). Experiment of nurture: Ablatio penis at 2 months, sex reassignment at 7 months and a psychosexual follow-up in young adulthood. *Pediatrics, 102,* 91–95.

Byne, W., Tobet, S. A., Mattiace, L. A., Lasco, M. S., Kemether, E., Edgar, M. A., et al. (2001). The interstitial nuclei of the human anterior hypothalamus: An investigation of variation with sex, sexual orientation, and HIV status. *Hormones and Behavior, 40,* 86–92.

Cattell, R. B., Eber, H. W., & Tatsuoka, M. M. (1970). *Handbook for the sixteen factor questionnaire.* Champaign, IL: Institute for Personality and Ability Testing.

Cohen, J. (1988). *Statistical power analysis for the behavioral sciences* (2nd ed.) Hillsdale, NJ: Erlbaum.

Collaer, M. L., Geffner, M., Kaufman, F. R., Buckingham, B., & Hines, M. (2002). Cognitive and behavioral characteristics of Turner syndrome: Exploring a role for ovarian hormones in female sexual differentiation. *Hormones and Behavior, 41,* 139–155.

Collaer, M. L., & Hines, M. (1995). Human behavioral sex differences: A role for gonadal hormones during early development? *Psychological Bulletin, 118,* 55–107.

de Lacoste-Utamsing, C., & Holloway, R. L. (1982). Sexual dimorphism in the human corpus callosum. *Science, 216,* 1431–1432.

De Vries, G. J., & Simerly, R. B. (2002). Anatomy, development, and function of sexually dimorphic neural circuits in the mammalian brain. In D. W. Pfaff, A.

P. Arnold, A. M. Etgen, S. E. Fahrbach, & R. T. Rubin (Eds.), *Hormones, brain and behavior* (4th ed., pp. 137–191). San Diego: Academic Press.

Diamond, M., & Sigmundson, H. K. (1997). Sex reassignment at birth: Long-term review and clinical implications. *Archives of Pediatric and Adolescent Medicine, 151,* 298–304.

Dittman, R. W., Kappes, M. E., & Kappes, M. H. (1992). Sexual behavior in adolescent and adult females with congenital adrenal hyperplasia. *Psychoneuroendocrinology, 17,* 153–170.

Ehrhardt, A. A., & Baker, S. W. (1974). Fetal androgens, human central nervous system differentiation, and behavior sex differences. In R. C. Friedman, R. M. Richart, & R. L. van de Wiele (Eds.), *Sex differences in behavior* (pp. 33–52). New York: Wiley.

Ehrhardt, A. A., Epstein, R., & Money, J. (1968). Fetal androgens and female gender identity in the early-treated adrenogenital syndrome. *Johns Hopkins Medical Journal, 122,* 165–167.

Finegan, J. K., Niccols, G. A., & Sitarenios, G. (1992). Relations between prenatal testosterone levels and cognitive abilities at 4 years. *Developmental Psychology, 28,* 1075–1089.

Fitch, R. H., & Denenberg, V. H. (1998). A role for ovarian hormones in sexual differentiation of the brain. *Behavior and Brain Sciences, 21,* 311–352.

Geschwind, N., & Galaburda, A. M. (1985). Cerebral lateralization: Biological mechanisms, associations, and pathology: II. A hypothesis and a program for research. *Archives of Neurology, 42,* 521–552.

Golombok, S., & Rust, J. (1993). The measurement of gender role behavior in preschool children: A research note. *Journal of Child Psychology and Psychiatry, 34,* 805–811.

Gould, S. J. (1981). *The mismeasure of man.* New York: Norton.

Goy, R. W., & McEwen, B. S. (1980). *Sexual differentiation of the brain.* Cambridge, MA: MIT Press.

Green, R., & Blanchard, R. (1995). Gender identity disorders. In H.I. Kaplan & B. J. Sadock (Eds.), *Comprehensive textbook of psychiatry VI* (pp. 1347–1360). Baltimore: Williams & Wilkins.

Grimshaw, G. M., Sitarenios, G., & Finegan, J. K. (1995). Mental rotation at 7 years: Relations with prenatal testosterone levels and spatial play experiences. *Brain and Cognition, 29,* 85–100.

Gur, R. C., Alsop, D., Glahn, D., Petty, R., Swanson, C. L., Maldjian, J. A., et al. (2002). An fMRI study of sex differences in regional activation to a verbal and a spatial task. *Brain and Language, 74,* 157–170.

Helleday, J., Edman, G., Ritzen, E. M., & Siwers, B. (1993). Personality characteristics and platelet MAO activity in women with congenital adrenal hyperplasia (CAH). *Psychoneuroendocrinology, 18,* 343–354.

Helleday, J., Siwers, B., Ritzen, E. M., & Hugdahl, K. (1994). Normal lateralization for handedness and ear advantage in a verbal dichotic listening task in women with congenital adrenal hyperplasia (CAH). *Neuropsychologia, 32,* 875–880.

Hines, M. (2002). Sexual differentiation of human brain and behavior. In D. W. Pfaff, A. P. Arnold, A. M. Etgen, S. E. Fahrbach, & R. T. Rubin (Eds.), *Hormones, brain and behavior* (4th ed., pp. 425–461). San Diego: Academic Press.

Hines, M. (2004). *Brain gender.* New York: Oxford University Press.

Hines, M., Ahmed, S. F., & Hughes, I. (2003). Psychological outcomes and gender-related development in complete androgen insensitivity syndrome. *Archives of Sexual Behavior, 32,* 93–101.

Hines, M., Brook, C., & Conway, G. S. (in press). Androgen and psychosexual development: Core gender identity, sexual orientation and recalled childhood gender role behavior in men and women with congential adrenal hyperplasia (CAH). *Journal of Sex Research.*

Hines, M., Fane, B. A., Pasterski, V. L., Mathews, G. A., Conway, G. S., & Brook, C. (2003). Spatial abilities following prental androgen abnormality: Targeting and mental rotations performance in individuals with Congential Adrenal Hyperplasia. *Psychoneuroendocrinology, 28,* 1010–1026.

Hines, M., Chiu, L., McAdams, L. A., Bentler, P. M., & Lipcamon, J. (1992). Cognition and the corpus callosum: Verbal fluency, visuospatial ability and language lateralization related to midsagittal surface areas of callosal subregions. *Behavioral Neuroscience, 106,* 3–14.

Hines, M., Golombok, S., Rust, J., Johnston, K., Golding, J., & the ALSPAC Study Team (2002). Testosterone during pregnancy and childhood gender role behavior: A longitudinal population study. *Child Development, 73,* 1678–1687.

Hines, M., & Gorski, R. A. (1985). Hormonal influences on the development of neural asymmetries. In D. F. Benson & E. Zaidel (Eds.), *The dual brain: Hemispheric specialization in humans* (pp. 75–96). New York: Guilford Press.

Hines, M., Johnston, K., Golombok, S., Rust, J., Stevens, M., Golding, J., et al. (2002). Prenatal stress and gender role behavior in girls and boys: A longitudinal, population study. *Hormones and Behavior, 42,* 126–134.

Hines, M., & Kaufman, F. R. (1994). Androgen and the development of human sex-typical behavior: Rough-and-tumble play and sex of preferred playmates in children with congenital adrenal hyperplasia (CAH). *Child Development, 65,* 1042–1053.

Hines, M., & Sandberg, E. C. (1996). Sexual differentiation of cognitive abilities in women exposed to diethylstilbestrol (DES) prenatally. *Hormones and Behavior, 30,* 354–363.

Hines, M., & Shipley, C. (1984). Prenatal exposure to diethylstilbestrol (DES) and the development of sexually dimorphic cognitive abilities and cerebral lateralization. *Developmental Psychology, 20,* 81–94.

Imperato-McGinley, J., Pichardo, M., Gautier, T., Voyer, D., & Bryden, M. P. (1991). Cognitive abilities in androgen-insensitive subjects: Comparison with control males and females from the same kindred. *Clinical Endocrinology, 34,* 341–347.

Jacklin, C. N., Wilcox, K. T., & Maccoby, E. E. (1988). Neonatal sex-steroid hormones and cognitive abilities at six years. *Developmental Psychobiology, 21,* 567–574.

Juraska, J. M. (1991). Sex differences in "cognitive" regions of the rat brain. *Psychoneuroendocrinology, 16,* 105–119.

Kelso, W. M., Nicholls, M. E. R., Warne, G. L., & Zacharin, M. (2000). Cerebral lateralization and cognitive functioning in patients with congenital adrenal hyperplasia. *Neuropsychology, 14,* 370–378.

Kester, P., Green, R. Finch, S. J., & Williams, K. (1980). Prenatal "female hormone" administration and psychosexual development in human males. *Psychoneuroendocrinology, 5,* 269–285.

Kimura, D. (1999). *Sex and cognition.* Cambridge, MA: MIT Press.

Lasco, M. S., Jordan, T. J., Edgar, M. A., Petito, C. K., & Byne, W. (2002). A lack of dimorphism of sex or sexual orientation in the human anterior commissure. *Brain Research, 936,* 95–98.

LeVay, S. (1991). A difference in hypothalamic structure between heterosexual and homosexual men. *Science, 253,* 1034–1037.

Leveroni, C. L., & Berenbaum, S. A. (1998). Early androgen effects on interest in infants: Evidence from children with congenital adrenal hyperplasia. *Developmental Neuropsychology, 14,* 321–340.

Loehlin, J. C. (2000). Group differences in intelligence. In R. J. Sternberg (Ed.), *Handbook of intelligence* (pp. 176–193). New York: Cambridge University Press.

Masica, D. N., Money, J., & Ehrhardt, A. A. (1971). Fetal feminization and female gender identity in the testicular feminizing syndrome of androgen insensitivity. *Archives of Sexual Behavior, 1,* 131–142.

Masters, J. C., Ford, M. E., Arend, R., Grotevant, H. D., & Clark, L. V. (1979). Modeling and labelling as integrated determinants of children's sex-typed imitative behavior. *Child Development, 50,* 364–371.

Mathews, G. A., Fane, B. A., Conway, G. S., Brook, C., & Hines, M. (2003). Prenatal androgen abnormality and personality development. Manuscript submitted for publication.

Mathews, G. A., Fane, B., Pasterski, V. L., Conway, G. S., Brook, C., & Hines, M. (in press). Androgenic influences on neural asymmetry: Handedness and language lateralization in congenital adrenal hyperplasia (CAH). *Psychoneuroendocrinology.*

Meyer-Bahlburg, H. F. L., Ehrhardt, A. A., Rosen, L. R., Gruen, R. S., Veridiano, N. P., Vann, F. H., et al. (1995). Prenatal estrogens and the development of homosexual orientation. *Developmental Psychology, 31,*12–21.

Meyer-Bahlburg, H. F. L., Ehrhardt, A. A., Whitehead, E. D., & Vann, F. H. (1987). Sexuality in males with a history of prenatal exposure to diethylstilbestrol (DES). In *Psychosexual and reproductive issues affecting patients with cancer* (pp. 79–82). New York: American Cancer Society.

Meyer-Bahlburg, H. F. L., Gruen, R. S., New, M. I., Bell, J. J., Morishima, A., Shimshi, M., et al. (1996). Gender change from female to male in classical congenital adrenal hyperplasia. *Hormones and Behavior, 30,* 319–332.

Money, J., & Daléry, J. (1976). Iatrogenic homosexuality: Gender identity in seven 46, XX chromosomal females with hyperadrenocortical hermaphroditism born with a penis, three reared as boys, four reared as girls. *Journal of Homosexuality, 1,* 357–371.

Money, J., & Ehrhardt, A. (1972). *Man and woman: Boy and girl.* Baltimore: Johns Hopkins University Press.

Money, J., & Lewis, V. (1966). IQ, genetics and accelerated growth: Adrenogenital syndrome. *Johns Hopkins Hospital Bulletin, 118,* 365–373.

Money, J., Schwartz, M., & Lewis, V. (1984). Adult erotosexual status and fetal hormonal masculinization and demasculinization: 46 XX congenital virilizing adrenal hyperplasia and 46 XY androgen-insensitivity syndrome compared. *Psychoneuroendocrinology, 9,* 405–414.

Nass, R., Baker, S., Speiser, P., Virdis, R., Balsamo, A., Cacciari, E., et al. (1987). Hormones and handedness: Left-hand bias in female congenital adrenal hyperplasia patients. *Neurology, 37,* 711–715.

O'Kusky, J., Strauss, E., Kosaka, B., Wada, J., Li, D., Druhan, M., et al. (1988). The corpus callosum is larger with right-hemisphere cerebral speech dominance. *Annals of Neurology, 24,* 379–383.

Perry, D. G., & Bussey, K. (1979). The social learning theory of sex difference: Imitation is alive and well. *Journal of Personality and Social Psychology, 37,* 1699–1712.

Plante, E., Boliek, C., Binkiewicz, A., & Erly, W. K. (1996). Elevated androgen, brain development and language/learning disabilities in children with congenital adrenal hyperplasia. *Developmental Medicine and Child Neurology, 38,* 423–437.

Reiner, W. G., Gearhart, J. P., & Jeffs, R. (1999). Psychosexual dysfunction in males with genital anomalies: Late adolescence, Tanner Stages IV to VI. *Journal of the American Academy of Child and Adolescent Psychiatry, 38,* 865–872.

Reinisch, J. M. (1981). Prenatal exposure to synthetic progestins increases potential for aggression in humans. *Science, 211,* 1171–1173.

Reinisch, J. M., & Sanders, S. A. (1992). Effects of prenatal exposure to diethylstilbestrol (DES) on hemispheric laterality and spatial ability in human males. *Hormones and Behavior, 26,* 62–75.

Rossell, S. L., Bullmore, E. T., Williams, S. C. R., & David, A. S. (2002). Sex differences in functional brain activation during a lexical visual field task. *Brain and Language, 80,* 97–105.

Schachter, S. C. (1994). Handedness in women with intrauterine exposure to diethystilbesterol. *Neuropsychologia, 32,* 619–623.

Scheirs, J. G. M., & Vingerhoets, A. J. J. M. (1995). Handedness and other laterality indices in women prenatally exposed to DES. *Journal of Clinical and Experimental Neuropsychology, 17,* 725–730.

Schober, J. M. (1998). Feminizing genitoplasty for intersex. In M. D. Stringer (Ed.), *Pediatric surgery and urology: Long term outcomes* (pp. 549–558). London: Saunders.

Schober, J. M., Carmichael, P. A., Hines, M., & Ransley, P. G. (2002). The ultimate challenge of cloacal exstrophy. *Journal of Urology, 167,* 300–304.

Shaywitz, B. A., Shaywitz, S. E., Pugh, K. R., Constable, R. T., Skudlarski, P., Fulbright, R. K., et al. (1995). Sex differences in the functional organization of the brain for language. *Nature, 373,* 607–609.

Sinforiani, E., Livieri, C., Mauri, M., Bisio, P., Sibilla, L., Chiesa, L., et al. (1994). Cognitive and neuroradiological findings in congenital adrenal hyperplasia. *Psychoneuroendocrinology, 19,* 55–64.

Slijper, F. M. E., Drop, S. L. S., Molenaar, J. C., & de Muinck Keizer-Schrama, S. M. P. F. (1998). Long-term psychological evaluation of intersex children. *Archives of Sexual Behavior, 27,* 125–144.

Smith, L. L., & Hines, M. (2000). Language lateralization and handedness in women prenatally exposed to diethylstilbestrol (DES). *Psychoneuroendocrinology, 25,* 497–512.

Swaab, D. F., & Hofman, M. A. (1990). An enlarged suprachiasmatic nucleus in homosexual men. *Brain Research, 537,* 141–148.

Tanner, J. M., Whitehouse, R. H., & Takaishi, M. (1966). Standards from birth to maturity for height, weight, height velocity and weight velocity: British children, 1965. *Archives of Disease in Childhood, 41,* 454–471.

Udry, J. R., Morris, N. M., & Kovenock, J. (1995). Androgen effects on women's gendered behaviour. *Journal of Biosocial Sciences, 27,* 359–368.

Vernon, P. A., Wickett, J. C., Bazana, P. G., & Stelmack, R. M. (2000). The neuropsychology and psychophysiology of human intelligence. In R. J. Sternberg (Ed.), *Handbook of intelligence* (pp. 245–264). New York: Cambridge University Press.

Voyer, D. (1996). On the magnitude of laterality effects and sex differences in functional lateralities. *Laterality, 1,* 51–83.

Wilcox, A. J., Maxey, J., & Herbst, A. L. (1992). Prenatal hormone exposure and performance on college entrance examinations. *Hormones and Behavior, 24,* 433–439.

Wilson, J. D. (2001). Androgens, androgen receptors and male gender role behavior. *Hormones and Behavior, 40,* 358–366.

Wisniewski, A. B., Migeon, C. J., Meyer-Bahlburg, H. F. L., Gearhart, J. P., Berkovitz, G. D., & Brown, T. R. (2002). Complete androgen insensitivity syndrome: Long-term medical, surgical, and psychosexual outcome. *Journal of Clinical Endocrinology and Metabolism, 85,* 2664–2669.

Witelson, W. F. (1989). Hand and sex differences in the isthmus and genu of the human corpus callosum: A postmortem morphological study. *Brain, 112,* 799–835.

Zhou, J., Hofman, M. A., Gooren, L. J. G., & Swaab, D. F. (1995). A sex difference in the human brain and its relation to transsexuality. *Nature, 378,* 68–70.

Zucker, K. J. (1999). Intersexuality and gender differentiation. *Annual Review of Sex Research, 10,* 1–69.

Zucker, K. J., Bradley, S. J., Oliver, G., Blake, J., Fleming, S., & Hood, J. (1996). Psychosexual development of women with congenital adrenal hyperplasia. *Hormones and Behavior, 30,* 300–318.

3

The Psychobiology of Gender

Cognitive Effects of Reproductive Hormones in the Adult Nervous System

ELIZABETH HAMPSON
SCOTT D. MOFFAT

One of the most novel approaches in the study of gender to emerge in the past 25 years is the neuroendocrine approach. This method is based on the observation that behavioral sex differences are not unique to humans. In fact, they occur in most species. Whereas some of these differences are learned, others are driven by the actions of reproductive hormones in the central nervous system. The neuroendocrine approach starts with the premise that at least some human sex differences stem from biological predispositions generated by *organizational* and *activational* effects of hormones in the brain. A key task facing researchers is to identify *which* cognitive and behavioral sex differences are rooted in biology, and to learn how factors in the social environment interact with these predispositions to accentuate or mitigate their impact. The neuroendocrine approach emphasizes biology, but it is not rigidly deterministic. The surface behavior we eventually see is a product not only of biology but also of the molding of biologically based predispositions by learning and experience.

The neuroendocrine approach is still fairly new in human studies, but it has been applied to the study of behavioral sex differences in other species since the 1950s. This chapter focuses on a class of hormone actions called *activational effects*, which are one of two major classes of steroid hormone actions in the nervous system. The other class includes organizational effects, described by Hines (Chapter 2, this volume). Activational effects differ from organizational effects in important ways. First, they occur in the adult brain, not the developing brain. Second, a critical period is not required. Activational effects are time-locked to the presence of active hormone in the bloodstream and dissipate when hormone levels decline. Therefore, unlike organizational effects, activational effects are reversible. Human studies only recently began to consider the effects of reproductive hormones in the adult brain. But already this approach has shed new light on sex differences in cognitive function. The approach can be extended to other areas of gender differentiation as well.

In this chapter, we review some of the research that has investigated the possibility of activational effects on cognition. Although this is of interest in its own right, the demonstration of activational effects on cognitive function has implications beyond the exact functions studied. First, it implies that, contrary to popular thinking, sex differences may be dynamic and variable, not fixed—waxing and waning in their expression with changes in the endocrine environment of the brain. The second implication is that if sex steroids dynamically modulate activity in some neural pathways, men and women may differ in their ways of perceiving and interacting with the world at the most basic phenomenological levels. Our perceptions, thoughts, moods, and characteristic ways of responding to the environment may be subtly influenced by the hormonal milieu.

BASIC PRINCIPLES OF HORMONE ACTION

The hormones secreted by the adult gonads are sexually differentiated. In women, high levels of estrogen, notably a form of estrogen called 17β-estradiol, are secreted by the ovaries during the fertile years. The amount of estrogen secreted into the bloodstream depends on the stage of the menstrual cycle. During menses, estradiol levels are not much higher than in postmenopausal women. But levels increase by five- to 12-fold during the 3 days preceding ovulation and in the second half of the menstrual cycle, after ovulation takes place. (Although progesterone secretion by the ovaries is also high in the second half of the cycle, this chapter focuses only on the estrogens). In men, the testes secrete high concentrations of testosterone (T) during the reproductive years. Although the change is often overlooked, men undergo a drop in T in late life akin to menopause in women. Between the ages of 40 and 80, plasma free testosterone decreases by about 50%. This is *andropause,* a topic of current interest among behavioral researchers and endocrinologists. There are also biological rhythms in T secretion that occur at younger ages. For example, in males of reproductive age, T release shows a diurnal rhythm, with levels of free testosterone 30–50% higher in early morning than in late afternoon or evening. There is also a seasonal rhythm, with higher T in autumn than in spring, although the precise timing depends on geographical locale. Both sexes also secrete small amounts of "opposite-sex" hormones—T in women, which comes mainly from the adrenal glands and ovaries, and estradiol in men, which mostly comes, not from the testes, but from peripheral conversion of T to estradiol by enzymes in fatty tissue.

Hormones circulating in the bloodstream can diffuse into the brain. There, they influence the activity of certain populations of neurons. Hormones are able to act only at sites where brain cells contain the proper receptors. Receptors for estrogens and for androgens are not distributed evenly over the whole brain but are densely expressed in some brain regions and sparsely or not at all in others. As a consequence, the effects of the hormones are selective. By diffusing out of the bloodstream and attaching to receptors inside neurons, various reproductive hormones are able to alter brain events. Binding to the receptors initiates changes in gene transcription, thereby changing the amounts or types of protein products produced by the cell. Although the mechanisms might seem arcane, the implications of hormone–brain interactions for function are profound. It has been discovered that numerous neurotransmitters, or their receptors, or the enzymes involved in their synthesis, release, and degradation, are influenced by the levels of sex hormones present in the bloodstream. For instance, estradiol has multiple effects on serotonin activity in the forebrain. These effects are of considerable interest considering serotonin's role in the regulation of mood and other functions. Circulating hormone levels can even influence the structural anatomy of the brain. For instance, Woolley and McEwen (1992) discovered a section of the hippocampus, a brain region believed to be involved in memory, in which the number of synapses covaries with the female rat's estrous cycle—rising when estradiol levels are high and falling when they are low. A single hormone, such as estradiol, can have effects in several different brain systems simultaneously and may either increase or decrease the capacities of neurons to transmit information. These sorts of molecular-level changes are called *activational effects* of hormones because they modify brain *activity.* Researchers also speak of activational effects on behaviors or facets of cognition, because these represent the functional end points of the cellular events. Whereas the effects of sex steroids on

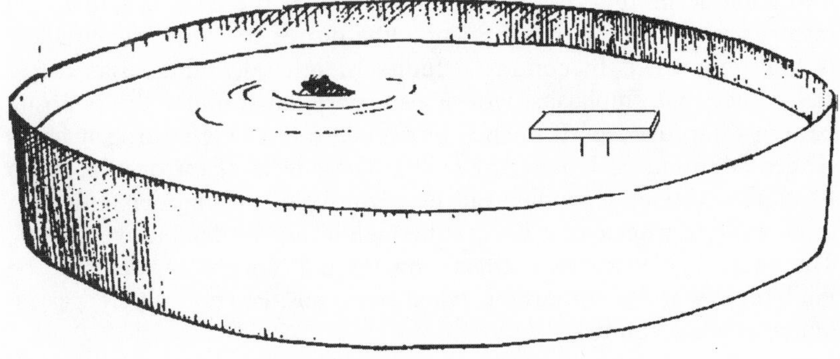

FIGURE 3.1. The Morris water maze is one example of a spatial task that elicits a sex difference in laboratory animals. Over a series of trials, the rat progressively learns to navigate to a platform hidden just beneath the surface of the water (shown raised here). The platform is always in the same position, so the rat must learn where the platform is located, and where to seek refuge from the water, by navigating relative to visual cues in the extramaze environment. The release point of the animal around the circumference of the maze is varied from trial to trial.

neurochemistry have been studied in some detail in laboratory animals, we are only beginning to appreciate the implications of these effects for behavior and cognitive processes, especially in humans.

Let us consider one example from comparative research before we go on to discuss human cognition. A sex difference has been found in the ability of laboratory animals to navigate, or learn the layout, of complex spatial mazes (Figure 3.1). In lab rats and mice, as well as wild species such as meadow voles, deer mice, and kangaroo rats, males acquire knowledge of such mazes faster than do females. Although the sex difference is not universal, it is found in many mammals, even if they are raised in laboratory housing, without any opportunity to gain experience in spatial ranging. The sex difference in spatial learning is not a matter of motor activity, because females are, if anything, more active in exploring the maze than males in most species. The expression of the behavioral sex difference turns out to be modified by the level of circulating hormones present in the bloodstream. When in a high-estrogen state, such as late pregnancy or just before ovulation during the rat's estrous cycle, female animals perform less accurately than they do when in a low-estrogen state (Galea et al., 2000; Warren & Juraska, 1997). In many studies, female animals perform at least as well as males, if they are tested at low-estrogen levels. This suggests that both sexes harbor brain circuitry equally capable of mediating accurate spatial navigation, but that the level of circulating estrogen is one factor that influences the degree to which the circuitry is fully expressed. In contrast, studies of other learning tasks, especially ones that emphasize working memory, have found the opposite pattern—improved performance by female rats at *high*-estrogen levels (Fader, Johnson, & Dohanich, 1999). The effects of estrogen seem to be quite selective; depending on the cognitive-processing demands of a given task, estrogen can have either inhibitory or facilitative effects. The fact that estrogen's effects on spatial cognition seem to be inhibitory will be important when we consider sex differences in human spatial abilities.

EFFECTS OF ESTROGEN ON COGNITIVE FUNCTIONS IN WOMEN

In most Western countries, it is considered unethical to administer hormones to humans unless there is some medical reason to do so. Therefore, it is generally infeasible for researchers to employ true experimental designs. Instead, they must rely on biological rhythms in hormone production, testing individuals during periods of high and low hormone release and contrasting their performance on cognitive tests in the two endocrine states. This approach has the advantage of being naturalistic and therefore readily generalizable outside the laboratory. Its major drawback is the difficulty in controlling extraneous influences that might covary with changes in hormone levels (e.g., changes in other hormones). Therefore, it is imperative to demonstrate convergent evidence from a number of different methodologies before we draw firm conclusions.

A second type of study involves hormones that are prescribed for some clinical purpose, for example, hormone supplements prescribed to remedy a medical condition. In this situation, problems that can arise are the necessity of generalizing from nonphysiological levels, types of hormones, or timings of exposure, and confounds introduced by the medical condition that required intervention in the first place. In the case of estrogen, its use for medical purposes is limited. The only major uses include synthetic estrogens in oral contraceptives and synthetic or natural estrogens in hormone replacement therapy after menopause. Minor medical uses involve the use of synthetic estrogens to treat transsexuals wishing to undergo a sex change and to induce secondary sexual characteristics in girls who have Turner syndrome. The study of girls with Turner syndrome presents extra problems because of the chromosome deletion that characterizes the condition. However, all the other methods for studying estrogen's effects have been used profitably in the last 10 years. We describe data from the various methodologies in the following sections.

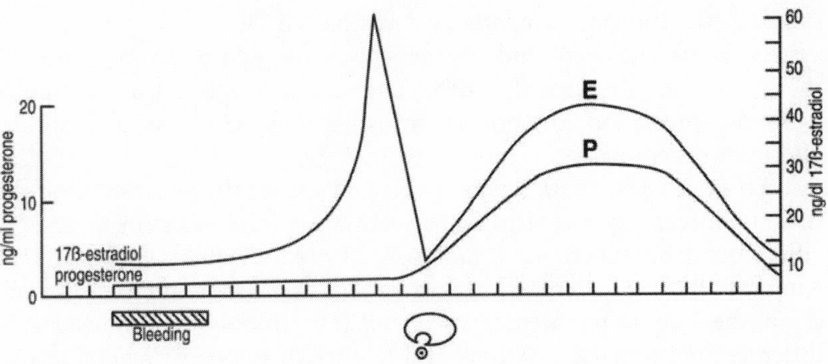

FIGURE 3.2. A simplified diagram of the changes in estradiol and progesterone that occur over the menstrual cycle. Onset of menstrual flow marks the beginning of a new cycle. Estradiol rises exponentially just prior to ovulation, then drops and undergoes a more gradual rise in the postovulatory portion of the cycle. The time period from ovulation to the start of a new cycle is the *luteal phase*. Progesterone, as well as estradiol, is high during the midluteal phase. Both are at their lowest ebb during menstruation. Adapted from Ganong (1977). Copyright 1977 by Lange Medical Books/McGraw-Hill. Adapted by permission.

Studies of Young Women

The activational approach to the study of sex differences in cognition began in the 1980s. Estrogen, specifically estradiol, was the first hormone implicated. The first data came from detailed studies of the menstrual cycle, in which repeated measure designs were used to evaluate an array of cognitive functions in healthy women tested at phases of the cycle characterized by low and high levels of estrogen (Figure 3.2). In parallel to these studies, but in a different context, the use of estrogen replacement in postmenopausal women was shown to have a visible effect on measures of explicit memory. We begin with a review of the menstrual cycle findings.

Prior to the mid-1980s, studies of the menstrual cycle were not designed to assess the activational hypothesis. Instead, the research focus was premenstrual syndrome (PMS) and its disruptive effects on mood and affective states. Conceptually, these studies tended to be atheoretical or to attribute premenstrual changes to social stereotypes about menstruation (May, 1976; Ruble, 1977). Social expectations do exaggerate some women's symptom reports, but the activational effects of ovarian hormones almost certainly play a role in triggering mood changes; PMS-like phenomena are seen in other female primates, not just humans (Hausfater & Skoblick, 1985). However, in the early 1980s, the concept of activational effects had not yet taken hold. Another group of studies tested a theory proposing that sex steroids alter the balance between the sympathetic and parasympathetic branches of the autonomic nervous system. Both androgens and estrogens were thought to promote sympathetic arousal. Although the theories were not supported, these studies were the precursors to modern investigations based on activational effects in other species.

From 1988 to 1990, several published studies demonstrated, for the first time, what appeared to be activational effects of estrogen on specific cognitive functions (Hampson, 1990a, 1990b; Hampson & Kimura, 1988). The research used a variety of tests known to elicit well-established sex differences, plus control tests that assessed nonsexually differentiated functions. A powerful feature of the experimental design was the use of repeated testing in the same groups of women. Their cognitive performance was evaluated in counterbalanced fashion at low and high levels of estradiol. Several findings emerged. First and foremost, modest fluctuations in performance were seen across the menstrual cycle on several, though not all, of the sexually differentiated tests. The largest fluctuations were found on tests of spatial abilities (d = .44), in which women had to perform mental transformations of objects or envision changes in positions of objects or their component parts (e.g., folding, rotation, or disembedding). On many spatial tests, males achieve higher average scores than do females. It was therefore of considerable interest that better performance on a set of spatial tests was found at the lowest estrogen levels, during the menstrual phase of the cycle. In contrast, no changes in scores over the menstrual cycle were observed on a control task. Even more interesting, several of the tests that assessed functions known to show a sex difference in favor of women showed a reverse effect—better scores at phases characterized by high estrogen. The fact that reciprocal changes were found simultaneously at high estrogen levels on tests showing a male versus female advantage suggested that the effects were selective and ruled out general shifts in arousal or attention, or other generalized processes in accounting for the effects.

In the initial studies, women were evaluated at the late menstrual and midluteal phases (Figure 3.2). These were chosen for practical reasons, because the preovulatory peak in estrogen is evanescent and difficult to target accurately. However, a possible confound was introduced, in that there is a rise in progesterone during the luteal phase that parallels the rise in estradiol. As it turns out, progesterone does not appear to be critical for the cognitive effects. Hampson (1990b) found the same effects on spatial ability, articulatory fluency, and manual coordination when testing a group of women at the preovulatory peak in estradiol, a time point when progesterone levels are still low and only estrogen is raised. High estradiol and low progesterone were confirmed by radioimmunoassays of blood serum, a widely used biochemical technique that allows researchers to quantify accurately the concentrations of steroids. Subsequent studies have failed to identify any significant correlations between circulating progesterone and cognitive test scores, although correlations with estradiol have consistently been observed (Hausmann, Slabbekoorn, Van Goozen, Cohen-Kettenis, & Güntürkün, 2000; Maki, Rich, & Rosenbaum, 2002).

The menstrual cycle studies were of great importance in demonstrating, for the first time, that activational effects of sex steroids were possible in humans. Sex steroids could exert visible effects at the behavioral level despite our complex brains and capacity to modify our behaviors through learning and experience. Moreover, because functions such as visuospatial abilities are mediated by cortical pathways, the studies implied that hormone–brain interactions can take place outside the hypothalamic–pituitary zone. It was previously believed that any hormone actions would be confined to this zone and its role in sexual behavior and motivation. The doors were now opened to investigating the possible role of sex steroids in a whole range of behaviors and functions that show sex differences.

Recent menstrual cycle studies have advanced our knowledge of these effects on several fronts. Nearly a dozen studies since 1990 have confirmed that spatial tests are susceptible to changes in estrogen levels. The range of tests has expanded and includes tests requiring folding or mental rotation of depicted items, accurate perception of spatial positions, and spatial bisection tasks. Tests of mental rotation have been particularly studied, yielding an average effect size of about $d = .65$. Many, but not all, spatial tasks show menstrual cycle variability. The reasons for this are not well understood. One suggestion is that tests with greater ecological validity are more likely to be sensitive to estrogen, because they tax problem-solving capabilities that evolved to cope with spatial problems in the natural environment (Phillips & Silverman, 1997).

The tendency of recent research to focus almost exclusively on visuospatial abilities has deemphasized the positive role of estrogen in promoting many functions. In a rare glimpse of other domains, Maki et al. (2002) were able to confirm that verbal fluency, or word generation, is improved at higher estrogen levels in healthy young women. This supports the idea that estrogen levels might contribute to sex differences, because women often score higher than men on measures of fluency. Improvement on an implicit memory task was also found and led to the suggestion that estrogen might facilitate the automatic activation of verbal representations.

The past 10 years have also brought evidence that activational effects on cognition occur in other primates, including rhesus monkeys and gorillas (Lacreuse, Verreault, & Herndon, 2001; Patterson, Holts,

TABLE 3.1. Motor Performance in Oral Contraceptive (OC) Users on High- and Low-Estrogen Pills

	Menses (n = 22)	Low OC (n = 24)	High OC (n = 32)
Demographics			
Age (yr)	22.45 (4.15)	22.29 (2.48)	22.25 (2.53)
Height (in)	65.00 (1.53)	65.61 (2.86)	65.00 (3.09)
Weight (lb)	131.89 (16.97)	126.87 (13.81)	128.41 (17.26)
Articulatory tests			
Syllable repetition (no. of syllables)			
Single	28.40 (3.26)*	29.00 (3.42)	30.40 (4.01)
Multiple	26.10 (5.45)*	26.54 (4.76)	29.23 (4.70)
Speeded counting (sec)[a]	17.79 (2.72)*	16.27 (2.30)	15.85 (2.84)
Reading color names (sec)	38.93 (4.12)	37.18 (3.64)	38.36 (5.19)
Speeded naming (sec)	51.05 (8.15)**	49.33 (7.21)	47.69 (7.58)
Tests of manual dexterity			
Manual sequence box (sec)			
Left hand	20.07 (15.16)*	15.85 (8.54)	14.81 (4.89)
Right hand	19.46 (10.81)*	14.85 (5.99)	16.11 (7.38)
Purdue pegboard (no. of pegs)			
Left hand	15.64 (1.70)*	16.50 (1.31)	16.39 (1.52)
Right hand	17.52 (1.43)	17.77 (1.76)	17.31 (1.67)
Assembly	41.11 (5.22)*	43.37 (3.90)	42.63 (4.44)
Finger tapping (no. of taps)			
Left hand	43.86 (3.97)	44.94 (5.03)	44.53 (3.91)
Right hand	47.15 (5.58)	48.48 (5.24)	48.29 (4.33)

Note. Data are from 22 non-OC users tested during menses and not reported previously. Women on OCs were classified as taking formulations low or high in estrogen potency according to ratings given in Dickey (1998) or related publications. Description of tasks and administration procedures can be found in Hampson (1990a or 1990b).

[a] For all timed measures, lower scores equal faster performance.

* Menses group significantly different from one or both OC groups, p<.05 one-tailed; **p<.06.

& Saphire, 1991), species that have a menstrual cycle much like our own. The evolutionary basis for these effects is still a mystery. One hypothesis is that the spatial abilities used for purposes of ranging and distance navigation may have come under the dynamic regulatory control of ovarian steroids, because they divert precious energy resources important for female reproductive success (Hampson, 2000; Sherry & Hampson, 1997). Briefly, the metabolic costs of reproduction in females are high; therefore, during periods of actual or impending reproductive investment, mechanisms may come into play to channel available energies preferentially into reproductive processes, and away from metabolically costly activities with low reproductive payoff, such as ranging or excess mobility. Down-regulation of spatial abilities may be one effect.

Although chiefly important during pregnancy and lactation, initiation of the same mechanisms may be evident over the menstrual cycle, if high levels of female hormones constitute a signal that denotes reproductive investment.

As compelling as the menstrual cycle studies are, they are still only correlational. If these are really effects of estradiol, the same cognitive outcomes should be found when estrogen levels are manipulated deliberately. Two types of studies speak to this issue. Oral contraceptives (OCs) are combinations of synthetic estrogens and progestins used to prevent pregnancy. They may also be used for therapeutic purposes. They suppress endogenous estrogen production but act as replacement hormones, and can bind to estrogen receptors. The estrogenic potency varies greatly from one brand to another. The OCs currently in widespread use are weak and do not always elicit effects on spatial functions (Hampson, 1990c; cf. Silverman & Phillips, 1993). Table 3.1 shows data on a set of motor and articulatory measures previously shown to be estrogen-sensitive, in two groups of OC users. The women were classified into Low and High groups based on the estrogen potency of their particular brand of OCs. There was a tendency for a mild facilitative effect in the OC users, as found at higher estrogen phases of the menstrual cycle, and some evidence of dose dependence. Although not always individually significant, women on the higher estrogen OCs showed the lowest mean scores on three tests that ordinarily show a male advantage (Figure 3.3). When the estrogen and progestin potencies of individual brands of pills were entered into regression equations predicting the cognitive test scores, estrogen potency showed a negative beta weight in all three cases. This emphasizes that the estrogen dose must be taken into account when assessing potential cognitive effects.

Ethinyl estradiol, the major estrogen in oral contraceptives, can also be used at high doses to induce the development of female secondary sex characteristics in transsexual men who wish to undergo a sex change. Antiandrogens are administered concurrently to suppress testosterone. Transsexualism is the only condition where opposite-sex hormones can be administered ethically and provides a powerful test of the ability of sex steroids to regulate cognitive function. Van Goozen, Cohen-Kettenis, Gooren, Frijda, and Van de Poll (1995) assessed cognitive performance in a group of transsexual men before and after 12 weeks of treatment with estrogen and antiandrogens. Relative to the men's performance at pretest, estrogen use was associated with deterioration in scores on a mental rotation test and with relative improvement in verbal fluency. Of course, attributing the changes to estrogen is complicated by the fact that the men were taking antiandrogens as well. Combined, however,

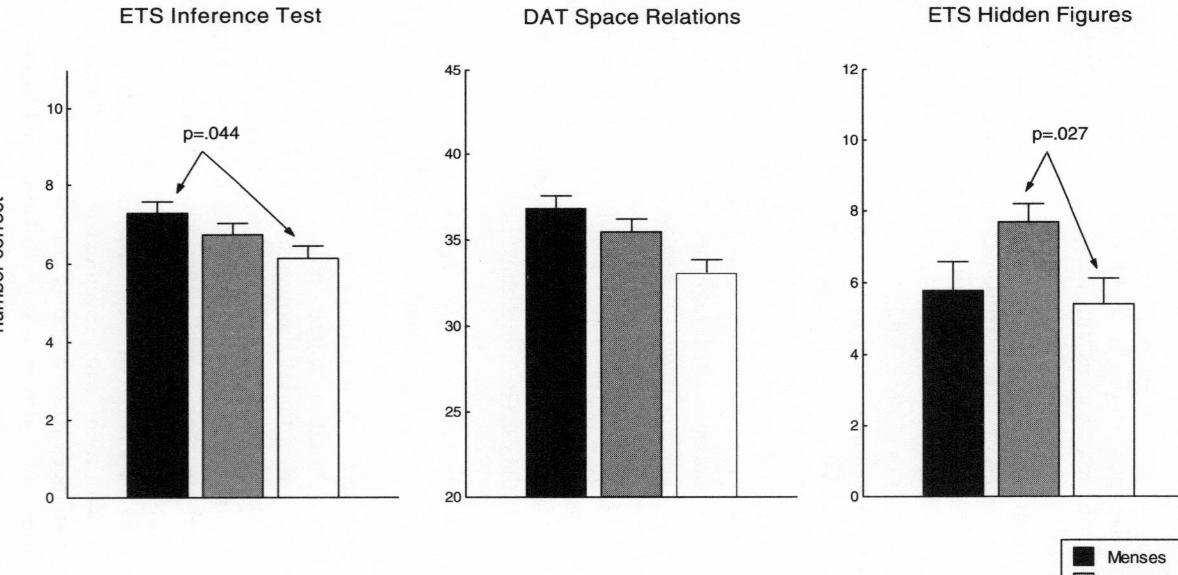

FIGURE 3.3. Performance of OC users and women at menses on a set of male-typed cognitive tests. Performance on the same tests varied over the menstrual cycle in Hampson (1990a). Consistent with the 1990 findings, OC users on higher estrogen pills achieved the lowest scores on the tests. Differences between menses and low estrogen pills were not statistically significant. The Rod and Frame test was administered but is not shown here, because the data were severely skewed. ETS, Educational Testing Service; DAT, Differential Aptitude Tests.

data from oral contraceptive users and from treated transsexuals support the view that estrogen exerts activational effects on some sexually differentiated cognitive functions.

Beyond the Reproductive Years: Studies of Postmenopausal Women

In parallel to the menstrual cycle work, researchers during the 1990s demonstrated that estrogen might have a regulatory effect on memory systems. The studies involved postmenopausal women, who were either taking or not taking various forms of hormone replacement therapy (HRT). These studies were motivated by clinical questions; therefore, the range of functions investigated was limited. Nevertheless, they are relevant to the activational hypothesis and extend our knowledge of the cognitive systems in which estrogen may be active.

Much of the work on menopause and cognition was stimulated by a set of well-controlled studies in which the impact of estrogen replacement was studied in women who had their ovaries removed by hysterectomy (Phillips & Sherwin, 1992; Sherwin, 1988). The studies convincingly implicated estrogen, because they used a double-blind, placebo-controlled design, the "gold standard" in medical studies. Following surgery, the onset of menopause is immediate, with a large, rapid decrease in circulating estrogen. Using a standardized memory scale, Sherwin discovered that surgery resulted in a decrease in the ability to recall factual details of short stories or to learn word pairs and retain them over a brief delay. The memory loss could be reversed by estrogen or, if estrogen was initiated right after the surgery, memory was maintained at its former levels. Later studies suggested that the benefits of HRT might extend to the ability to remember nonverbal material (e.g., geometric designs) and to women who are naturally menopausal due to age (Resnick, Maki, Golski, Kraut, & Zonderman, 1998; Resnick, Metter, & Zonderman, 1997). However, this is less certain because the effects on explicit memory tend to be small and are easily masked in observational studies, unless the groups are well-matched on other health-related variables.

Menopause researchers typically do not think of their work in terms of sex differences. However, there is a small female advantage on many tests of explicit memory (Herlitz, Airaksinen, & Nordström, 1999). Therefore, a positive effect of HRT supports the view that estrogen helps to promote a feminized cognitive profile. The effects on memory are of special interest because of animal studies showing facilitative effects of high estrogen levels on synaptic connections in the hippocampus. Although this is not the only possible route by which estrogen could lead to improved memory, it is one possible mechanism. The hippocampal region is widely believed to participate in memory encoding and retrieval processes.

Temporal lobe memory systems are probably not the only ones sensitive to estrogen. We know from animal studies that parts of the prefrontal cortex (PFC) are sites of estrogen activity. Recently, Duff and Hampson (2000) found that postmenopausal women taking estrogen scored significantly better than matched women not taking estrogen on verbal and spatial measures of working memory, a form of memory in which information must be actively held in mind or kept "on-line." This form of short-term memory depends heavily on the PFC. In our study, the women not on estrogen committed almost 40% more working memory errors. In young women asked to perform one of the same working memory tasks, we found poorer scores at the menstrual phase, when estrogen is low (Duff-Canning & Hampson, 2002; Figure 3.4), supporting the view that estrogen plays a regulatory role. Sex differences in working memory had not been investigated previously, but we discovered a robust sex difference in favor of women in three separate experiments using a demanding working memory task (Duff & Hampson, 2001). This line of research is very new, but already it suggests that sexual differentiation of the brain and the effects of HRT may extend to frontal lobe systems.

If there are cognitive benefits to be gained from the use of HRT after menopause, should all women be counseled to use HRT? Quality of life in old age rests on a number of factors, not just mental functioning. Because large-scale clinical trials have suggested that the long-term use of HRT has both risks and benefits for physical health (Writing Group for the Women's Health Initiative, 2002), decisions whether to use HRT must be individualized to each woman's lifestyle, needs, and risk factors. Cognitive outcomes are only one part of the mix.

EFFECTS OF ANDROGENS ON COGNITIVE FUNCTIONS IN MEN AND WOMEN

The existence of menstrual cyclicity and the widespread use of HRT in women provide powerful research tools for investigating the effects of gonadal steroids on cognitive function. Although these methods are not available in men, recent research has taken advantage of daily and seasonal changes in testosterone (T) levels to assess the impact of androgens on cognition. Another approach has been to study the relationship between individual differences in the levels of androgens in blood or saliva and scores on cognitive tests. Moreover, though not as common as HRT,

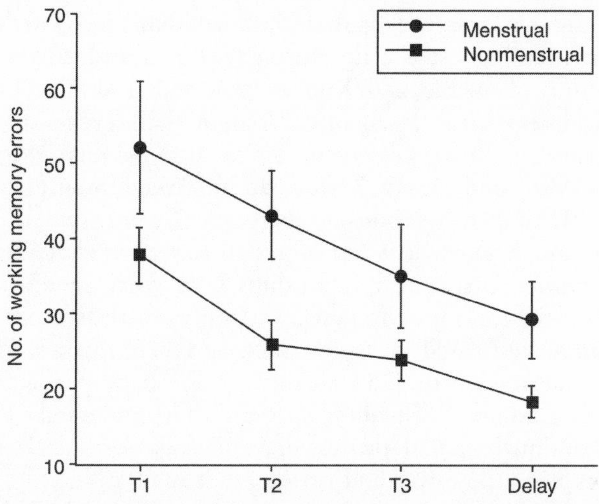

FIGURE 3.4. Performance of young women on a spatial working memory task. The task consisted of a spatial array of 20 doors behind which were hidden 20 colored dots. Participants were asked to find all 10 matching pairs of colors in as few moves as possible. The task resembles the card game "Concentration." We found that women tested at the menstrual phase of the cycle ($n = 8$) committed significantly more working memory errors than a mixed group of women not at the menstrual phase ($n = 19$) (Duff-Canning & Hampson, 2002). On average, estrogen levels would be lower in the menstrual group. T1, T2, T3, trials 1, 2, and 3; Delay, performance on the same task after a 30- to 40-minute delay.

androgen replacement is performed in older men. Studies of its effects on cognition are now being undertaken. We consider the findings from these approaches in the next section.

Circulating Androgens and Cognitive Performance in Young Adults

A common approach to investigating the effects of T on cognitive performance has been to measure circulating androgen levels in blood or saliva and to relate these values to scores on standardized neuropsychological tests. As with the menstrual cycle studies in women, the tests used in this research tend to be those that reveal sex differences. Although the results from these studies are somewhat variable, the available data suggest that an inverted-U-shaped function may best describe the relationship between T and spatial cognition, with optimum spatial performance at *moderately* high T. In support of this, Gouchie and Kimura (1991) found that men with lower T performed better on tests of spatial abilities than men with high T. Women with the highest T outperformed women with lower T on the same measures. Gouchie and Kimura reported a similar finding for mathematical reasoning, a cognitive domain that reveals male advantages similar to those observed for spatial ability. Moffat and Hampson (1996) and Neave, Menaged, and Weightman (1999) found an inverted-U-shaped relationship between T and spatial scores in young men and women. It is important to recognize that these studies observed inverted-U-shaped relationships only when men and women were assessed in the same analysis, and only on tests of spatial processing. Language-related measures, such as verbal fluency, showed no significant relationship to T. In all these studies, the participants were healthy young adults. Such findings imply that moderately high levels of T may optimize spatial processing, and suggest that the optimum level of T is near the lower end of the adult male range.

Although males do not show any temporal changes in T that resemble the menstrual cycle, T concentrations do vary substantially throughout the day and over the course of the year. Male T concentrations show a circadian rhythm, with T peaking in the early morning hours and declining sharply thereafter, until the trough is reached approximately 12 hours later (Nieschlag, 1974). The waxing and waning of T levels over the course of the day allow researchers to examine whether there are corresponding circadian changes in men's cognitive performance. Moffat and Hampson (1996) took advantage of the diurnal rhythm by administering verbal and spatial tests to men and women assigned to either early morning or late morning sessions. The diurnal change in T over the time course of the experiment was verified using radioimmunoassays. Men tested in early morning performed more poorly on the spatial tests than men tested later, when T levels were lower. Among females, the reverse pattern was observed. (This is consistent with the optimal level hypothesis, since T levels in women, as in men, are highest first thing in the morning.) These findings were specific to the spatial tests; verbal performance showed no diurnal changes. Paralleling the findings from the menstrual cycle, the results suggest that spatial performance may change dynamically over a relatively short time span, in concert with the diurnal change in T. Although a number of other biological and social factors besides T levels fluctuate throughout the day, the fact that the results were specific to the spatial tests and were opposite in men and women makes explanations based on more general factors, such as fatigue, less likely.

In addition to the circadian rhythm, male T concentrations exhibit circannual variability. T levels are higher in the autumn than the spring (Meriggiola, Noonan, Paulsen, & Bremner, 1996). It has been speculated that this circannual pattern of T secretion may have had ecological advantages for our ancestors, making births more likely in the spring and summer months, when environmental circumstances were more favorable to the rearing of newborns (Sherry & Hampson, 1997). Kimura and Hampson (1994) found that in young men, spatial performance was better in the spring, when T concentrations were lower, than in the fall, when they were higher. Once again, the effect was specific to spatial tasks. Other cognitive measures showed no seasonal fluctuations.

Exogenous T is not given to young men under normal conditions. This limits our options for studying the effects of T in intervention trials. However, T is used in the medical treatment of hypogonadism—a condition of low testicular output that can result from several causes. Hypogonadal men may have severe learning disabilities or other CNS anomalies, but they are of interest for two reasons: (1) It is conceivable that despite the complicating factors, we might still see improvement in spatial abilities if T is restored to the normal range; (2) two recent studies of hypogonadal men included control groups of healthy men who agreed to receive T, bringing androgens into the supranormal range (Alexander et al., 1998; O'Connor, Archer, Hair, & Wu, 2001). Although neither study was able to demonstrate a significant improvement in hypogonadal men, O'Connor et al. (2001) found that supranormal T in controls was associated with reduced scores on a spatial visualization test. This is consistent with the optimal level theory. Treatment of young *women* with androgens is even rarer. Transsexual females who desire to be males and are treated with androgens experience increased spatial abilities (Van Goozen, Cohen-Kettenis, Gooren, Frijda, & Van de Poll, 1994).

Although it is not a "normal" condition, there is one situation in which healthy young men self-administer androgens: the use of anabolic steroids to improve athletic performance. Steroid use for this purpose is illegal and contravenes the ethical guidelines of college athletics. Doses tend to be high, and some of the hormones used are veterinary preparations. Almost nothing is known about cognitive functioning in steroid users, but there are anecdotal reports of mood changes and even the precipitation of psychiatric symptoms in susceptible individuals (Pope & Katz, 1988). This suggests the steroids do have central nervous system actions. In the first placebo-controlled prospective study of anabolic steroids in healthy male volunteers, adverse effects on mood and behavioral variables were identified, including increased cognitive impairment on self-ratings of distractibility, forgetfulness, and confusion (Su et al., 1993). Performance on spatial tests was not assessed.

Much of the evidence pertaining to androgens and spatial abilities is from correlational studies. Therefore, a logical question to ask is whether spatial performance might alter T levels, instead of vice versa. Under some conditions, hormones can be recruited in anticipation of, or in response to, psychological stimuli. With respect to T, studies have found increases in T in males in response to competition situations, specifically in response to the perception of winning or achieving dominance (Gladue, Boechler, & McCaul, 1989; Rose, Bernstein, & Gordon, 1975). Might T therefore rise in response to performing cognitively demanding tasks? At present, we have no evidence to suggest this occurs. In fact, the "winners" (the males who achieve the highest spatial scores) are not the ones found to have the highest T levels.

Although work on the relationship between T and cognition is sparse compared to research on estrogen, a consistent pattern of results is beginning to emerge. Correlational studies relating individual differences in T to cognitive abilities reliably implicate spatial ability. They suggest that in young adults, the relationship between T and spatial cognition is nonlinear. Intermediate T concentrations, not the top of the male range, seem to be maximally beneficial to performance. Data from circadian and circannual variations provide convergent support for the possibility that higher spatial processing is observed when T is at or near the low end of the male T distribution. Only a few studies have investigated cognitive variables in males receiving exogenous T. There is some support for the optimal level theory, but treatment studies are few and far between, and the results are still mixed (cf. Alexander et al., 1998).

Why would lower levels of T be associated with higher spatial ability in men? Men who live in Western, industrialized nations turn out to have quite high T. This is probably due to diet and lifestyle factors, but whatever the reason, these levels are almost certainly not typical of our evolutionary past. In fact, these high levels might help to explain why some hormone-stimulated cancers, such as prostate cancer, occur at such high rates in Western countries. Many non-Western groups living today, such as the !Kung San, Aché, or other subsistence or hunter–gatherer groups, have been reported to have lower T, though still within the range we consider normal (Ellison & Panter-Brick, 1996; Winkler & Christiansen, 1993). Perhaps spatial ability is optimized under the range of physiological T levels that would have been expected to occur in our human ancestors.

Cognitive Effects of Androgen Loss and Supplementation in Older Adults

Older age is associated with functional declines in multiple body systems, including some aspects of cognitive performance. However, there are large individual differences, with some individuals showing dramatic changes and others maintaining excellent cognitive faculties well into old age. The factors that contribute to this variability are the subject of considerable interest in the biomedical and social sciences. In particular, recent evidence that age-related alterations in the endocrine environment may modulate cognitive changes has generated great interest.

Testosterone and Cognitive Function in Older Adults

As we noted earlier, in women there is evidence that postmenopausal estrogen replacement therapy may exert beneficial effects on specific cognitive functions, and may reduce the incidence and delay the onset of Alzheimer's disease. In men, total T declines by as much as 50% from ages 30 to 80 (Lamberts, van den Beld, & van der Lely, 1997), and as many as 68% of men over age 70 can be classified as hypogonadal based on their free T concentrations (Harman, Metter, Tobin, Pearson, & Blackman, 2001). These observations raise the question of whether the loss of androgens with age, known as the *male andropause,* is associated with age-related declines in some cognitive functions. Conversely, we can ask whether the replacement of T might result in some recovery of cognitive function in older men.

A few recent studies suggest that, indeed, androgen loss and/or its subsequent replacement may in fact modulate cognitive processing in both older men and women. Barrett-Connor, Goodman-Gruen, and Patay (1999) measured androgen levels and neuropsychological performance in 547 men, ages 59–89 years. Higher T concentrations predicted better scores on measures of short-term memory and concentration. Nonlinear relationships were also found, in which moderately high T levels were associated with better scores on tests of mental control and long-term verbal memory. In a second study, the relationship between endogenous steroid levels and cognitive performance was investigated in 383 women, ages 55–89 years (Barrett-Connor & Goodman-Gruen, 1999). Women with higher scores on mental status had significantly higher total and bioavailable T levels. These studies are hard to interpret, because higher T may simply be an index of better health. Unfortunately, measures of spatial cognition were not included in these studies, making direct comparisons with studies of younger adults difficult. Nevertheless, these data are consistent with the possibility that T may continue to modulate neuropsychological performance in elderly men and women.

In the most comprehensive study of the effects of androgen loss on cognitive function in older men, Moffat et al. (2002) investigated age-associated decreases in endogenous serum T concentrations and declines in neuropsychological performance among 407 men ages 50–91 years.

The men in the study were followed longitudinally for an average of 10 years, with assessments of multiple cognitive domains and contemporaneous determination of serum total T, sex hormone binding globulin, and free T. Longitudinal research is important in the study of cognitive aging, because it allows for the assessment of the *rate of change* in cognitive skills, a measure that is thought to be an important predictor of later life neuropsychological outcomes. In this study, higher free T was associated with higher scores on visual and verbal memory, and visuospatial functioning, and with a reduced rate of longitudinal decline in visual memory. No relations were observed between T and measures of verbal knowledge, general mental status, or depressive symptoms.

In a second component to the study, men were classified as either hypogonadal or eugonadal (normal T levels) based on their free T concentrations. Comparison of the two groups of men revealed higher spatial and memory function among the eugonadal men and a reduced rate of decline in visual memory. The effect sizes from these comparisons were substantial. For example, the difference between hypogonadal and eugonadal men on spatial ability was $d = .52$. The results suggest a possible beneficial relationship between circulating free T concentrations in older men and specific domains of cognitive performance and cognitive decline.

As noted earlier, a drawback of correlational studies is that one cannot confirm that T concentrations per se caused the cognitive effects. As with estrogen replacement therapy in women, testosterone replacement therapy (TRT) is now performed in older men, albeit less frequently. In a double-blind, placebo-controlled study, Janowsky, Oviatt, and Orwoll (1994) investigated cognitive performance in older men who were given TRT to treat androgen deficiency. Men who received T had selectively enhanced Wechsler Adult Intelligence Scale—Revised (WAIS-R) Block Design scores compared to men receiving a placebo, demonstrating that TRT may improve spatial–constructional abilities. In a more recent placebo-controlled trial, Janowsky, Chavez, and Orwoll (2000) found that men who received T supplementation showed a reduction in working memory errors compared to placebo-treated men. In the most recent intervention study, Cherrier et al. (2001) found improved verbal memory, improved spatial ability, and improved route recall in men who received 6 weeks of TRT. At first glance, these studies might seem inconsistent with prior investigations reporting that higher T in young men is detrimental to spatial performance. However, older men in whom the T replacement trials are performed have already undergone substantial T depletion. Thus, the T supplementation may be returning T levels in these men to the optimal range.

The results of correlational studies, together with recent, small-scale

T intervention trials in elderly men, suggest that the progressive physiological decline in T secretion with aging contributes to selective losses in cognitive function. These can be reversed, at least in part, by T supplementation. Interestingly, in older men, *nonspatial* measures of cognition, such as verbal and visual memory, seem also to be T-sensitive. It is not clear whether this represents an actual change in the function of T over the lifespan or researchers' neglect of memory as a possible androgen-responsive set of functions in younger adults. Studies in young adults tend to have been guided by research on sex differences, and thus have focused on spatial cognition, whereas studies in older adults that stress cognitive functions susceptible to age have emphasized verbal and visual memory. It will be interesting to discover whether the memory capacities of men and women are under hormonal influence in young adulthood.

Dehydroepiandrosterone and Cognitive Function in Older Adults

Another source of androgen depletion in both males and females is the progressive, age-related decline in dehydroepiandrosterone (DHEA). DHEA is a weak androgen secreted by the adrenal gland and may be converted to estradiol and T, thus making it an indirect source of both steroids. DHEA has recently received considerable popular and scientific attention due in part to the fact that it was made available in the United States as an over-the-counter food supplement in 1994. Some elderly individuals currently self-administer DHEA because of its reputed antiaging effects in a variety of physiological and psychological systems. Empirical support for the cognition-enhancing effects of DHEA comes primarily from an extensive animal literature demonstrating that DHEA improves long-term memory and has neuroprotective properties (Bologa, Sharma, & Roberts, 1987; Roberts, Bologa, Flood, & Smith, 1987).

However, in humans, similar benefits have not been demonstrated. Barrett-Connor and Edelstein (1994) found that baseline DHEA levels did not predict measures of mental status and verbal or visual memory in men or women. Similarly, Yaffe et al. (1998) found no significant correlation between DHEA concentrations and cognitive performance in elderly women. Most recently, Moffat et al. (2000), in a longitudinal study, followed 883 men for a mean duration of 12 years, sampling both serum DHEA and a wide range of cognitive abilities every 2 years. This design allowed long-term changes in DHEA levels to be quantified in direct temporal association with longitudinal changes in neuropsychological outcomes. Neither the DHEA concentration nor the rate of change of DHEA over time predicted cognitive decline in this sample of men. Currently, the evidence from large population studies suggests that although both DHEA concentrations and neuropsychological performance decline with age, the phenomena appear to occur independently of one another.

Despite the negative results from population studies, researchers have begun to assess the possible cognitive benefits of DHEA supplementation. These trials have failed to provide strong evidence of a cognition-enhancing role for DHEA. Wolf and colleagues performed two placebo-controlled clinical trials examining the efficacy of DHEA replacement therapy on cognition (Wolf, Naumann, Hellhammer, & Kirschbaum, 1998; Wolf et al., 1997). In both trials, DHEA supplementation of 50 mg/day for 2 weeks failed to exert cognitive effects in either men or women. In another study, Wolf et al. (1998) assessed the effects of DHEA on cognitive function following the application of a stressor. It has been hypothesized that DHEA may have antistress effects and, hence, may exert beneficial effects only under conditions of stress. Consistent with this hypothesis, Wolf et al. found that under stressful conditions, DHEA supplementation improved attention/concentration compared with placebo. However, they also found that DHEA impaired recall of previously learned material. Although controlled trials of DHEA supplementation have yielded largely negative results, it should be noted that these trials sampled only a limited range of cognitive abilities in relatively small samples of subjects over a short duration. Larger, placebo-controlled clinical trials will be needed to evaluate conclusively the effects of exogenous DHEA on cognition.

It is not entirely clear why studies of DHEA have produced negative results, whereas studies investigating the cognitive effects of T and estrogen have yielded positive findings. One possibility is that the DHEA : cortisol ratio may be a more critical measure than DHEA levels alone (Hechter, Grossman, & Chatterton, 1997). This is based on the antistress effects of DHEA that have been observed in rodents (Kalimi, Shafagoj, Loria, Padgett, & Regelson, 1994). Still another possibility is that, to our knowledge, no DHEA receptor has been identified in the brain of any mammal (see Wolf & Kirschbaum, 1999). This suggests that DHEA may exert cognitive effects only if converted to other substances, or via interactions with specific neurotransmitter systems (Wolf & Kirschbaum, 1999). It is possible that DHEA supplementation does not produce a large enough change in circulating T or estrogen to affect cognition appreciably. Moreover, studies to date have assessed cognitive outcomes that are not particularly sensitive to sex differences. It is possible that tests of spatial cognition might yield different results.

To summarize, a variety of studies and methodologies support the theory that androgens exert detectable effects on cognition in men and, more tentatively, women. The studies suggest that in young adults, moderately high levels of T are optimal for the performance of visuospatial tasks. In elderly men, who have already experienced age-related T depletion, T loss appears to be associated with cognitive decline, and T supplementation may benefit spatial performance and memory. Although earlier studies suggested that T effects may be limited to spatial cognition, recent epidemiological studies and clinical trials demonstrate broader correlations with cognitive performance, at least in the elderly. Larger scale investigations are warranted to assess whether T treatment is able to prevent or attenuate cognitive loss in healthy aging men and/or men with Alzheimer's disease. Moreover, understanding whether T exerts its cognitive effects chiefly via androgenic or estrogenic mechanisms will be an important issue to resolve. As well as providing possible practical treatments for cognitive loss in older adults, such studies will contribute to our basic understanding of the effects of hormones on cognitive sex differences and brain aging.

CONCLUSIONS

Research on the activational effects of reproductive hormones supports a very different view of sex differences. Historically, sex differences in cognitive function have been viewed as static, stemming largely from the differential experiences of the two sexes. It was not anticipated that metabolic state at the time of testing would have such large and consistent effects. Although only a small subset of abilities has been shown so far to be subject to the activational effects of sex steroids, it is unclear how prevalent activational effects may be. Certainly, they may extend to other behavioral domains that show sex differences, beyond the realm of cognitive functions. Finding activational effects is one more piece to the puzzle of how sex differences originate. It does not in any way negate the possibility that organizational effects also play a role in generating differences, nor does it negate the possibility of nonbiological influences. Many genetic, social, developmental, cultural, and contextual factors, not just the level of circulating hormones, interact to influence cognitive performance at any particular point in time. Environmental factors can either accentuate or act to mitigate the differences induced by hormones, and this is fertile ground for new research. The existence of activational effects does mean, however, that sex differences may be more dynamic entities than previously appreciated. The question, "How big is the sex difference?," cannot be answered without reference to specific conditions that exist at the time.

The activational approach can shed light on how biology contributes to sexual differentiation, and can help to identify functions that were once so basic to human survival that Mother Nature etched into our genes a mechanism for ensuring that the "proper" sex differences come about. Like all sex differences based in evolutionary selection, the cognitive adaptations must have provided a competitive advantage. If we are to understand fully the scope and limits of social and cultural influences on our sexual identities, it is important to identify the biological differences between the sexes.

REFERENCES

Alexander, G. M., Swerdloff, R. S., Wang, C., Davidson, T., McDonald, V., Steiner, B., et al. (1998). Androgen–behavior correlations in hypogonadal men and eugonadal men: II. Cognitive abilities. *Hormones and Behavior, 33,* 85–94.

Barrett-Connor, E., & Edelstein, S. L. (1994). A prospective study of dehydroepiandrosterone sulfate and cognitive function in an older population: The Rancho Bernardo Study. *Journal of the American Geriatric Society, 48,* 420–423.

Barrett-Connor, E., & Goodman-Gruen, D. (1999). Cognitive function and endogenous sex hormones in older women. *Journal of the American Geriatric Society, 47,* 1289–1293.

Barrett-Connor, E., Goodman-Gruen, D., & Patay, B. (1999). Endogenous sex hormones and cognitive function in older men. *Journal of Clinical Endocrinology and Metabolism, 84,* 3681–3685.

Bologa, L., Sharma, J., & Roberts, E. (1987). Dehydroepiandrosterone and its sulfated derivative reduce neuronal death and enhance astrocytic differentiation in brain cell cultures. *Journal of Neuroscience Research, 17,* 225–234.

Cherrier, M. M., Asthana, S., Plymate, S., Baker, L., Matsumoto, A. M., Peskind, E., et al. (2001). Testosterone supplementation improves spatial and verbal memory in healthy older men. *Neurology, 57,* 80–88.

Dickey, R. P. (1998). *Managing contraceptive pill patients* (9th ed.). Durant, OK: EMIS Medical Publishers.

Duff, S. J., & Hampson, E. (2000). A beneficial effect of estrogen on working memory in postmenopausal women taking hormone replacement therapy. *Hormones and Behavior, 38,* 262-276.

Duff, S. J., & Hampson, E. (2001). A sex difference on a novel spatial working memory task in humans. *Brain and Cognition, 47,* 470–493.

Duff-Canning, S., & Hampson, E. (2002, May). *Working memory performance varies across the menstrual cycle in young women.* Paper presented at the meeting of the Canadian Society for Brain, Behavior, and Cognitive Science, Vancouver, BC.

Ellison, P. T., & Panter-Brick, C. (1996). Salivary testosterone levels among Tamang and Kami males of central Nepal. *Human Biology, 68,* 955–965.

Fader, A. J., Johnson, P. E. M., & Dohanich, G. P. (1999). Estrogen improves working but not reference memory and prevents amnestic effects of scopolamine on a radial-arm maze. *Pharmacology, Biochemistry, and Behavior, 62,* 711–717.

Galea, L. A. M., Ormerod, B. K., Sampath, S., Kostaras, X., Wilkie, D. M., & Phelps, M. T. (2000). Spatial working memory and hippocampal size across pregnancy in rats. *Hormones and Behavior, 37,* 86–95.

Ganong, W. F. (1977). *Review of medical physiology* (8th ed.). Los Altos, CA: Lange Medical Publications.

Gladue, B. A., Boechler, M., & McCaul, K. D. (1989). Hormonal response to competition in human males. *Aggressive Behavior, 15,* 409–422.

Gouchie, C., & Kimura, D. (1991). The relationship between testosterone levels and cognitive ability patterns. *Psychoneuroendocrinology, 16,* 323–334.

Hampson, E. (1990a). Variations in sex-related cognitive abilities across the menstrual cycle. *Brain and Cognition, 14,* 26–43.

Hampson, E. (1990b). Estrogen-related variations in human spatial and articulatory–motor skills. *Psychoneuroendocrinology, 15,* 97–111.

Hampson, E. (1990c). Influence of gonadal hormones on cognitive function in women. *Clinical Neuropharmacology, 13*(Suppl. 2), 522–523.

Hampson, E. (2000). Sexual differentiation of spatial functions in humans. In A. Matsumoto (Ed.), *Sexual differentiation of the brain* (pp. 279–300). Boca Raton, FL: CRC Press.

Hampson, E., & Kimura, D. (1988). Reciprocal effects of hormonal fluctuations on human motor and perceptual–spatial skills. *Behavioral Neuroscience, 102,* 456–459.

Harman, S. M., Metter, E. J., Tobin, J. D., Pearson, J., & Blackman, M. R. (2001). Longitudinal effects of aging on serum total and free testosterone levels in healthy men. Baltimore Longitudinal Study of Aging. *Journal of Clinical Endocrinology and Metabolism, 86,* 724–731.

Hausfater, G., & Skoblick, B. (1985). Perimenstrual behavior changes among female yellow baboons: Some similarities to premenstrual syndrome (PMS) in women. *American Journal of Primatology, 9,* 165–172.

Hausmann, M., Slabbekoorn, D., Van Goozen, S. H. M., Cohen-Kettenis, P. T., & Güntürkün, O. (2000). Sex hormones affect spatial abilities during the menstrual cycle. *Behavioral Neuroscience, 114,* 1245–1250.

Hechter, O., Grossman, A., & Chatterton, R. T. (1997). Relationship of dehydroepiandrosterone and cortisol in disease. *Medical Hypotheses, 49,* 85–91.

Herlitz, A., Airaksinen, E., & Nordström, E. (1999). Sex differences in episodic memory: The impact of verbal and visuospatial ability. *Neuropsychology, 13,* 590–597.

Janowsky, J. S., Chavez, B., & Orwoll, E. (2000). Sex steroids modify working memory. *Journal of Cognitive Neuroscience, 12,* 407–414.

Janowsky, J. S., Oviatt, S. K., & Orwoll, E. S. (1994). Testosterone influences spatial cognition in older men. *Behavioral Neuroscience, 108,* 325–332.

Kalimi, M., Shafagoj, Y., Loria, R., Padgett, D., & Regelson, W. (1994). Antiglucocorticoid effects of dehydroepiandrosterone (DHEA). *Molecular and Cellular Biochemistry, 131,* 99–104.

Kimura, D., & Hampson, E. (1994). Cognitive pattern in men and women is influenced by fluctuations in sex hormones. *Current Directions in Psychological Science, 3,* 57–61.

Lacreuse, A., Verreault, M., & Herndon, J. G. (2001). Fluctuations in spatial recognition memory across the menstrual cycle in female rhesus monkeys. *Psychoneuroendocrinology, 26,* 623–639.

Lamberts, S. W., van den Beld, A. W., & van der Lely, A. J. (1997). The endocrinology of aging. *Science, 278,* 419–424.

Maki, P. M., Rich, J. B., & Rosenbaum, R. S. (2002). Implicit memory varies across the menstrual cycle: Estrogen effects in young women. *Neuropsychologia, 40,* 518–529.

May, R. R. (1976). Mood shifts and the menstrual cycle. *Journal of Psychosomatic Research, 20,* 125–130.

Meriggiola, M. C., Noonan, E. A., Paulsen, C. A., & Bremner, W. J. (1996). Annual patterns of luteinizing hormone, follicle stimulating hormone, testosterone and inhibin in normal men. *Human Reproduction, 11,* 248–252.

Moffat, S. D., & Hampson, E. (1996). A curvilinear relationship between testosterone and spatial cognition in humans: Possible influence of hand preference. *Psychoneuroendocrinology, 21,* 323–337.

Moffat, S. D., Zonderman, A. B., Harman, S. M., Blackman, M. R., Kawas, C., & Resnick, S. M. (2000). The relationship between longitudinal declines in dehydroepiandrosterone sulfate concentrations and cognitive performance in older men. *Archives of Internal Medicine, 160,* 2193–2198.

Moffat, S. D., Zonderman, A. B., Metter, E. J., Blackman, M. R., Harman, S. M., & Resnick, S. M. (2002). Longitudinal assessment of serum total and free testosterone concentrations predicts memory performance and cognitive status in elderly men. *Journal of Clinical Endocrinology and Metabolism, 87,* 5001–5007.

Neave, N., Menaged, M., & Weightman, D. R. (1999). Sex differences in cognition: The role of testosterone and sexual orientation. *Brain and Cognition, 41, 245–262.*

Nieschlag, E. (1974). Circadian rhythm of plasma testosterone. In J. Aschoff, F. Ceresa, & F. Halberg (Eds.), *Chronobiological aspects of endocrinology* (pp. 117–128). Stuttgart, Germany: Schattaquer Verlag.

O'Connor, D. B., Archer, J., Hair, W. M., & Wu, F. C. W. (2001). Activational effects of testosterone on cognitive function in men. *Neuropsychologia, 39,* 1385–1394.

Patterson, F. G. P., Holts, C. L., & Saphire, L. (1991). Cyclic changes in hormonal, physical, behavioral, and linguistic measures in a female lowland gorilla. *American Journal of Primatology, 24,* 181–194.

Phillips, K., & Silverman, I. (1997). Differences in the relationship of menstrual cycle phase to spatial performance on two- and three-dimensional tasks. *Hormones and Behavior, 32,* 167–175.

Phillips, S. M., & Sherwin, B. B. (1992). Effects of estrogen on memory function in surgically menopausal women. *Psychoneuroendocrinology, 17,* 485–495.

Pope, H. G., & Katz, D. L. (1988). Affective and psychotic symptoms associated with anabolic steroid use. *American Journal of Psychiatry, 145,* 487–490.

Resnick, S. M., Maki, P. M., Golski, S., Kraut, M. A. & Zonderman, A. B. (1998). Effects of estrogen replacement therapy on PET cerebral blood flow and neuropsychological performance. *Hormones and Behavior, 34,* 171–182.

Resnick, S. M., Metter, E. J., & Zonderman, A. B. (1997). Estrogen replacement therapy and longitudinal decline in visual memory: A possible protective effect? *Neurology, 49,* 1491–1497.

Roberts, E., Bologa, L., Flood, J. F., & Smith, G. E. (1987). Effects of dehydroepiandrosterone and its sulfate on brain tissue in culture and on memory in mice. *Brain Research, 406*(1–2), 357–362.

Rose, R. M., Bernstein, I. S., & Gordon, T. P. (1975). Consequences of social conflict on plasma testosterone levels in rhesus monkeys. *Psychosomatic Medicine, 37,* 50–61.

Ruble, D. N. (1977). Premenstrual symptoms: A reinterpretation. *Science, 197,* 291–292.

Sherry, D. F., & Hampson, E. (1997). Evolution and the hormonal control of sexually dimorphic spatial abilities in humans. *Trends in Cognitive Sciences, 1,* 50–56.

Sherwin, B. B. (1988). Estrogen and/or androgen replacement therapy and cognitive functioning in surgically menopausal women. *Psychoneuroendocrinology, 13,* 345–357.

Silverman, I., & Phillips, K. (1993). Effects of estrogen changes during the menstrual cycle on spatial performance. *Ethology and Sociobiology, 14,* 257–270.

Su, T. P., Pagliaro, M., Schmidt, P. J., Pickar, D., Wolkowitz, O., & Rubinow, D. R. (1993). Neuropsychiatric effects of anabolic steroids in male normal volunteers. *Journal of the American Medical Association, 269,* 2760–2764.

Van Goozen, S. H. M., Cohen-Kettenis, P. T., Gooren, L. J. G., Frijda, N. H., & Van de Poll, N. E. (1994). Activating effects of androgens on cognitive performance: Causal evidence in a group of female-to-male transsexuals. *Neuropsychologia, 32,* 1153–1157.

Van Goozen, S. H. M., Cohen-Kettenis, P. T., Gooren, L. J. G., Frijda, N. H., & Van de Poll, N. E. (1995). Gender differences in behavior: Activating effects of cross-gender hormones. *Psychoneuroendocrinology, 20,* 343–363.

Warren, S. G., & Juraska, J. M. (1997). Spatial and nonspatial learning across the rat estrous cycle. *Behavioral Neuroscience, 111,* 259–266.

Winkler, E. M., & Christiansen, K. (1993). Sex hormone levels and body hair growth in !Kung San and Kavango men from Namibia. *American Journal of Physical Anthropology, 92,* 155–164.

Wolf, O. T., & Kirschbaum, C. (1999). Dehydroepiandrosterone replacement in elderly individuals: Still waiting for the proof of beneficial effects on mood or memory. *Journal of Endocrinological Investigations, 22,* 316.

Wolf, O. T., Naumann, E., Hellhammer, D. H., & Kirschbaum, C. (1998). Effects of dehydroepiandrosterone replacement in elderly men on event-related brain potentials, memory and well-being. *Journal of Gerontology, 53A*(5), M385–M390.

Wolf, O. T., Neumann, O., Hellhammer, D. H., Geiben, A. C., Strasburger, C. J., Dressendorfer, R. A., Pirke, K. M., & Kirschbaum, C. (1997). Effects of a two-week physiological dehydroepiandrosterone substitution on cognitive performance and well-being in healthy elderly women and men. *Journal of Clinical Endocrinology and Metabolism, 82,* 2363–2367.

Woolley, C. S., & McEwen, B. S. (1992). Estradiol mediates fluctuation in hippocampal synapse density during the estrous cycle in the adult rat. *Journal of Neuroscience, 12,* 2549–2554.

Writing Group for the Women's Health Initiative Investigators. (2002). Risks and benefits of estrogen plus progestin in healthy postmenopausal women: Principal results from the Women's Health Initiative randomized controlled trial. *Journal of the American Medical Association, 288,* 321–333.

Yaffe, K., Ettinger, B., Pressman, A., Seeley, D., Whooley, M., Schaefer, C., & Cummings, S. (1998). Neuropsychiatric function and dehydroepiandrosterone sulfate in elderly women: A prospective study. *Biological Psychiatry, 43,* 694–700.

4

Sex Roles as Adaptations

An Evolutionary Perspective on Gender Differences and Similarities

DOUGLAS T. KENRICK
MELANIE R. TROST
JILL M. SUNDIE

FBI crime reports provide an interesting starting point to consider evolved psychological mechanisms and how they interact with societal norms. Whether there are sex differences or similarities depends on the crime being considered (Federal Bureau of Investigation, 2000). For example, 50% of those arrested for embezzlement in the year 2000 were women and 50% were men. Women slightly outnumbered men in the category of runaways (59% women), and commercialized vice and prostitution (61% women). For the remaining categories, women constituted less than half of those arrested. The discrepancy was small for fraud (46% women) and larger for violent crimes such as aggravated assault (20% women) and murder (11% women). The largest gap was in the category of forcible rape, where only 1% of arrestees were women.

Perhaps these crime statistics reflect not only actual differences in behavior but also differences in societal norms about appropriate behavior for women and men. For example, maybe women commit as many assaults as do men, but are less likely to be arrested for them. Indeed, although men are more likely to be arrested for domestic violence, women are more likely to report striking a partner (Archer, 2000). Sex differences in both behaviors and societal rules are interesting from an evolutionary perspective. Furthermore, the sex similarities may be as informative as the differences. From an evolutionary perspective, sex differences and similarities in norms and behaviors reflect adaptational problems regularly faced by our male and female ancestors (e.g., Alcock, 2001; Geary, 1998; Pinker, 2002). Evolutionary theorists presume that the design of any animal now living is ultimately linked to what its ancestors did to survive and reproduce. To understand the design of *Homo sapiens,* it helps to look beyond one's own society to the wider context of different human cultures and different animal species. This wider view can help us to understand how our own species and culture are unique, and how they are not.

In this chapter, we review basic evolutionary concepts, such as sexual selection and parental investment, focusing on how those concepts have been applied to understanding sometimes puzzling sex differences and similarities. We then consider how these concepts reflect on several behavioral consistencies across human cultures, as well as several cross-cultural variations. We explore gene–culture interactions and consider how researchers might finally move beyond the oversimplified nature–nurture debate to collect data on these more complex interactions.

Human behavior represents an amalgam of influences. Since its inception, the evolutionary approach to understanding these influences has often aroused controversy (see Conway & Schaller, 2002). Educated criticism can be useful, ultimately fueling the motor of scientific progress. Today's evolutionary models have been expanded and modified in the face of logical argument and new data. Those models now emphasize issues such as female choice, male parental investment, gender similarities as well as differences, and environmental variability in human behavior (e.g., Gangestad & Simpson, 2000; Geary, 1998; Kenrick, Li, & Butner, 2003). The view of behavioral predispositions as adaptations to recurrent problems of survival and reproduction is complementary to other perspectives. It is neither necessary nor appropriate to choose between models emphasizing evolution *or* culture *or* learning *or* cognition. The human brain was designed by the same natural forces that shaped other natural phenomena, but it is a brain designed to think, to learn, and to construct cultures. To isolate or ignore any of these facets limits our understanding of human behavior. The psychology of gender is perhaps the best domain in which to appreciate the importance of an integrative biosocial approach (Kenrick, 1987; Wood & Eagly, 2002).

EVOLUTION AND BEHAVIOR: BASIC PRINCIPLES

Evolutionary theory consists, at base, of three simple assumptions, outlined in Darwin's (1859) *The Origin of Species*. The first assumption is that all animals are involved in a *struggle for existence*. Even slowly reproducing animals multiply rapidly enough to overrun the earth in a few centuries. Limited resources prevent this: When the giraffe population grows too large, its members begin to exhaust the supply of arboreal vegetation, limiting the number of giraffes that can survive and reproduce. Given that other members of a species are the main competitors for resources, animals within a species struggle against *one another* to survive. Giraffes must beat other giraffes to the limited treetop greens, and lions must beat other lions to the giraffes.

The second assumption of evolutionary theory is that of *heritable variation within a species*. This assumption, quite controversial when Darwin first advanced it, is that members of any species are not all the same but differ in many ways and pass some of those differences to their offspring. Darwin showed how such variations were exploited by pigeon breeders to produce a diverse array of birds, many of which appeared very unlike their common ancestral rock pigeons. Likewise, all domesticated dogs come from common ancestors, but some strains are notoriously aggressive, such as pit bulls; others are notoriously good-natured, such as golden retrievers; and still others are notoriously jittery, such as Irish setters.

The third assumption, *natural selection,* follows from the other two. If animals compete with one another to survive, and vary on traits that can be inherited, then some variants will produce more offspring. Over generations, the strains best suited to their environments will replace those that are less well adapted. Imagine a pond that can support 100 catfish. If one catfish inherits a mutated gene that enlarges his mouth, he may eat faster, hence maturing more quickly, reproducing sooner, and staying alive longer than his small-mouthed cousins. His offspring will tend to share his physical advantage, thus outeatting the next generation of small-mouthed catfishes. Given that the larger mouth does not carry some hidden cost, the pond will eventually consist entirely of large-mouthed catfish.

Most psychologists understand how Darwin's theory of natural selection applies to physical characteristics, but the theory's behavioral implications are not always as well understood. As Darwin later clarified in *The Expression of Emotions in Man and Animals* (1873), behavioral predispositions evolve according to the same rules as physical features. A simple logical chain reveals why. Seals are closely related to dogs, but if a seal inherited a brain programmed to run a dog's body and tried to run down large mammals on dry land, it would not last much longer than a dog that attempted to swim out to sea and dive for fish. Along with their bodily structures, seals, dogs, bats, giraffes, and cobras inherit brains designed to run their particular bodies. Thus, evolution applies to survival-related behaviors in much the same way that it applies to physical characteristics. Animals with behavioral variations suited to their bodies and their environments will survive and outreproduce those with less well-adapted behavioral tendencies.

Life History Strategies

Although some traits are fixed at birth, many inherited tendencies affect development in more flexible and environmentally contingent ways. A *life history* is a genetically organized developmental plan—a set of general strategies and specific tactics by which an organism allocates energy to survival, growth, and reproduction (Stearns, 1976). Depending on a number of contingencies in ancestral environments, animals may be designed to reach reproductive maturity rapidly or very slowly. Once mature, they may devote all of their resources to one short reproductive burst or spread their reproductive efforts over several months or years. Some may not allocate any further resources to caring for offspring, whereas others may care for their offspring for days, weeks, months, or years.

Life histories can be divided into two broad categories: *somatic effort* and *reproductive effort* (Alexander, 1987). Somatic effort, the energy expended to build the body, is analogous to building a bank account. Reproductive effort is analogous to spending the money in that bank account to replicate one's genes and may include mating effort, parental care, and investment in relatives sharing common genes. Somatic and reproductive effort may peak during different phases of the life cycle, but the general developmental trajectory was designed to allocate energy in ways that tended to enhance ancestors' fitness.

Organisms show an amazing array of life history patterns. One small mammal from Madagascar reaches sexual maturity 40 days after birth (Quammen, 1996). Female elephants take 100 times that long to mature, then carry their fetuses for over a year (Daly & Wilson, 1983). Pacific salmon also take several years of somatic effort to mature, then expend all their reproductive effort in a brief period—laying several thousand eggs in one burst just before dying.

These variations in development are keyed to ecological conditions, such as climate, presence of predators, and availability of food or shelter. For example, wildebeest newborns are vulnerable to heavy predation, so calves are born *en masse* on one day of each year. Communal birthing reduces the risk of losing offspring, because predatory hyenas cannot eat all of the newborns in a huge herd before they are strong enough to protect themselves (Estes, 1976). Mosquitoes, whose life history is linked to temperature, run through their life cycle in 10 days at 80°F, but 14 days at 70°F (Floore, 2002). Thus, ecological pressures can shape or change the life course.

Although the name of the evolutionary game is reproduction, animals frequently *restrain* reproduction. The fulmar petrel reaches full size in one season but typically waits 9 years to begin nesting (Ollason & Dunnet, 1978). Unlike many birds that lay up to a dozen eggs in a season, petrels reliably lay only one. The reason for restraint is that rampant reproduction is not always successful reproduction. In many bird species, the probability of raising any offspring drops if the clutch size increases beyond a critical point (Lack, Gibb, & Owen, 1957). Similarly, animals that begin reproducing too early in life may not have the experience to provide for their young. Compared with younger female elephant seals, for example, older, experienced, female seals are less likely to lose their pups (Reiter, Panken, & LeBoeuf, 1981). Reproductive effort is analogous to spending money in a bank account, and there is a direct cost to parenting. Female elephant seals lose body fat in direct proportion to that gained by their pups (Reiter et al., 1981), and a female red deer's chance of surviving from one season to the next decreases if she has a fawn (Clutton-Brock, 1984). On the other side, male fruit flies that are experimentally prevented from mating survive longer than those given free access to mates (Partridge & Farquhar, 1981). Under natural circumstances, strategically limiting reproduction may ultimately be more adaptive than unrestrained breeding.

Considering an organism's life history aids us in understanding not only ancestral evolution but also current behavior and development. The strategies that determine an organism's somatic and reproductive effort have been shaped by adaptation to particular pressures in the environment, leading to particular progressions in both physiological development and behavioral expression.

Different Strategies within and between Species

Which behavioral strategy works best in the struggle for survival and differential reproduction? As discussed, the answer depends partly on the animal's body type and partly on the physical environment. It also depends in part on the social environment. Evolutionary theorists often use the metaphor of "hawks and doves" to explicate the importance of social ecology (e.g., Dawkins, 1976). When nonaggressive doves predominate in an environment, it pays to be an aggressive hawk that preys on other birds. As the number of hawks increases, however, attacking other birds becomes increasingly dangerous. Under these circumstances, a pacifist dove that flees conflict will fare better. Evolutionary theorists assume that different species within an ecosystem often maintain equilibrium. If hawks become too numerous, they begin to destroy the dove population. Hawks then begin to starve and die, and the dove population increases. As doves proliferate, hawks have more to eat and their population increases again. Eventually, this interdependence stabilizes at some mutually limiting equilibrium.

Such a reciprocal equilibrium can also occur *within* a species. For instance, there are two types of adult male blue-gilled sunfish (Gross, 1984): a larger, colorful male that is highly attractive to females; and a smaller, drab male that acts as a "sneak-copulator." Rather than investing nutritional energy in developing a large, gaudy physique, the smaller males develop enormous sperm-producing organs. When a large male is mating with a female, the smaller male darts in and releases his sperm. Obviously, the ratio of competitors is important. A sneak copulator's success depends on the existence of a larger neighbor to attract females, but too many sneak-copulators in the vicinity causes them to put one another out of business. *Polymorphism* (different body types within a species) can take even more interesting twists. Female cleaner wrasse congregate in harems around a large-territoried male. If the male dies, the largest female in his harem goes through a series of physiological changes and transforms into a male (Warner, 1984). Thus, the success of a particular combination of body type and behavior is linked to variations in the environment, and some species have evolved to change body types as the environment changes.

The most prevalent morphological and physical divisions within species are based on sex. Males and females frequently differ in size and behavior. Some of these differences are unique: the differences between a peacock and peahen are not the same as those between a walrus bull and cow. However, some generalizations in sex differences can be found across a wide range of vertebrate species. Darwin (1859) noted that males tend to be relatively larger and more ornate than females. If one member of a species has more decorative fins (as in Siamese fighting fish), or more colorful plumage (as in peacocks), or larger antlers (as in elk), then it tends to be the male. There are also fairly general sex differences in behavior. Males are more likely to be aggressive and inclined toward dominance competitions. These sex differences in physiology and behavior are correlated with sex differences in mating strategies (Geary, 1998). Two general principles are often used to explain these relationships: differential parental investment and sexual selection.

Differential Parental Investment and Sexual Selection

Differential parental investment refers to the fact that males and females differ in the amount of resources they invest in offspring (Trivers, 1972). Eggs are generally more costly to produce than sperm. In mammals, this small initial difference is compounded by a lengthy internal gestation. A mammalian female carries a fetus that requires a large amniotic sac and takes first priority on her nutritional intake for several months. Following birth, the female nurses the newborn, again sacrificing her own nutritional intake to feed her progeny. In some species, such as humans, offspring must be fed and cared for even after they are weaned. Therefore, the minimum parental investment for female mammals is quite large.

Males can father young with much less investment—the amount of energy required for one act of intercourse. Consider the Xavante, a hunter–gatherer group. The average number of offspring for males and females was 3.6. However, the variance was 3.9 for women, whereas it was 12.1 for men. In other words, some Xavante men had many offspring and others had few. Only 1 of 195 Xavante women was childless at age 20, but 6% of men were still childless at age 40. One man fathered 23 children, whereas for a woman the highest number of children was 8 (Salzano, Neel, & Maybury-Lewis, 1967). This pattern holds for most species; females, compared to males, tend to have fewer offspring and a greater investment in them.

Some of the physical differences between males and females are due simply to natural selection based on differential parental investment. The female body needs to produce eggs, and in mammals, to nurture the fetus and the newborn baby. Why are male mammals usually larger, when a relatively larger body would seem to be of more use to females that must directly contribute bodily resources to the young (Ralls, 1976)? Why are males more likely to have decorative features such as antlers or brilliant feathers, and to use some of those features (e.g., antlers) to compete with one another? To explain such differences, Darwin (1859) used the concept of *sexual selection,* a term that encompasses two separable processes. *Intrasexual selection* refers to the pressure one sex exerts on other members of the same sex via competition. In a species such as bighorn sheep, in which males compete for access to females by butting their heads, those males with the boniest heads, the largest shoulder muscles, and the largest antlers are more likely to win dominance competitions and survive. *Epigamic selection* refers to influence one sex exerts by choosing partners with certain features, such as large antlers or bright feathers. Andersson (1982) has demonstrated that female widowbirds are more likely to mate with males whose tails were experimentally elongated, and to reject males whose tails were experimentally shortened. If only one sex shows such a preference, such features eventually become more characteristic of one sex than the other.

Darwin suspected that epigamic sexual selection could explain why male vertebrates tend to be larger, showier, and more dominance-oriented. The mechanism seems to link back to differential parental investment. Because females invest more in any given offspring, an ill-chosen mating is more costly for a female than for a male. Thus, females, compared to males, tend to be relatively more selective in choosing mates. An extreme example of this sex difference occurs in fallow deer, which mate in an arena, or *lek*. All males in the herd compete for a limited number of choice territories. Female deer mate with only the relatively few bucks that make it to the top of this territorial hierarchy. Male fallow deer are essentially nonselective, but the females mate with only the most dominant males (Clutton-Brock, 1991). In other mammalian species (such as humans), males invest more in the young and exercise greater discrimination in mating.

Male Parental Investment

This general mammalian model of differential parental investment explains the behaviors of species such as fallow deer and peacocks but must be qualified in talking about humans (Kenrick, Sadalla, Groth, & Trost, 1990). Human males invest heavily in their offspring, and without paternal investment, human offspring have lower survival rates (Geary, 1998). Consider Maharajah Bhupinder Singh, who had a harem of 350 women (Collins & LaPierre, 1975). Although he may have spent little quality time with any one of his mates, he did provide food, care, and shelter for each woman, and for their offspring. A monogamous man may provide resources for his one partner and their offspring for his entire life. Because human males heavily invest in their children, we would also expect them to be selective about choosing a mate. Sex differences tend to be smaller when males invest more in their offspring (Geary, 1998). Accordingly, men and women are relatively similar in size and decoration, in contrast to peacocks and peahens. In some species, the typical "sex roles" are completely reversed. In phalaropes and a few other bird species, for example, larger and more colorful females compete for sexual access to males. Consistent with parental investment theory, males in those species invest relatively more in offspring care than do females.

Even though human males and females both invest in their offspring, the two sexes do not necessarily play the same mating game. Because men and women contribute fundamentally different resources to produce offspring, the characteristics they desire in mates are also different. Women directly invest their bodily resources in offspring. Their reproductive potential peaks in the mid-20s, then declines, until it ends with menopause (Dunson, Colombo, & Baird, 2002). Consistently, men's judgments of female attractiveness have been linked to indicators of youth and physical health (Alley, 1992; Symons, 1979). Men, on the other hand, invest indirect resources (e.g., food, money, and protection) that do not necessarily diminish as men get older. Thus, women would be expected to value the ability to provide those resources more than youth per se. We consider these differences further when we discuss mate selection.

Environmentally Contingent Strategizing

We mentioned earlier that the same rules apply to the evolution of physical traits and behavioral predispositions. There is an important difference, however. Many physical traits do not vary from situation to situation, whereas virtually all behavioral predispositions can and must vary. The length of a turtle's head and neck bones, and the dimensions of its shell, do not change when the turtle is threatened, but the tendency to tuck its head and neck inside the shell does. Likewise, human eye color does not change from situation to situation, but we may or may not blink our eyes depending on what is coming toward our faces. Hence, the way animals move their bodies (or behave) varies according to adaptive contingency rules, some of which are strictly inherited (as in the blinking reflex), yet many of which can be modified by learning. For example, the human fear response appears to be innate but can be elicited by very rapid acquisition of novel threat cues (Öhman & Mineka, 2001). Similarly, the capacity for language is innate, but the specific words we speak depend on inputs learned over several years (Pinker, 1994). An evolutionary perspective does not assume that human behavior is based in rigid reflexes and closed instincts, but it does assume domain-specific biases relative to what is learned and how information is connected. Research on humans and other animals has revealed different learning biases adapted to recurrent problems faced by the animals' ancestors. The way a bird learns its song follows different rules than those for the way it learns where food is stored, and still different rules for the way it learns to avoid poisonous substances (Sherry & Schacter, 1987).

Mothering is particularly sensitive to environmental constraints. Contrary to the notion that females are warm and nurturing to a fault, Sarah Hrdy (1999) argues that mothers are strategic actors that respond to environmental conditions in ways that enhance the chances of their own survival and that of their offspring. This behavior can appear ruthless at times. We all know that mothers will kill attackers to protect their offspring; but in rare circumstances, mothers might desert offspring to protect limited resources. In a case from South American Aché foragers, one mother's newborn was left behind, because its father had died during the pregnancy, and the mother's new husband would not provide for the child. For others, when a close birth interval between two children threatened the older child's milk supply, the newborn was killed (Hill & Hurtado, 1996). Lest these behaviors be solely ascribed to "primitive" cultures, infanticide has been documented on all continents. For example, in Denmark, all instances of female–female homicide between 1933 and 1961 were infanticide (Daly & Wilson, 1988). These examples illustrate very real trade-offs that mothers must make between somatic and reproductive effort within environmental constraints. In primates (including humans), these strategic choices can lead to acts that seem contrary to common concepts of mothering, including favoring one child over another, abandonment, or even infanticide (Hrdy, 1999).

Evolutionary pressures are also linked to sex differences in attention, learning, and decision making. In cognitive terms, we can think about these differences as variations in decision-rules (Kenrick et al., 2003). For example, both men and women make distinctions between friendly and flirtatious gestures. But the threshold at which a friendly gesture is interpreted as flirtation is different for men and women, and is consistent with parental investment principles (Haselton & Buss, 2000). For men, casual mating carries relatively fewer costs and possibly high benefits, so it makes sense that men have a lower threshold for interpreting social cues as sexual (unless the person emitting those cues is the man's sister). Similarly, although men and women have different boundaries for choosing a monogamous or promiscuous mating strategy, both sexes can act in either manner, depending on the behaviors of others in their dating pool (Gangestad & Simpson, 2000).

Over time, subtle differences in decision-rules used by local members of one sex interact dynamically with those of the opposite sex to result in very different local norms. With even random variation in the initial behaviors of individuals in a local community (e.g., female freshmen at one college), very different local norms for sexual behavior can emerge due to simple principles of spatial dynamics (Kenrick et al., 2003). Because a given person's decision-rules are tuned to other people in the social environment, radically divergent behavioral norms can persist over time (e.g., sexual promiscuity vs. strict monogamy), even though the individuals who comprise the different populations are not very different from one another. Very small variations in individual decision-rules can influence a whole community's norms to tip in one direction or the other (e.g., a few local women who slightly shift to more unrestricted behavior can move a whole community toward unrestricted behavior). For example, a man or woman who initially is slightly inclined toward forming a single, monogamous relationship may instead end up "dating around," if he or she attends a small college at which most members of the opposite sex are adamantly unattached. The reverse may occur for someone inclined toward unrestricted dating but who attends a small college at which most students are monogamously attached. Hence, there are important links between the underlying predispositions of the individual men and women making up a community and the norms that emerge in that community. However, the causal relationships between individual traits and community-level outcomes are dynamic and bidirectional. Evolutionary psychologists have historically adopted individual-based models of behavior. Such models are easier to grasp but, unfortunately, do not capture the real world's complexity. New theories of complex systems have begun to explore how preferences in different individuals can combine into patterned behavior at the group level (Vallacher, Read, & Nowak, 2002). An integration of evolutionary models of individual decision-making with dynamical systems approaches holds great promise for understanding organism–environment interactions at all levels, including the emergence of culture (Kenrick et al., 2002).

CROSS-CULTURAL COMMONALITIES IN GENDER-LINKED BEHAVIOR

One advantage to adopting an evolutionary perspective on gender is that it leads to questions regarding universal issues: Are there cross-cultural regularities in the behaviors of human males and females? Do those regularities reflect different problems faced by the two sexes across different species, or are they unique to humans? How do those regularities fit with general evolutionary models (e.g., parental investment theory)? Taking this broader perspective can help to clarify some seemingly arbitrary features of sex-linked behavior (Kenrick, 1987).

In many ways, men and women within any culture are more alike than they are different. On most behavioral dimensions, there are probably more differences within a sex than between the sexes. This holds true for spatial abilities, verbal intelligence, friendliness, and many other characteristics. Some women are better than most men at solving spatial problems; some men have higher verbal intelligence than most women. At first glance, such overlap makes it difficult to imagine universal sex differences in behavior that compare to the universal sex differences in morphology (e.g., having testicles or a uterus). Even many of the morphological sex differences show overlap. Although men are typically about 10% taller and 30% heavier than women, there are, nevertheless, women within any culture who are taller than most of the men.

Our perspective assumes that sex-linked behaviors arose as adaptations to the problems of survival and reproduction faced by our ancestors. When ancestral men and women met similar demands in a given domain, we would expect small or nonexistent sex differences. When they faced different demands, we would expect larger differences. Given a similar diet and family background, the average man is slightly taller, heavier, and more muscular in his upper body than a woman. Behavioral differences are more like these differences in height and weight than the morphological differences in male and female sex organs. Because reproductive competition is central to evolutionary theory, evolutionary theorists have been particularly interested in the relationships between sex and behaviors related to social dominance, aggression, and mating.

Dominance Competition

As of 2002, women held just under 14% of seats in the United States Congress. Worldwide, the representation of women in national governing bodies varies, with the largest female representation found in Nordic countries (39%). Most nations' levels are more similar to the U.S. level, with less than 18% average representation in all other regions of the world (Inter-Parliamentary Union, 2002). Similar differences in leadership attainment are found in situations ranging from ad hoc groups formed in the laboratory to play groups on the kindergarten playground. Although men constitute 50% of jury members, they are elected as foremen 90% of the time (Kerr, Harmon, & Graves, 1982). Such differences are typically explained in terms of cultural pressures and biases in our society.

A look across cultures does reveal some variations in women's economic and decision-making power (Eagly & Wood, 1999). Nevertheless, across diverse cultures, terms related to dominance are universally considered more applicable to males (Williams & Best, 1986). These differences are muted in that most studies of sex differences in competitiveness have been conducted in the more egalitarian North American and northern European countries. Even in societies organized by the mother's lineage, men are still the chiefs (Daly & Wilson, 1983). As with physical differences, the range of dominance-related behaviors among men and women forms overlapping distributions. There are individual women in most cultures who are socially dominant over most of the men. For example, Margaret Thatcher was elected Prime Minister of one of the world's most powerful countries. Even so, she was preceded and succeeded by men, and over 80% of the British Parliament remains male (Inter-Parliamentary Union, 2002). Thus, even in relatively egalitarian cultures, men tend to compete more for social dominance.

A sex difference in competitiveness is not unique to humans, but it tends to characterize most vertebrate species. As noted earlier, differential parental investment creates differences in competition for access to mates. When males invest relatively more in offspring, females tend to compete more with one another, and vice versa. Although human females make an initially larger, direct investment, human males also invest heavily in their offspring. For this reason, one would expect some degree of intrasexual competitiveness among human females, and there is ample evidence of such competition (Buss & Dedden, 1990). Furthermore, social dominance has advantages in a group-living species other than access to mates. Although there are reasons to assume more adaptive payoff for male–male competitiveness, it would be a mistake to portray women as being selected for noncompetitiveness. Researchers are just starting to examine how women's dominance hierarchies differ from, and resemble, those of men.

Aggressive and Antisocial Behavior

As noted earlier, men committed 90% of homicides in the United States in the year 2000. This ratio varies slightly from year to year but persisted throughout the last century in North America; FBI reports indicate that women never commit more than 15% of homicides in the United States. Daly and Wilson (1988) examined homicide rates for various societies across different time periods and reliably found that same-sex murderers were much more likely to be committed by males than by females across all those societies. For example, the proportion of Uganda's Alur males murdering males was .97 of all same-sex murders between 1945 and 1954. Among the Bhil of India between 1971 and 1975, the proportion was .99. Among the Belo Horizonte of Brazil, between 1961 and 1965, 97% of male murders were committed by other males. The ratios were similar for the Gros Vendre between 1850 and 1885, and the residents of Oxford, England, from 1296 to 1398. Of the 35 cultures examined, the Danish posted the lowest ratio (.85). In providing reasons for same-sex murder, a predominant motive for male–male homicides is "saving face," linked to competitions over dominance. This motive is rarely found in female–female homicides (Wilson & Daly, 1985).

Men similarly outnumber women in murdering members of the opposite sex, although this difference is somewhat less pronounced because women are more likely to kill men than to kill other women. However, the motives for cross-sex homicides do differ for men and women. A woman most commonly murders a man in self-defense: Women tend to kill men who have been threatening and/or abusing them. On the other hand, a man is more likely to murder a woman who has deserted him or been sexually unfaithful (Daly & Wilson, 1988).

Behaviors related to the technology of aggression show similar sex discrepancies (Crabb, 2000). In a classic examination of the division of labor, Murdock (1935) found considerable overlap between the sexes. For example, manufacturing leather products was the sole province of men in 29 cultures, the usual province of men in 3 societies, acceptable for either sex in 9 societies, the usual province of women in 3 societies, and the exclusive province of women in 32 societies. However, weapon making was the exclusive domain of men in 121 societies and the usual domain of men in 1 society. Women were not the predominant, usual, or equal weapon makers in any society.

One recent meta-analysis examined a wide range of behaviors that might be defined as risky (Byrnes, Miller, & Schafer, 1999). Across 16 categories of risky behavior, one effect size was nonsignificantly negative (-.02, suggesting that females may smoke slightly more than do males). All others were positive (14 of 16 significantly so). The largest sex differences were found for risks involving physical skills (.43), and willingness to engage in experiments that involved the possibility of physical or psychological harm (.41). Wilson and Daly (1985) argue that males are generally more likely to engage in risky and dangerous behaviors that carry the potential benefit of increased social status, and they link this difference to differences in mating behavior (which we discuss next).

Mating Behavior and Sexuality

Before we consider some of the more obvious sex differences in human mating, it is worth noting several similarities. These similarities become more salient in light of mating practices of other mammals. In over 90% of mammalian species, males and females do not form long-lasting bonds, and males contribute little or nothing but sperm to their offspring (Geary, 1998). Although maternal care is found in all mammals, most males do not bond to their mates or offspring. Human males, on the other hand, universally form enduring emotional bonds to their mates and to their children (Daly & Wilson, 1983; Zeifman & Hazan, 1997).

Cross-cultural variation in mating arrangements masks this human universal of pair-bonding. Some human societies (e.g., India) are *polygynous* (one man marrying several women), others (e.g., the Tibetan Tre-ba) are *polyandrous* (one woman marrying several men), and still others (e.g., Victorian England) are *monogamous* (one man marrying one woman). Alongside this variation is the singular fact that all societies have some form of marital alliance between men and women. In contrast, most mammals' mating arrangements involve radical polygyny, not monogamy. Most female mammals do not need males to help care for their young and have benefited from prioritizing males' genetic characteristics over bonding tendencies. Do humans show any vestiges of the mammalian tendency toward polygyny? Data from 849 cultures suggest that they do (Daly & Wilson, 1983). Of the 849 cultures, only 4 were polyandrous, whereas 708 were polygynous and 137 were monogamous. Moreover, the 4 cultures listed as polyandrous also allowed polygyny. Among the Pahari of Northern India, for instance, several brothers pool resources to obtain one wife. If they accumulate more wealth, they typically marry additional women. Hrdy (2000) notes that although there are very few cultures that officially permit polyandry, there is, across cultures, some degree of de facto polyandry as a result of extramarital affairs, a shortage of women, husbands sharing wives with kin, or serial monogamy over the lifespan.

Thus, depending on resources and other ecological factors, there are variable benefits to both sexes in monogamous versus polygamous matings. On the other hand, even in nominally monogamous cultures, men are more likely to engage in unrestricted sexual behaviors and show a desire for multiple partners. For example, 20% of American men and 10% of women in one survey reported having had an extramarital affair, whereas 48% of men, but only 5% of women, reported a desire to engage in extramarital relations in the future (Johnson, 1970). In a survey of Germans with steady dating partners, 46% of the men, but only 6% of the women, reported a willingness to have casual sex with someone they found attractive (Sigusch & Schmidt, 1971). These findings are interesting, because they were gathered at the peak of the so-called "sexual revolution" when traditional ideas about fidelity were at an all-time low in popularity. More recent surveys of "post-sexual-revolution" Americans continue to reveal large discrepancies in the permissiveness of men and women (e.g., Astin, Green, Korn, & Schalit, 1987).

Other studies reveal consistent sex differences. For example, men and women in one study indicated their minimum criteria for partners at several levels of relationship involvement (e.g., a date, marriage; Kenrick et al., 1990). When rating partners for a sexual liaison, men reliably indicated lower criteria than did women. Men specified a minimum 51st percentile for intelligence in a date, but only a 43rd percentile for a sexual partner. Women, on the other hand, specified a minimum intelligence level at the 49th percentile for a date, and a higher minimum for a sexual partner (55th percentile). In a subsequent study, students were also asked about their criteria for partners for a "one-night stand" in which they would never see the person again (Kenrick, Groth, Trost, & Sadalla, 1993). Considering all levels of relationship commitment, the sex differences were strongest for this explicitly low-commitment relationship: Men were very nondiscriminating, whereas women tended to be relatively more selective.

Partner Preferences

In most mammalian species, females are more discriminating about the qualities of a desirable mate (Daly & Wilson, 1983). In contrast, both men and women are highly selective when choosing long-term mates (Kenrick et al., 1990, 1993). Nevertheless, men and women differ in selection criteria in ways linked to the different resources each sex invests in the offspring. Women show a relative preference for wealth, social status, and seniority in a partner, whereas men show a relative preference for youth and attractiveness (Buss & Barnes, 1986).

Evolutionary theorists generally explain male preferences for youth and physical attractiveness as following from age variations in the human reproductive cycle (Daly & Wilson, 1983). As women age beyond their 20s, they gradually become less fertile, until they reach menopause by their early 50s (Dunson, Colombo, & Baird, 2002). Although a man's fertility also decreases with age, the decline is less dramatic, and even men well above 50 retain the capacity to procreate, if they can attract a woman of reproductive age (see Kenrick & Keefe, 1992, for an extended discussion of these issues). This age-related variation has important implications for mate selection behaviors. Men are most attracted to women in their peak years of fertility—the mid-20s. Men in their 20s tend to seek and marry women about their own age, whereas older men seek progressively younger women (relative to their own age) (Kenrick & Keefe, 1992). Teenage males' preferences provide the clearest differential support for a life history model (Kenrick, Gabrielidis, Keefe, & Cornelius, 1996). Teenage males find women in their early 20s more attractive than girls their own age. This preference does not mesh with sex role norms or with reciprocation of interest by older women: Teenage men are not very desirable as partners in any part of the world (Kenrick & Keefe, 1992; Kenrick et al., 1996).

Social scientists have traditionally explained these sex differences as being a result of American culture (e.g., Cameron, Oskamp, & Sparks, 1977; Deutsch, Zalenski, & Clark, 1986). Indeed, there is some variation across cultures in the magnitude of these sex differences (Eagly & Wood, 1999). However, sex differences in mate preferences persist even in the most egalitarian societies. For instance, older men in North America, as well as in Europe, Asia, Africa, and the South Pacific, show the same preference for relatively younger women as mates, whereas younger men marry women closer to their own age (Kenrick & Keefe, 1992). Similarly, women across 37 cultures showed a relatively greater interest in having a partner with resources than did men, whereas men across the different cultures placed more emphasis on physical attractiveness (Buss, 1989).

The sex similarities and differences summarized here make sense in light of the perspective provided by comparing human behavior with that of other animal species. Sex differences in competitiveness and violence, as well as differential desires for casual relationships, are consistent with general mammalian sex differences in parental investment. Similarities between men and women in familial bonding and standards for long-term relationships are consistent with the fact that human males, unlike most other mammalian species, form enduring pair-bonds and make substantial contributions to their young.

GENE–ENVIRONMENT INTERACTIONS

The Construction of Culture

How do evolved genetic predispositions and cultural influences interact with one another? At the most obvious level, human cultures are likely to be affected by the abilities, limitations, preferences, and aversions of our species (Janicki & Krebs, 1998). For example, Pentecost Islands adolescents jump from tall towers with vines tied to their legs. They start with small towers and short vines, and some eventually construct towers nearly 100 feet high. Because they study the technology of jumping and vine tying quite carefully, very few youth die. But the sport is dangerous, and there is an occasional fatal mishap. This sport is actually a form of competition for status among adolescent males. Whereas "land diving" is a unique and somewhat arbitrary cultural custom, its adoption follows the universal need for males to display dominance. One would expect that, across cultures, males and females frequently adopt unique cultural practices that express evolved preferences and capacities. For example, males are more likely to occupy social roles related to warfare and fighting with outgroups, whereas females are more likely to occupy social roles related to infant care (Brown, 1991; Wrangham & Peterson, 1996). However, the exact nature of the norms surrounding warfare and infant care varies across societies as a function of technology, resource availability, and historical factors (e.g., Hrdy, 1999).

Cultural customs and evolved predispositions can be linked in different ways. Culture may exaggerate evolved predispositions, act against them, or be irrelevant. For instance, if a society creates training experiences for athletics or military defense that exclude females, then any inherent sex differences will be exaggerated. Boys who are initially inclined to be pacific and sensitive and girls who appear aggressive and competitive may be the targets of especially strong sanctions. Eventually, the small average differences between the two sexes could transform into two nonoverlapping distributions. It has frequently been argued that this constraint is the status quo in modern American society: Women and men are forced into tightly configured roles that promote differences, not similarities. But the evidence does not support the assumption that these pressures are unique to American culture. Cross-cultural studies reveal that many societies are much more sex typed than America (Daly & Wilson, 1988; Kenrick & Keefe, 1992). Cultural pressures can also act *against* biological predispositions. Rules against violence, exploitation, and sexuality fall into this category. Campbell (1975) reasoned that the existence of strong social rules may point to an underlying selfish genetic tendency. We do not need as many rules to instruct people to feed themselves or take care of their children as we need rules to keep them from cheating or exploiting strangers (Jones, 2001). To some extent, some of the differential cultural pressures on men and women may be designed to counter unpleasant biological defaults. Boys are more likely to be disciplined for competitiveness than are girls, for example, and the laws against rape are designed to check men's, not women's, compulsions.

The road between genes and culture is not a one-way street. Over time, cultural pressures might shape natural selection. For example, cultural institutions may select individuals with particular genetic predispositions for specific roles. If the tallest males are most often chosen as group leaders, and if leader status affords more mating opportunities (e.g., more wives in a polygynous society), then over time, these cultural institutions could enhance any preexisting sex difference in physical size. Such cultural forces are not out of line with existing evidence. For example, taller men are more likely to be chosen as, and perceived as, leaders (Simonton, 1994), and high-status men in polygynous societies have more wives (Hill, 1984). It therefore makes sense to posit that the choices of human cultural groups over the millennia have affected the natural selection of today's human characteristics.

Although it is interesting to speculate about the evolutionary past, it is very difficult to study how the social customs in ancestral cultures may have affected human evolution. Archaeological records leave hard evidence about cooking implements and weapons, but clues about social structure and organization only seldom emerge from petroglyphs and artwork. Evolutionary anthropologists do sometimes attempt to shed light on human origins by examining existing hunter–gatherer cultures, on the assumption that our ancestors spent most of their years in such cultures (e.g., Brown, 1991). Evolutionary psychology may be informed by the findings in fields such as anthropology, archaeology, and zoology, but ultimately psychologists are not themselves in the business of reconstructing the ancestral history of our species. Many of the most powerful generalizations we have discussed, such as differential parental investment theory, come instead from comparative studies of existing animal species. Like all psychologists, those who adopt an evolutionary framework are more interested in studying how ongoing behavioral choices, thoughts, and emotions are influenced by environmental variations that unfold over the course of a few minutes, days, or years of the lifespan. Next, we consider how gene–environment interactions might be related to such ongoing processes.

The Environmental Construction of the Individual

Some evolved behavioral predispositions, such as the suckling response in newborn mammals, arise independent of environmental inputs. However, rigid instincts are rare in humans and in other vertebrates. Instead, genetic predispositions interact with the environment throughout the animal's life. For instance, adult males in one species of African cichlid fish take two forms—one large and colorful, the other small and colorless (Davis & Fernald, 1990). Whether a male matures rapidly into the larger version depends on his neighbors. If there are no large males around, a young male shows noticeable development in the hypothalamic area, linked to rapid development of the gonads and testes. However, a large male neighbor inhibits development of smaller males. If the local territorial male is removed, smaller males compete for dominance, and the highest ranking male goes through the series of hypothalamic and gonadal changes, accompanied by a sudden increase in size and coloration. This type of adaptive interplay between physiology and the environment has been observed in other vertebrate species (e.g., Lehrman, 1964).

Do humans exhibit a similar interplay between genes and the environment? Evidence indicates that the answer is sometimes "yes." For example, Frisch (1988) found a relationship between a woman's amount of body fat and onset of menarche. Young girls do not enter puberty until they reach a critical ratio of body fat to muscle; mature women stop menstruating if that ratio goes too low. This effect is independent of other indices of health; menstrual termination is often found in highly fit athletes. Frisch argues that a correlation between menstruation and body fat would have been adaptive for our ancestors, who often faced uncertain food supplies. Infants require reliable feedings. Without an ample reserve of nutrition stored as fat, a hunter–gatherer's offspring would not likely survive. Thus, the fat–menstruation relationship serves as an innate insurance policy on a mother's reproductive investment.

In addition to influencing the pace of physical development and the flow of hormones in response to the environment, genetic predispositions may influence psychological events, from momentary cognitions to long-term learning. Differences in physical size provide a simple example of how a genetically influenced sex difference might lead to different life experiences. The larger size and upper-body development of males make it more likely that certain types of competitive or aggressive behavior will result in rewarding outcomes. All other things being equal, a tall man with a weightlifter's body is likely to be treated with greater deference and respect by other men than one with a slight stature. Two men with divergent physiques will thus have different learning histories, and develop different self-concepts and schemas for interpreting social situations. Physical size likewise affects everyday experiences for both sexes. Few women are likely to have experienced a stranger crossing the street to avoid contact with them on a dark night, but many men have had it happen. On the other hand, women would more likely have developed a lower threshold for feeling fear and learning to avoid single males walking down the street.

Ongoing cognitive processes ranging from attention, encoding, and retrieval to problem solving may also be influenced by evolved mechanisms (Kenrick, 1994; Öhman & Mineka, 2001). A number of studies indicate that incoming information about men and women is processed differently, and in ways that involve adaptive constraints. For example, contextual effects on judgments related to mating are consistent with the sex differences in mate preferences discussed earlier. In making self-judgments of their own desirability as a mate, for example, women are more schematic for beauty than for status (Gutierres, Kenrick, & Partch, 1999). In making decisions about commitment to a current mate, on the other hand, women are more sensitive to availability of highly successful and dominant men than to availability of physically attractive men (Kenrick, Neuberg, Zierk, & Krones, 1994). Men show the reverse patterns in both these domains. At this point, preliminary evidence indicates that ongoing thoughts about oneself and members of the opposite sex are influenced by evolved heuristics in interaction with the current environment. Incorporating more rigorous methods from experimental psychology will facilitate a richer and more articulated approach to questions raised by evolutionary models of cognition (Kenrick, 1994).

Some General Theoretical Issues

A crucial assumption of evolutionary approaches to behavior is that our brains are well suited not to current environments, but to past ones. Humans reproduce slowly, and it can take thousands of generations for a recurrent selection pressure to shape physiology or behavior. For example, currently, birth control is widely available. Over a number of generations, this could affect the distribution of genes related to mating preferences. However, our assessments of the costs and benefits of mating opportunities are likely to be less than completely "rational" in the current environment (Jones, 2001). Our ancestors faced many generations of selection in which the costs of sex were very different for males and females (indeed, this applies to all our mammalian ancestors). Evolutionary theorists do not assume that calculations involving inclusive fitness and parental investment are the results of conscious deliberation, any more than is the assessment that ripe peaches taste better than raw turnips. Indeed, female selectivity is found in most vertebrate species, including all other mammals and most birds. Hence, it is not surprising that, as demonstrated in numerous studies, even modern university females with easy access to birth control nevertheless continue to be relatively more careful in their choice of sexual partners (e.g., Kenrick, Sundie, Nicastle, & Stone, 2001; Kenrick et al., 1990, 1993).

Partly because evolutionary hypotheses implicate historical processes that are difficult or impossible to observe directly, they are sometimes regarded as "untestable" (see Conway & Schaller, 2002; Ketelaar & Ellis, 2000). One way around the problem posed by having to make guesses about a particular species' ancestral past is to focus on patterns of behavior found across a wide range of different species (e.g., sex differences in parental investment). It is important to note that evolutionary psychological hypotheses are subject to all the same rules of logic and empirical verification that apply to hypotheses generated with any other theoretical framework. Hypotheses (evolutionary or otherwise) are guesses based on existing evidence, whose validity depends on their ability to generate new findings, and to integrate the network of other relevant evidence. For example, we discussed earlier the finding that women in American society often marry older males (Kenrick & Keefe, 1992). As noted, that could simply reflect the norms of modern American society (e.g., Cameron et al., 1977). To state simply that the same pattern instead seems to fit with lifespan changes in human fertility would not have advanced our understanding much. To reflect on the evolutionary life history hypothesis, data were collected from different societies from around the world at different historical periods. Those data were not consistent with the hypothesis that American society was to blame (Kenrick & Keefe, 1992). However, this does not prove the evolutionary explanation once and for all. An alternative hypothesis might be that, across all societies, men and women are assigned to different roles, and age differences across societies flow from this (Eagly & Wood, 1999). Consistent with the social role hypothesis, data suggest that the magnitude of the sex difference in age preferences is larger in more traditional societies. However, the social role hypothesis has difficulty explaining several features of the overall data pattern: why teenage males are interested in older females, for example, or why men across societies are more likely to compete for status or to prefer youthful females in the first place (Kenrick & Li, 2000; Kenrick et al., 1996). Within the United States, there is evidence that women who gain social status do not shift to male-like preferences for relative youth and attractiveness, but instead continue to prefer older and higher status partners (Kenrick & Keefe, 1992; Wiederman & Allgeier, 1992).

These issues therefore continue to provide the grounds for productive controversy and highlight the fact that generating a plausible hypothesis is only the beginning of the scientific process. The evolutionary perspective has proved immensely useful in understanding the behavior of other animal species and has suggested a number of fruitful empirical questions regarding human behavior (e.g., Alcock, 2001; Geary, 1998; Pinker, 2002). Like all scientific theories, the evolutionary psychological approach to human behavior will ultimately stand or fall based on its capacity to inspire novel and elucidating hypotheses that stand up to empirical verification.

CONCLUSIONS

The concepts of sexual selection and differential parental investment connect human sex differences in competition, aggressiveness, sexuality, and mate choice criteria with a vast literature on life history strategies in other animals. Our evolutionary heritage is expressed through genetic predispositions that interact with the social environment. Genetic predispositions have a direct influence on biochemical and structural differences between men and women, and also indirectly influence learning experiences and cognitions. Cultural influences can oppose or exaggerate biological differences between men and women. However, those cultural influences are themselves the products of interactions between human genetic predispositions and past conditions of human existence.

REFERENCES

Alcock, J. (2001). *The triumph of sociobiology.* New York: Oxford University Press.

Alexander, R. D. (1987). *The biology of moral systems.* New York: Aldine de Gruyter.

Alley, T. R. (1992). Perceived age, physical attractiveness, and sex differences in preferred mates' ages. *Behavioral and Brain Sciences, 15,* 92.

Andersson, M. (1982, October 28). Female choice selects for extreme tail length in a widowbird. *Nature,* pp. 818–820.

Archer, J. (2000). Sex differences in aggression between heterosexual partners: A meta-analytic review. *Psychological Bulletin, 5,* 651-680.

Astin, A. W., Green, K. C., Korn, W. S., & Schalit, M. (1987). *The American freshman: National norms for fall 1987.* Los Angeles: Higher Education Research Institute, UCLA.

Brown, D. E. (1991). *Human universals.* New York: McGraw-Hill.

Buss, D. M. (1989) Sex differences in human mate preferences: Evolutionary hypotheses tested in 37 cultures, *Behavioral and Brain Sciences, 12,* 1–49.

Buss, D. M., & Barnes, M. F. (1986). Preferences in human mate selection. *Journal of Personality and Social Psychology, 50,* 559–570.

Buss, D. M., & Dedden, L. A. (1990). Derogation of competitors. *Journal of Social and Personal Relationships, 7,* 395–422.

Byrnes, J. P., Miller, D. C., & Schafer, W. D. (1999). Gender differences in risk taking: A meta-analysis. *Psychological Bulletin, 125,* 367–383.

Cameron, C., Oskamp, S., & Sparks, W. (1977). Courtship American style—Newspaper ads. *Family Coordinator, 26,* 27–30.

Campbell, D. T. (1975). On the conflicts between biological and social evolution and between psychology and moral tradition. *American Psychologist, 30,* 1103–1126.

Clutton-Brock, T. H. (1984). Reproductive effort and terminal investment in iteroparous animals. *American Naturalist, 123,* 212–229.

Clutton-Brock, T. (1991, October). Lords of the *lek. Natural History,* pp. 34–41.

Collins, L., & LaPierre, D. (1975). *Freedom at midnight.* New York: Avon.

Conway, L. G., & Schaller, M. (2002). On the verifiability of evolutionary psychological theories: An analysis of the psychology of scientific persuasion. *Personality and Social Psychology Review, 6,* 152–166.

Crabb, P. B. (2000). The material culture of homicidal fantasies. *Aggressive Behavior, 26,* 225–234.

Daly, M., & Wilson, M. (1983). *Sex, evolution, and behavior* (2nd ed.). Belmont, CA: Wadsworth.

Daly, M., & Wilson, M. (1988). *Homicide.* New York: Aldine de Gruyter.

Darwin, C. (1958/1859). *The origin of species by natural selection.* New York: Mentor. (Original work published 1859)

Darwin, C. (1873). *The expression of emotions in man and animals.* London: Murray.

Davis, M. R., & Fernald, R. D. (1990). Social control of neuronal soma size. *Journal of Neurobiology, 21,* 1180–1188.

Dawkins, R. (1976). *The selfish gene.* Oxford, UK: Oxford University Press.

Deutsch, F. M., Zalenski, C. M., & Clark, M. E. (1986). Is there a double standard of aging? *Journal of Applied Social Psychology, 16,* 771–775.

Dunson, B. D., Colombo, B., & Baird, D. D. (2002). Changes with age in the level and duration of fertility in the menstrual cycle. *Human Reproduction, 17,* 1399–1403.

Eagly, A. H., & Wood, W. (1999). The origins of sex differences in human behavior: Evolved predispositions versus social roles. *American Psychologist, 54,* 408–423.

Estes, R. D. (1976). The significance of breeding synchrony in the wildebeest. *East African Wildlife Journal, 14,* 135–152.

Federal Bureau of Investigation. (2000). *Crime in the United States 2000: Uniform crime reports (Table 37, p. 225).* Washington, DC: Author.

Floore, T. (2002, June 22). *Mosquito information.* Retrieved August 20, 2002 from the American Mosquito Control Association website: *http://www.mosquito.org/mosquito.html*

Frisch, R. E. (1988, March). Fatness and fertility. *Scientific American,* pp. 88–95.

Gangestad, S. W., & Simpson, J. A. (2000). The evolution of human mating: Trade-offs and strategic pluralism. *Behavioral and Brain Sciences, 23,* 573–644.

Geary, D. C. (1998). *Male, female: The evolution of human sex differences.* Washington, DC: American Psychological Association.

Gross, M. (1984). Sunfish, salmon, and the evolution of alternative reproductive strategies and tactics in fishes. In G. Potts & R. Wootton (Eds.), *Fish reproduction: Strategies and tactics* (pp. 55–75). New York: Academic Press.

Gutierres, S. E., Kenrick, D. T., & Partch, J. J. (1999). Beauty, dominance and the mating game: Contrast effects in self-assessment reflect gender differences in mate selection. *Personality and Social Psychology Bulletin, 25,* 1126–1134.

Haselton, M. B., & Buss, D. M. (2000). Error management theory: A new perspective on biases in cross-sex mind reading. *Journal of Personality and Social Psychology, 78,* 81–91.

Hill, J. (1984). Prestige and reproductive success in man. *Ethology and Sociobiology, 5,* 77–95.

Hill, K., & Hurtado, A. M. (1996). *Aché life history: The ecology and demography of a foraging people.* Hawthorne, NY: Aldine de Gruyter.

Hrdy, S. B. (1999). *Mother Nature.* New York: Pantheon.

Hrdy, S. B. (2000). The optimal number of fathers: Evolution, demography, and history in the shaping of female mate preferences. *Annals of the New York Academy of Sciences, 907,* 75–96.

Inter-Parliamentary Union. (2002). *Women in national parliaments.* Retrieved Sep. 1, 2002 from *http://www.ipu.org/wmn-e/classif.htm.*

Janicki, M., & Krebs, D. L. (1998). Evolutionary approaches to culture. In C. Crawford & D. L. Krebs (Eds.), *Handbook of evolutionary psychology* (pp. 163–208). Mahwah, NJ: Erlbaum.

Johnson, R. E. (1970). Some correlates of extramarital coitus. *Journal of Marriage and the Family, 32,* 449–456.

Jones, O. D. (2001). Time-shifted rationality and the law of law's leverage: Behavioral economics meets behavioral biology. *Northwestern University Law Review, 95,* 1141–1198.

Kenrick, D. T. (1987). Gender, genes, and the social environment: A biosocial interactionist perspective. In P. Shaver & C. Hendrick (Eds.), *Review of personality and social psychology* (Vol. 7, pp. 14–44). Newbury Park, CA: Sage.

Kenrick, D. T. (1994). Evolutionary social psychology: From sexual selection to social cognition. In M. P. Zanna (Ed.), *Advances in experimental social psychology* (Vol. 26, pp. 75–121). San Diego: Academic Press.

Kenrick, D. T., Gabrielidis, C., Keefe, R. C., & Cornelius, J. S. (1996). Adolescents' age preferences for dating partners: Support for an evolutionary model of life-history strategies. *Child Development, 67,* 1499–1511.

Kenrick, D. T., Groth, G. R., Trost, M. R., & Sadalla, E. K. (1993). Integrating evolutionary and social exchange perspectives on relationships: Effects of gender, self-appraisal, and involvement level on mate selection criteria. *Journal of Personality and Social Psychology, 64,* 951–969.

Kenrick, D. T., & Keefe, R. C. (1992). Age preferences in mates reflect sex differences in human reproductive strategies. *Behavioral and Brain Sciences, 15,* 75–91.

Kenrick, D. T., & Li, N. (2000). The Darwin is in the details. *American Psychologist, 55,* 1060–1061.

Kenrick, D. T., Li, N. P., & Butner, J. (2003). Dynamical evolutionary psychology: Individual decision-rules and emergent social norms. *Psychological Review, 110,* 3–28.

Kenrick, D. T., Maner, J. K., Butner, J., Li, N. P., Becker, D. V., & Schaller, M. (2002). Dynamical evolutionary psychology: Mapping the domains of the new interactionist paradigm. *Personality and Social Psychology Review, 6,* 347–356.

Kenrick, D. T., Neuberg, S. L., Zierk, K. L., & Krones, J. M. (1994). Evolution and social cognition: Contrast effects as a function of sex, dominance, and physical attractiveness. *Personality and Social Psychology Bulletin, 20,* 210–217.

Kenrick, D. T., Sadalla, E. K., Groth, G., & Trost, M. R. (1990). Evolution, traits, and the stages of human courtship: Qualifying the parental investment model. *Journal of Personality, 58,* 97–116.

Kenrick, D. T., Sundie, J. M., Nicastle, L. D., & Stone, G. O. (2001). Can one ever be too wealthy or too chaste?: Searching for nonlinearities in mate judgment. *Journal of Personality and Social Psychology, 80,* 462–471.

Kerr, N. L., Harmon, D. L., & Graves, J. K. (1982). Independence of multiple verdicts by jurors and juries. *Journal of Applied Social Psychology, 12,* 12–29.

Ketelaar, T., & Ellis, B. J. (2000). Are evolutionary explanations unfalsifiable?: Evolutionary psychology and the Lakatosian philosophy of science. *Psychological Inquiry, 11,* 1–21.

Lack, D., Gibb, J., & Owen, D. F. (1957). Survival in relation to brood-size in tits. *Proceeding of the Zoological Society of London, 128,* 313–324.

Lehrman, D. S. (1964, November). The reproductive behavior of ring-doves. *Scientific American, 211,* 48–54.

Murdock, G. (1935). Comparative data on the division of labor by sex. *Social Forces, 15,* 551–553.

Öhman, A., & Mineka, S. (2001). Fears, phobias, and preparedness: Toward an evolved module of fear and fear learning. *Psychological Review, 108,* 483–522.

Ollason, J. C., & Dunnet, G. M. (1978). Age, experience, and other factors affecting the breeding success of the fulmar, *Fulmarus glacialis,* in Orkney. *Journal of Animal Ecology, 47,* 961–976.

Partridge, L., & Farquhar, M. (1981). Sexual activity reduces lifespan of male fruit flies. *Nature, 294,* 580–582.

Pinker, S. (1994). *The language instinct.* New York: Morrow.

Pinker, S. (2002). *The blank slate: The modern denial of human nature.* New York: Viking.

Quammen, D. (1996). *The song of the dodo: Island biogeography in an age of extinctions.* New York: Scribner.

Ralls, K. (1976). Mammals in which females are larger than males. *Quarterly Review of Biology, 51,* 245–276.

Reiter, J., Panken, K. J., & LeBoeuf, B. J. (1981). Female competition and reproductive success in northern elephant seals. *Animal Behavior, 29,* 670–687.

Salzano, F. M., Neel, J. V., & Maybury-Lewis, D. (1967). Further studies on the Xavante Indians: I. Demographic data on two additional villages: Genetic structure of the tribe. *American Journal of Human Genetics, 19,* 463–489.

Sherry, D. F., & Shachter, D. L. (1987). The evolution of multiple memory systems. *Psychological Review, 94,* 439–454.

Sigusch, V., & Schmidt, G. (1971). Lower-class sexuality: Some emotional and social aspects in West German males and females. *Archives of Sexual Behavior, 1,* 29–44.

Simonton, D. K. (1994). *Greatness: Who makes history and why.* New York: Guilford Press.

Stearns, S. C. (1976). Life-history tactics: A review of ideas. *Quarterly Review of Biology, 51,* 3–47.

Symons, D. (1979) *The evolution of human sexuality.* Oxford, UK: Oxford University Press.

Trivers, R. L. (1972). Parental investment and sexual selection. In B. Campbell (Ed.), *Sexual selection and the descent of man* (pp. 136–179). Chicago: Aldine.

Vallacher, R. R., Read, S. J., & Nowak, A. (2002). The dynamical approaches in personality and social psychology. *Personality and Social Psychology Review, 6,* 264–273.

Warner, R. R. (1984). Mating behavior and hermaphroditism in coral reef fishes. *American Scientist, 72,* 128–134.

Wiederman, M. W., & Allgeier, E. R. (1992). Gender differences in mate selection criteria: Sociobiological or socioeconomic explanation? *Ethology and Sociobiology, 13,* 115–124.

Williams, J. E., & Best, D. L. (1986). Sex stereotypes and intergroup relations. In S. Worchel & W. G. Austin (Eds.), *Psychology of intergroup relations* (pp. 244–259). Chicago: Nelson-Hall.

Wilson, M., & Daly, M. (1985). Competitiveness, risk taking, and violence: The young male syndrome. *Ethology and Sociobiology, 6,* 59–73.

Wood, W., & Eagly, A. H. (2002). A cross-cultural analysis of the behavior of women and men: Implications for the origins of sex differences. *Psychological Bulletin, 128,* 699–727.

Wrangham, R., & Peterson, D. (1996). *Demonic males.* Boston: Houghton Mifflin.

Zeifman, D., & Hazan, C. (1997). A process model of adult attachment formation. In S. Duck (Ed.), *Handbook of personal relationships* (2nd ed., pp. 179–195). Chichester, UK: Wiley..

5

Social Cognitive Theory of Gender Development and Functioning

KAY BUSSEY
ALBERT BANDURA

In this chapter, we address the psychosocial determinants and mechanisms by which society socializes male and female infants into masculine and feminine adults. Gender development is a fundamental issue, because some of the most important aspects of people's lives, such as the talents they cultivate, the conceptions they hold of themselves and others, the societal opportunities and constraints they encounter, and the social life and occupational paths they pursue, are heavily prescribed by societal gender typing. It is the primary basis on which people get differentiated, with pervasive effects on their daily lives.

Gender differentiation takes on added importance, because many of the attributes and roles selectively promoted in males and females tend to be differentially valued, with those ascribed to males generally being regarded as more powerful, effectual, and of higher status (Berscheid, 1993). Although some gender differences are biologically founded, most of the stereotypical attributes and roles linked to gender arise more from cultural design than from biological endowment (Bandura, 1986; Beall & Sternberg, 1993; Epstein, 1997). This chapter provides an analysis of gender role development and functioning within the framework of social cognitive theory.

Over the years, several major theories have been proposed to explain gender development, including psychoanalytic theories (Freud, 1916), cognitive-developmental theory (Kohlberg, 1966), gender schema theory (Martin, 2000; Martin & Halverson, 1981), biological theories (e.g., Buss, 1995; Gould, 1987; Simpson & Kenrick, 1997), and social psychological theories (e.g., Eagly, Wood, & Diekman, 2000; West & Zimmerman, 1991). Social cognitive theory includes biological, cognitive, and social factors; however, it differs from the alternate theories in that it focuses on the interplay of diverse factors within the larger social context in gender development. In social cognitive theory, gender development is neither totally shaped and regulated by environmental forces or biological imperatives nor by socially disembodied intrapsychic processes. Rather, gender development is explained in terms of triadic reciprocal interaction among personal, behavioral, and environmental factors (Bussey & Bandura, 1999). Moreover, most theories of gender development have centered on the early years of development (Freud, 1916; Kohlberg, 1966), or have focused on adults (Deaux & Major, 1987). Social cognitive theory adopts a lifespan perspective. Therefore, analysis of the social cognitive determinants of gender orientations spans the entire life course.

Elsewhere, we have discussed in some detail the need to broaden the nature and scope of theories about gender development and functioning (Bussey & Bandura, 1999). For example, in traditional psychological theories, the role of cognitive detereminants of gender development and functioning have been largely confined to gender concepts such as gender schemas and stereotypical knowledge about gender attributes. In social cognitive theory, the regulatory mechanisms governing development and functioning encompass a much richer array of cognitive determinants. These self-regulatory mechanisms are rooted in personal standards linked to self-evaluative sanctions. They operate in concert with beliefs about personal efficacy in the management of one's life circumstances; behavioral outcome expectations that vary conditionally across different pursuits, situational circumstances, and structured relationships; and belief systems about institutional opportunities and constraints (Bandura, 1986). Clearly, there is more to gender development and functioning than fitting conduct to a stereotypical gender schema. The dynamic interplay of the diverse cognitive determinants is socially situated and changes as different periods of life present new demands for self-renewal, adaption, and change. In this agentic perspective of social cognitive theory (Bandura, 2001, 2002), people are self-organizing, proactive, self-regulating, and self-reflecting.

The sections that follow present the basic structure of social cognitive theory, the main determinants it posits, and the mechanisms through which they operate. Later sections analyze how these determinants operate within the network of influences of societal subsystems—familial, educational, mass media, organizational, and sociopolitical—in shaping the nature of gender development and functioning.

SOCIAL COGNITIVE THEORY: AN AGENTIC PERSPECTIVE

Causal Structure

In the model of triadic reciprocal causation, personal factors, in the form of cognitive, affective, and biological events; behavior patterns; and environmental events all operate as interacting determinants that influence each other bidirectionally (Bandura, 1986). The *personal* contribution includes biological endowments, gender-linked conceptions, values, personal standards, and belief systems; *behavior* refers to styles of behavior that tend to be linked to gender; the *environmental* factor refers to the broad network of social and institutional influences that organize, guide, and regulate human affairs.

In this model of triadic causation, there is no fixed pattern or strength of reciprocal influence. Rather, the relative contribution of the constituent influences depends on activities, situations, and environmental constraints and opportunities. For example, under low environmental dictates, as in egalitarian social systems with equitable opportunity structures, personal factors serve as major influences in the self-regulation of developmental paths. Under social conditions in which social roles, lifestyle patterns, and opportunity structures are rigidly prescribed, personal factors have less leeway in which to operate. Bidirectional causation does not mean that the interacting factors are of equal strength. Their relative impact may fluctuate over time, situational circumstances, and activity domains.

Sociocognitive Modes of Influence

Gendered roles and conduct involve intricate competencies, interests, and value orientations. A comprehensive theory of gender differentiation must, therefore, explain the determinants and mechanisms through which gender-linked roles and conduct are acquired. In social cognitive theory, gender development is promoted by three major modes of influence and the way in which the information they convey is cognitively processed (Bandura, 1986). These include social modeling, performance experiences in which gendered conduct is linked to evaluative social reactions, and direct tutelage.

Modeling Influences in Gender Development

Modeling is one of the most pervasive and powerful means of transmitting values, attitudes, and patterns of thought and behavior (Bandura, 1986; Rosenthal & Zimmerman, 1978). A great deal of gender-linked information is conveyed by models in one's immediate environment in transactions with parents, siblings, peers, and significant persons in social, educational, and occupational contexts. In addition, the mass media provide pervasive modeling of gendered roles, conduct, and power relations.

Modeling is not simply a process of response mimicry, as is commonly believed. Modeled activities convey the rules and structures embodied in the exemplars for generating new variants of a behavior. This higher level of learning is achieved through abstract modeling. Rule-governed behavior patterns differ in specific content and other details, but they embody the same underlying rule. For example, children can extract the moral standards governing models' judgments of particular ethical predicaments, then use those standards to judge different types of ethical dilemmas. Once observers extract the rules and structure underlying the modeled activities, they can generate new patterns of behavior that conform to the structural properties but go beyond what they have seen or heard. Hence, social cognitive theory characterizes learning from exemplars as a generative social construction, not just mimicking the particular actions exemplified.

Most theories of gender development assign a major role to modeling in gender role learning (Bandura, 1969; Kohlberg, 1966; Mischel, 1970). However, Maccoby and Jacklin (1974) questioned whether modeling is influential in the development of gender-linked roles. They pointed to findings that, in laboratory situations, typically with a single male and female model, children do not consistently pattern their behavior after same-gender models. In everyday life, of course, children observe multiple models in both their immediate environments and media representations of gender roles. The power of modeling is enhanced by the typicalness in role behavior exhibited by male and female models. Indeed, in a set of studies, Bussey and Perry (1982; Perry & Bussey, 1979) varied the degree of gendered similarity by using multiple models. The propensity of children to pattern their behavior after same-gender models increases as the percentage of same-gender models displaying the same conduct increases. Thus, the past findings of no consistent same-sex modeling reflected deficiency of experimentation, not limitation of modeling influence.

According to cognitive-developmental theory (Kohlberg, 1966), it is only after children have achieved gender constancy—the belief that their own gender is fixed and irreversible—that they prefer to emulate models of the same gender. Gender constancy is viewed as an antecedent of modeling rather than as a product of it. In social cognitive theory, repeated modeling of gender-typed behavior in the home, in schools, in workplaces, and in televised portrayals serves as a major conveyer of gender-role information. Through modeling and the social structuring of everyday activities, children learn the prototypical behaviors associated with each sex. In this view, gender constancy is the product, rather than an antecedent, of the emulation of same-sex models. This is verified in research using multiple models (Bussey & Bandura, 1984). When children observe models of their gender collectively exhibiting stylistic behaviors that diverge from those displayed by other-gender models, they pattern their behavior more after same-gender than other-gender models. This preference for same-gender models occurs regardless of children's level of gender constancy. After a more abstract conception of gender coupled with expected social reactions is formed, gender conceptions and gender-typed learning can operate as bidirectional influences.

Enactive Experience

The second mode is through enactive experience involving behavior and how others respond to it. People discern gender linkages of conduct from the results that actions produce. Gender-linked behavior is heavily socially sanctioned in most societies. Therefore, evaluative social reactions are important sources of information for constructing gender conceptions. People differ in how they respond to the same gender-linked conduct displayed by children. They can develop and refine gendered orientations by observing the positive and negative consequences accompanying certain patterns of behavior. Moreover, some people are more concerned about and reactive to gender-linked conduct. Fathers, for example, react more negatively than mothers to their sons' feminine toy play (Idle, Wood, & Desmarais, 1993). The wider the array of people and social systems to which children are exposed and with which they interact, the more diverse the array of outcomes they experience for various types of gender-linked conduct. The same behavior can meet with different reactions from different people in different contexts within the child's social milieu. Children extract, weigh, and integrate this diverse behavior-outcome information in constructing guides for conduct.

Direct Tutelage

People have views about what is appropriate conduct for each sex. The third mode of influence is through direct tutelage in which children are instructed in the behavior appropriate for their gender. It serves as a convenient way of informing people about different styles of conduct and their linkage to gender. Moreover, instructional guidance is often used to draw general lessons from specific instances of modeled behavior and the effect it evokes.

As in other forms of influence, direct tutelage is most effective when it is based on shared values and receives widespread social support. Models, of course, often do not practice what they preach. The impact of tuition is weakened when what is being taught is contradicted by what is modeled (Rosenhan, Frederick, & Burrowes, 1968). Discordances between the styles of behavior modeled by adults and peers add further to the complexity of modeling processes (Bandura, Grusec, & Menlove, 1967). Children vary in the relative weight they give to these divergent sources of influence.

As is evident from the preceding analysis, people do not passively absorb gender role conceptions from whatever influences that happen to impinge on them. Rather, they construct generic conceptions from the diversity of styles of conduct that are modeled, evaluatively prescribed, and taught by different individuals, or even by the same person for different activities in different contexts. In short, the development of gender role conceptions is a construction rather than simply a wholesale incorporation of what is socially transmitted.

The different forms of social influence affect four major aspects of gender role development and functioning. They affect the development of gender-linked knowledge and competencies, and the three major sociocognitive regulators of gendered conduct, which include outcome expectations concerning gendered conduct and roles, self-evaluative standards, and self-efficacy beliefs.

REGULATORS OF GENDERED CONDUCT AND ROLE BEHAVIOR

The discussion thus far has centered on the acquisition of gender conceptions and competencies. Social cognitive theory also addresses the factors that regulate gender-linked conduct and how their relative influence changes developmentally. As previously noted, these factors include personal standards, self-efficacy beliefs, self-evaluative sanctions, outcome expectancies, and beliefs about the practices of societal systems.

Gender-Linked Social Sanctions

Children have to gain predictive knowledge about the likely social outcomes of gender-linked conduct in different settings, toward different individuals, and for different pursuits. The three basic modes of influence already reviewed similarly promote learning about the incentive structures of the social environment. Children acquire predictive knowledge about likely behavioral effects from observing the outcomes experienced by others, from the outcomes they experience firsthand, and from what they are told about the likely consequences of behaving in different ways for their sex.

In the gender domain, most gender-linked outcomes are socially prescribed rather than intrinsic to the action, and include socially based consequences such as approval, praise, and reward for activities traditionally linked to the same gender, and disapproval, or even punishment, for those linked to the other gender. It is not naturally foreordained that the same behavior enacted by females should produce different outcomes than those produced when enacted by males. These normative sanctions are socially constructed.

In social cognitive theory, evaluative social outcomes influence behavior mainly through their informational and motivational functions (Bandura, 1986). Outcomes convey information about the social norms and the system of sanctions governing gender-linked behavior. Anticipated outcomes serve as incentives and disincentives for action. Forethought converts foreseeable outcomes into current motivators of behavior (Bandura, 1991a). People pursue courses of action that they believe will bring valued outcomes, and refrain from those that they believe will give rise to aversive outcomes.

Regulatory Self-Sanctions

Social cognitive theory posits that, in the course of development, the regulation of behavior shifts from predominately external sanctions and mandates to gradual substitution of self-sanctions and self-direction grounded in personal standards (Bandura, 1986, 1991b). After self-regulatory functions are developed, children guide their conduct by sanctions they apply to themselves. Self-regulation operates through a set of psychological subfunctions that must be developed and mobilized for self-directed influence. These subfunctions include self-monitoring of gender-linked conduct, judgment of conduct in relation to personal standards and environmental circumstances, and self-evaluative reactions. Judgments of one's behavior against personal standards set the occasion for self-reactive influence. The standards give direction to behavior; the anticipatory self-sanctions provide the motivators for it. These self-sanctions include self-approving reactions for behaving in ways that measure up to personal standards, and self-disapproval for behaving in ways that violate those standards.

Both gender constancy and gender schema theory focus on conception matching as the primary regulative process (i.e., children strive to match the customary gender conception). Social cognitive theory posits both the standard-matching function and the motivating function rooted in self-evaluative influences. Both functions are necessary in the motivation and regulation of conduct (Bandura, 1991a).

The development of self-influence does not eliminate the sway of social influence. After children have developed self-regulatory capabilities, their behavior usually produces two sets of outcomes: self-evaluative reactions and social reactions. These may operate as complementary or as opposing influences on behavior. The way that gender roles are orchestrated is largely determined by the interplay between personal and social sources of influence.

Perceived Self-Efficacy in the Development and Regulation of Gender Role Conduct

In the agentic social cognitive theory (Bandura, 1997, 1999), beliefs of personal efficacy are the foundations of human agency. Unless people believe they can produce desired effects by their actions, they have little incentive to act or to persevere in the face of difficulties. Efficacy beliefs affect whether individuals think in self-enhancing or self-debilitating ways, how well they motivate themselves and preserve in the face of difficulties, the quality of their emotional life and vulnerability to stress and depression, and the life choices they make, which set the course of life paths (Bandura, 1997).

The theoretical analysis and growing body of research on how efficacy beliefs are formed, the processes through which they operate, their diverse effects, and their modification have been extensively reviewed elsewhere (Bandura, 1995, 1997; Maddux, 1995; Schwarzer, 1992). Eight meta-analyses conducted on findings from studies with diverse experimental and analytical methodologies applied across diverse spheres of functioning and cultural milieus with both children and adults attest to the positive impact of efficacy beliefs on human self-development and functioning (Bandura, 2002).

The power of efficacy beliefs to affect the life paths of men and women through selection processes is clearly revealed in studies of career choice and development (Bandura, 1997; Hackett, 1995). Occupational choices are of considerable importance, because they structure a major part of people's everyday reality, provide them with a source of personal identity, and determine the satisfaction and quality of their worklife. Efficacy beliefs set the slate of options for serious consideration. For example, people rapidly eliminate from consideration entire classes of vocations on the basis of perceived efficacy, regardless of the benefits the vocations may hold. Those who have a strong sense of personal efficacy consider a wide range of career options, show greater interest in them, prepare themselves better for different careers, and have greater staying power in their chosen pursuits (Lent, Brown, & Hackett, 1994).

Occupational pursuits are extensively gendered. The pervasive stereotypical practices of the various societal subsystems, which we examine later, eventually leave their mark on women's beliefs about their occupational efficacy. Male students have a comparable sense of efficacy for both traditionally male-dominated and female-dominated occupations. In contrast, female students judge themselves more efficacious for the types of occupations traditionally held by women, but have a weaker sense that they can efficaciously master the educational requirements and job functions of traditionally male-gendered occupations, even though they do not differ in actual verbal and quantitative ability (Betz & Hackett, 1981). The disparity in perceived efficacy for male- and female-dominated occupations is greatest for women who view themselves as highly feminine, distrust their quantitative capabilities, and believe that there are few successful female models in traditionally male-dominated occupations (Matsui, Ikeda, & Ohnishi, 1989).

Gender differences disappear, however, when women judge their efficacy to perform the same activities in everyday situations in stereotypically feminine tasks rather than in the context of male-dominated occupations (Betz & Hackett, 1983; Junge & Dretzke, 1995; Matsui & Tsukamoto, 1991). Such findings suggest that gender-related efficacy impediments arise from stereotypical linkage rather than actual capabilities.

SOCIAL COGNITIVE ANALYSIS OF GENDER DEVELOPMENT AND FUNCTIONING

Pregender Identity Regulation of Gender Conduct

Because societies are extensively organized around gender, it takes on special importance from birth. Children learn to categorize people on the basis of their gender from a very early age. By 7 months, infants can discriminate between male and female faces and voices. Infants use hair length and voice pitch as the distinguishing features for gender differentiation (Leinbach, 1990). By 9 months, infants begin to link male and female faces with their respective voices. When presented with pairs of male and female faces, they attend more to female faces when they hear female voices (Poulin-Dubois, Serbin, Kenyon, & Derbyshire, 1994), and by 18 months, they attend more to male than female faces when they hear male voices (Poulin-Dubois, Serbin, & Derbyshire, 1998).

As children's receptive language skills develop, by 18 months, infant girls match the gender labels "man" and "lady" with male and female faces, and both boy and girl infants match the gender label "boy" with male faces (Poulin-Dubois et al., 1998). Because of the pervasiveness of gender stereotyping, gender labels are among the first labels that children understand. At this age, they also begin to match stereotyped, gender-linked activities to male and female faces. However, boys do not show any understanding of the gender-stereotyping of activities, and girls show gender-stereotypical understanding in some contexts and not in others (Serbin, Poulin-Dubois, Colburne, Sen, & Eichstedt, 2001).

None of this research has shown that knowing gender labels or gender stereotypes is a prerequisite for preferential attention to same-sex activities. It is noteworthy that over the age range of 12–24 months, when boys are increasing their preferential attention to same-sex activities, girls are not increasing their same-sex preferences to the same extent, yet they show more knowledge of the gender linkage of activities. Obviously, the stronger correlative effects associated with attention to same-sex activities for boys rather than for girls are helping to guide boys' greater developing interest in same-sex activities.

Consider the pervasive social forces that are brought to bear on the development of gender orientation from the very beginning of life. Parents do not suspend influencing gender orientations until children can identify themselves as girls and boys. On the contrary, parents begin the task at the very outset of development. They do so by the way they structure the physical environment and by their social reactions toward different activities. From the moment of birth, when infants are categorized as either male or female, many of the social influences that impinge on them are determined by their gender (Rheingold & Cook, 1975). For most children, both their physical and social environments are highly gendered. Names, clothing, and decoration of infants' rooms are all influenced by their categorization as either female or male. Boys are adorned in blue and girls in pink. Boys are attired in rugged trousers, girls in pastel jeans or skirts. They are given different hairstyles as well

(Shakin, Shakin, & Sternglanz, 1985). Children come to use differential physical attributes, hairstyles, and clothing as indicators of gender.

Much early role learning occurs in play. The forms that play takes are structured and channeled by social influences. Parents stereotypically stock their sons' rooms with educational materials, machines, vehicles, and sports equipment, and their daughters' rooms with baby dolls, doll houses, domestic items, and floral furnishings (Pomerleau, Bolduc, Malcuit, & Cossette, 1990). Boys are provided with a greater variety of toys than girls. These play materials orient boys' activities and interests to gender roles usually performed outside the home. By contrast, girls are given toys directed toward domestic roles such as homemaking and child care. Thus, the gender-linked play materials arranged for children channel their spontaneous play into traditionally feminine or masculine roles (Etaugh & Liss, 1992).

The differentiation of the sexes extends beyond the realm of attire, make-believe play, and other play activities. Whenever appropriate occasions arise, parents and adults instruct children in the kinds of behavior expected of girls and boys, and provide evaluative feedback when these are performed. Mothers respond more negatively when their children engage in gender-atypical rather than gender-typical activities (Leaper, Leve, Strasser, & Schwartz, 1995). Although not all parents are inflexible gender stereotypers in all activities, most accept, model, and teach the sex roles traditionally favored by the culture.

Social sanctions bear heavily on gender-linked conduct even in the earliest years. Parents convey to their children positive and negative sanctions through affective reactions and evaluative comments. Although preverbal children cannot label their own sex or that of others, or even the gender linkage of objects, parental affective reactions and communications about the objects are sufficient to sway children's play. Parents are excited, smile, and comment approvingly when their children engage in activities considered appropriate for their gender, but they are likely to show and voice disapproval when their children take up activities deemed appropriate for the other gender. These affective reactions, depending on their nature, create positive and negative orientations to gender-linked objects and activities (Caldera, Huston, & O'Brien, 1989; Fagot & Leinbach, 1991). These findings are in accord with a great deal of evidence from other spheres of functioning on parental affective regulation of children's approach and avoidance reactions to ambiguous and novel objects (Bandura, 1992; Feinman, 1992). Modeled affective reactions also shape behavioral orientations and even alter the valence of the activities themselves (Bandura, 1986). Objects and activities thus get gendered through such reactive, instructive, and modeled modes of influence.

Apart from parental evaluative reactions and direct tutelage concerning gender-linked conduct, children also notice the various activities modeled by their parents and peers. Modeling influences are important even in children's early gender development. Because gender is a category carrying consequential outcomes, girls attend closely to female models, and boys to male models, before they can label themselves or others according to gender (Kujawski & Bower, 1993; Lewis & Brooks-Gunn, 1979).

The ability to differentiate the two sexes and to link them to different activities and their associated social sanctions is all that is necessary for children to begin to learn gender role stereotypes. Children choose activities consistent with gender-linked stereotypes from having observed certain activities linked to the two sexes, before they have a conception of gender. This level of gender understanding precedes gender self-identity, which already involves abstraction of a set of gender attributes integrated into a more general knowledge structure. When exposed to a female model engaging in male- and female-stereotyped activities, boys of 25 months emulate male-stereotyped activities to a greater extent than they do female-stereotyped ones. In contrast, girls of this age show no differential emulation of the female- and male-stereotyped activities. It is evident that the stronger gender-typing pressures for boys lead them to favor male-stereotypical activities, even before they acquire gender-stereotypical knowledge (Bauer, 1993).

Self-Categorization and Acquisition of Gender Role Knowledge

As children become more cognitively adept, their knowledge of gender extends beyond nonverbal categorization of people and objects and attending more to male and females faces that match auditorily presented gender labels, to explicit labeling of people, objects, and styles of behavior according to gender. As children begin to comprehend speech, they notice that masculine and feminine verbal labeling are used extensively by those around them. It does not take them long to learn that children are characterized as boys and girls, and adults as mothers and fathers, women and men. Gender labeling gives salience not only to sorting people on the basis of gender, but it also clusters the features and activities that characterize each gender.

Gender labeling highlights gender not only as important for viewing the world but also as the basis for categorizing oneself. Once such self-categorization occurs, the label takes on added significance, especially as children increasingly recognize that the social world around them is heavily structured around this differentiation. One's gender status makes a big difference. It carries enormous significance not only for dress and play but also for the skills cultivated, the occupations pursued, the functions performed in family life, and the nature of one's leisure pursuits and social relationships.

Social cognitive theory posits that, through cognitive processing of direct and vicarious experiences, children come to categorize themselves as girls or boys, to gain substantial knowledge of gender attributes and roles, and to extract rules as to what types of behavior are considered appropriate for their gender. However, unlike the gender constancy and schema theories, it does not invest gender conceptions with automatic directive and motivating properties. Acquiring a conception of gender and valuing the attributes defining that conception are separable processes governed by different determinants. In the preceding sections, we have demonstrated how self-regulatory mechanisms operate through perceived self-efficacy, anticipated social sanctions, self-sanctions, and perceived environmental facilitators and impediments rather than gender labeling itself motivating and directing gender-linked conduct.

Just as having a conception of one's own gender does not drive one to personify the stereotype it embraces, neither does the self-conception of gender necessarily create positive valuation of the attributes and roles traditionally associated with it. For example, self-conception as an elderly person does not motivate one to behave like the negative stereotype of old age, and to value and take pride in matching it closely. Both the valuation of certain attributes and roles, and the eagerness to adopt them, are influenced by the value society places on them. Societies that subordinate women may lead many women to devalue their own gender identity. Boys clearly favor male models, but girls, who are fully cognizant of their gender constancy, do not display the exclusive, same-gender modeling that the cognitivistic theories would have us believe (Bussey & Bandura, 1984, 1992). Little conflict exists between boys' own valuation of their gender and societal valuation of it. However, although girls may value being girls, and value gender-linked activities, they very early recognize the differential societal valuation of male and female roles (Kuhn, Nash, & Brucken, 1978; Meyer, 1980). Consequently, women have some incentive to attempt to raise their status by mastering activities and interests traditionally typed as masculine. Even at the preschool level, girls show greater modeling after the other gender than do boys.

From Social Sanctions to Self-Sanctions

The developmental changes posited by social cognitive theory are concerned not only with attributes and activities that get gendered but also with the mechanisms through which such conduct is regulated (Bandura, 1986, 1991a). With development of self-reactive capabilities, the regulation of conduct gradually shifts from external direction and sanctions to self-sanctions governed by personal standards. On the basis of direct and vicarious experiences, young children gain increasing knowledge about the likely outcomes of gender-linked conduct and regulate their actions accordingly. Children eventually adopt personal standards linked to self-reactive guides and motivators that enable them to exercise influence over their own conduct.

Research by Bussey and Bandura (1992) provides evidence for socially guided control of gender-linked conduct in early development, with emergence of self-regulatory control with increasing age. Both 3- and 4-year-old children reacted in a gender-stereotypical manner to conduct by peers that did not conform to their gender. They disapproved of boys feeding, diapering, and comforting dolls, and girls driving dump trucks. They also expected the peer's friends to react in the same disapproving way. However, the 3-year-olds did not exhibit differential self-evaluative reactions to engaging in masculine- and feminine-typed activities. Nor did their self-reactions predict their gender-linked conduct. By contrast, the 4-year-olds exhibited substantial self-regulatory guidance on the basis of personal standards. They expressed anticipatory self-approval for conduct linked to their gender, but self-criticism for conduct deemed appropriate to the other gender. Moreover, their anticipatory self-sanctions predicted their actual gender-linked conduct.

The findings of this study also have an important bearing on gender constancy and gender schema theories. Children who had not even attained gender identity, let alone gender constancy, demonstrated clear preference for engaging in same-gender rather than other-gender activities. Although they could not label objects as gender-linked, they were quite aware of the social standards associated with gender-linked objects and disapproved of peers' conduct that did not conform to their gender. Even the youngest children behaved toward peers in a gender-stereotypical manner, despite their limited gender-linked knowledge. They regulated their own conduct by the reactions they expected from others, pursuing same-gender activities but shunning activities linked to the other gender. Neither children's gender identity, stability, and constancy nor gender classificatory knowledge predicted gender-linked conduct.

From Gender Categorization to Gender Role Learning

Gender role learning requires broadening gender conceptions to include not only appearances but also clusters of behavioral attributes and interests that form lifestyle patterns, and social and occupational roles. Knowledge about gender roles involves a higher level of organization and abstraction than simple categorization of persons, objects, and activities in terms of gender. To complicate matters further, the stylistic and role behaviors that traditionally typify male and female orientations are not uniformly gender linked. For example, many men are mild mannered and some females are aggressive. As a result, children have to rely on the relative prevalence of exemplars and the extent to which given activities covary with gender. If children routinely see women performing homemaking activities, and males only occasionally try their hand at it, homemaking readily gets gender typed as a woman's role. However, if children often observe both men and women gardening, then the task is not as easily linked to gender.

As children mature, not only are they more cognitively adept at discerning the gender linkage of interests and activities, and integrating diverse information into more composite conceptions, but their social worlds also expand. They are increasingly exposed to a broader range of social influences outside the home. Before examining how this expanded range of social influences affects children's gender development and functioning, we analyze the changing role of parents in gender differentiation over the course of development.

Parental Impact on Subsequent Gender Development

In an earlier section, we showed that parents play an active role in setting the course of their children's gender development by structuring, channeling, modeling, labeling, and reacting evaluatively to gender-linked conduct. As children's verbal and cognitive capabilities increase, parents broaden the conception of gender by instructing their children about gender-linked styles of conduct and roles that extend beyond merely classifying objects, people, and discrete activities into male and female categories. Behavioral styles represent clusters of attributes organized in a coherent way. Girls are encouraged to be nurturant and polite, and boys, to be adventuresome and independent (Huston, 1983; Zahn-Waxler, Cole, & Barren, 1991).

We have seen in the previous analysis that parents promote sharper differentiation of gendered conduct with boys than with girls. This extends to cross-gender conduct, which is more negatively regarded for boys than for girls (Sandnabba & Ahlberg, 1999). Parents view feminine toys and activities as more gender stereotypical than masculine toys and activities. This contributes to their greater acceptance of cross-gender conduct by girls than by boys (Campenni, 1999). The gender dichotomization and asymmetry of acceptance is stronger for fathers, who continue this differential treatment throughout childhood (Fagot & Hagen, 1991; Maccoby, 1998; Siegal, 1987). As a result, boys are more likely than girls to expect censure from their fathers for engaging in female-typical activities. The more strongly boys hold these expectations, the more likely they are to engage in male-typical activities, especially in situations where gender is salient (Raag & Rackliff, 1998).

Despite the extensive findings reported earlier, the influence of parents on children's gender development and functioning has been the subject of empirical dispute. Maccoby and Jacklin (1974) concluded that there is little support for parents' differential treatment of boys and girls. More recently, Lytton and Romney (1991) came to the same conclusion in a meta-analysis of findings. This conclusion was challenged by other theorists (Block, 1983; Collins & Russell, 1991; Siegal, 1987). A more comprehensive analysis that includes the findings of research on early family practices (Bussey & Bandura, 1999) shows that parents contribute to their children's gender orientation.

Impact of Peers on Gender Development

As children's social world expands outside the home, peer groups become another agency of gender development. Peers are sources of much social learning. They model and sanction styles of conduct and serve as comparative references for appraisal and validation of personal efficacy (Bandura, 1997; Schunk, 1987). In the social structuring of activities, children selectively associate with same-gender playmates pursuing gender-typed interests and activities (Huston, 1983). Gender segregation can increase the influence exerted by peers by creating highly differentiated environments for boys and girls. For school-age children, the segregation occurs not only in playgroups but in also the choice of friends (Hayden-Thomson, Rubin, & Hymel, 1987).

In these peer interactions, children reward each other for gender-appropriate activities and punish gender conduct considered inappropriate (Lamb, Easterbrooks, & Holden, 1980). They apply the same negative sanctions for playing with peers of the other gender (Thorne, 1986). Consistent with parental practices, peers' negative sanctions for other-gender conduct and playmates are stronger for boys than for girls (Zucker, Wilson-Smith, Kurita, & Stem, 1995). Both boys and girls generally respond more positively to members of their own sex, but boys differ from girls, in that they are less approving of boys who engage in female-linked conduct. Moreover, boys are much more likely to be criticized for activities considered to be feminine than are girls for engaging in male-typical activities (Fagot, 1985). Evaluative reactions from boys, such as "You're silly, that's for girls," "Now you're a girl," and "That's dumb. Boys don't play with dolls," provide strong disincentives to do things linked to girls or to spend much time playing with them. The mere presence of other boys is sufficient to heighten preschool boys' preferences for male-typed activities (Banerjee & Lintern, 2000).

In some of the current theorizing, the peer group is singled out as the prime socializing agency of gender development (Leaper, 1994; Maccoby, 1990, 1998). The peer group is not an autonomous agency, untouched by familial and other social influences. Indeed, the findings quite consistently show that all of the social subsystems—parents, teachers, peers, mass media, and the workplace—engage in a great deal of gender differentiation, and that the differential treatment is stronger for boys than for girls. Clearly, the peer group is neither the originator of societal gender stereotypes nor the unique player in the process of gender differentiation. Both gender differentiation and stereotyping have a much earlier and socially pervasive source.

In social cognitive theory, the peer group functions as an interdependent subsystem in gender differentiation, not a socially disembodied one (Bandura, 1986; Bandura & Walters, 1959). Peers are both the product and the contributing producers of gender differentiation. Children learn at a very early age what gets socially linked to gender, as well as the values and incentive systems relative to the type of conduct considered proper for their gender. The socially instilled orientations lead peers to promote further the gender differentiation by favoring same-gender playmates and making sure that their peers conform to the conduct expected of their gender.

Once subgroups are formed, the group dynamics of mutual modeling, social sanctioning, activity structuring, and social and psychological territoriality come into play. Social influences from interdependent social systems are important not only in the initial subgroup formation but also in the maintenance of gender differentiation. Experimental and field studies graphically reveal that group-stereotypical dynamics can be powerfully activated through subgroup formation on the basis of even an arbitrary characteristic, such as the color of shirts, socially invested with superior or inferior value (Elliott, 1977; Peters, 1971). The commercial stereotyping and exploitation of gender in the media pop culture, which holds great attraction for youth, is but one example of another gendering social force that must be considered in analytical efforts to disentangle the unique contribution of peers.

Media Representations of Gender Roles

Superimposed on the differential modeling, tutelage, and social sanctioning by parents and peers, which leave few aspects of children's lives untouched, is a pervasive cultural modeling of gender roles. Children are continually exposed to models of gender-linked behavior in readers, storybooks, video games, and representations of society on the television screen of every household (Dietz, 1998; Thompson & Zerbinos, 1997; Turner-Bowker, 1996). Males are generally portrayed as directive, venturesome, enterprising, and in pursuit of engaging occupations and recreational activities. In contrast, women are usually shown as acting in dependent, unambitious, and emotional ways. These stereotypical portrayals of gender roles are not confined to North America. Similar stereotyping of gender roles has been reported in the televised fare of Great Britain, Australia, Mexico, and Italy (Bussey & Bandura, 1999; Furnham & Mak, 1999). Male and female televised characters are also portrayed as differing in agentic capabilities. Men are more likely to be shown exercising control over events, whereas women tend to be more at the mercy of others, especially in the coercive relationships that populate the prime-time fare.

The exaggerated gender stereotyping extends to the portrayal of occupational roles in the televised world. Men are often shown pursuing careers of high status, whereas women are largely confined to domestic roles or employed in low-status jobs (Durkin, 1985). The gender stereotypes are replicated in television and radio commercials as well. Women are usually shown in the home as consumers of advertised products. Men, in contrast, are more likely to be portrayed as authoritative salesmen for the advertised products (Coltrane & Messineo, 2000; Furnham & Mak, 1999; Mazzella, Durkin, Cerini, & Buralli, 1992). Gender-stereotypical portrayals are also typical of commercials and cartoons targeting children. Boys are shown as dominant, assertive, and athletic, whereas girls are portrayed as subservient, affectionate, and domestic (Browne, 1998; Thompson & Zerbinos, 1995).

From the early preschool years, children watch a great deal of television day in and day out (Wright & Huston, 1983). Given the media representations of gender in diverse spheres of life, heavy viewers of television are exposed to a vast amount of stereotypical gender role modeling. It is not surprising that those who have a heavy diet of the televised fare display more stereotypical gender role conceptions than do light viewers (McGhee & Frueh, 1980). The more children remember gender-stereotypical portrayals, the more strongly they prefer traditional gender-stereotypical occupations (Thompson & Zerbinos, 1997).

Studies in which females are portrayed in a counterstereotypical way attest to the influence of modeling on gender role conceptions. Nonstereotypical modeling expands children's aspirations and the range of role options they deem appropriate to their gender. Repeated symbolic modeling of egalitarian role pursuits by males and females enduringly reduces gender role stereotyping in young children (Ochman, 1996; Thompson & Zerbinos, 1997).

Impact of Educational Practices on Gender Development

The school functions as another primary agency for developing gender orientations. Teachers criticize children for engaging in play activities considered inappropriate for their gender, which further serves to link gender attributes with social normative sanctions (Fagot, 1977). As in the case of parents and peers, teachers foster, through their social sanctions, sharper gender differentiations for boys than for girls.

Teachers also pay more attention to boys than to girls, and interact with them more extensively (Morse & Handley, 1985). From nursery school through to the early elementary school years, boys receive both more praise and more criticism from teachers than girls (Simpson & Erickson, 1983). The nature of the social sanctions also differs across gender. Boys are more likely to be praised for academic success and criticized for misbehavior, whereas girls tend to be praised for tidiness and compliance, and criticized for academic failure. This differential pattern of social sanctions, which can enhance the perceived self-efficacy of boys but undermine that of girls, continues throughout the school years (Eccles, 1987).

School is the place where children expand their knowledge and competencies, and form the sense of intellectual efficacy essential for participating effectively in the larger society. The self-beliefs and competencies acquired during this formative period carry especially heavy weight, because they shape the course of career choices and development. Even as early as middle school, children's beliefs in their occupational efficacy, which are rooted in their patterns of perceived efficacy, have begun to crystallize and steer their occupational considerations in directions congruent with their efficacy beliefs (Bandura, Barbarnelli, Caprara, & Pastorelli, 2001). Stereotypical gender occupational orientations are very much in evidence and closely linked to the structure of efficacy beliefs. Girls' perceived occupational efficacy centers on service, clerical work, caretaking, and teaching pursuits, whereas boys judge themselves more efficacious for careers in science, technology, computer systems, and physically active pursuits.

The gender bias in the judgment and cultivation of competencies operates in classrooms, as well as in homes. Teachers often convey in many subtle ways that they expect less of girls academically, and are inclined to attribute scholastic failures to social and motivational problems in boys but to deficiencies of ability in girls (Dweck, Davidson, Nelson, & Enna, 1978). Girls have higher perceived efficacy and valuation of mathematics in classrooms in which teachers emphasize the usefulness of quantitative skills, encourage cooperative or individualized learning rather than competitive learning, and minimize social comparative assessment of students' ability (Eccles, 1989).

Even for teachers who do not share the gender bias, unless they are proactive in providing equal gender opportunities to learn quantitative and scientific subjects, the more skilled male students dominate the instructional activities, which only further entrenches differential development of quantitative competencies. Thus, for example, computer coursework for children, designed to reduce gender differences in computer literacy, superimposed on a pervading gender bias, raises boys' self-efficacy about computer use but lowers girls' self-efficacy and interest in computers (Collis, 1985). Clearly, concerted effort is required to counteract the personal effects of stereotypical gender role socialization and the social perpetuation of those effects.

Despite the lack of gender differences in intelligence, there are differences in the courses boys and girls select, and how they judge their capabilities in these varied academic domains (Hyde, Fennema, & Lamon, 1990; Hyde & Linn, 1988; Walkerdine, 1989). Females enroll in significantly fewer higher level mathematics, science, and computer courses, have less interest in these subjects, and view them as less useful to their lives than do their male counterparts.

The channeling of interests into different academic domains has a profound impact on career paths. Inadequate preparation in mathematics is an especially serious barrier, because it filters out a large number of career options requiring this competency (Sells, 1982). The differential precollege preparation stems not from differences in ability, but from differences in support and encouragement from teachers, peers, and parents to children who pursue quantitative and scientific coursework.

Negatively biased practices not only constrain career aspirations and options but also undermine a sense of personal agency. Ancis and Phillips (1996) examined the extent to which college women experience a negatively biased academic environment in which they are regarded to be less serious and capable than male students, are given fewer academic opportunities and less support, and have fewer female academic models and mentors. White, female students experience such academic inequities, and female students of color experience them to an even greater degree. The more that students perceive academic inequities, the lower they perceive their agentic self-efficacy to take proactive charge of their educational and occupational advancement. The impact of academic bias on agentic efficacy remains when the influence of egalitarian gender role orientation, academic major, and race are controlled.

The Gendered Practices of Occupational Systems

Occupational activities make up a major part of daily living and serve as important sources of personal identity. The gendered practices of familial, educational, peer, and media subsystems are essentially replicated in organizational structures and practices, including extensive segregation of jobs along gender lines, concentration of women in lower level positions, inequitable wages, limited opportunities for upper level mobility, and power imbalances in work relationships, that erect barriers to equitable participation in organizational activities (Stockard & Johnson, 1992).

Recent years have witnessed vast changes in the roles women perform, but the institutional practices lag far behind (Bandura, 1997; Riley, Kahn, & Foner, 1994). Low birthrate and increased longevity creates the need for purposeful pursuits that provide satisfaction to women's lives long after the offspring have left home (Astin, 1984). Women are educating themselves more extensively, which creates a wider array of options than was historically available for women. Women are entering the workforce in large numbers, not just for economic reasons but as a matter of personal satisfaction and identity. Many have the personal efficacy, competencies, and interests to achieve distinguished careers in occupations traditionally dominated by men. Although the constraints to gaining entry into such careers have eased, many impediments to achieving progress at the higher levels within them remain (Jacobs, 1989).

Changing gender roles pose challenges on how to strike a balance between family and job demands for women who enter the workforce. The effects of juggling dual roles are typically framed negatively on how competing interrole demands breed distress and discordance. Much has been written on the negative spillover that women's job pressures have on family life but little on how job satisfaction may enhance family life. Research by Ozer (1995) speaks to this issue. Married women who pursued professional, managerial, and technical occupations were tested before the birth of their first child for their perceived self-efficacy to manage the demands of their family and occupational life. Their physical and psychological well-being and the strain they experienced over their dual roles were measured after they had returned to work. Neither family income, occupational workload, nor division of child care responsibility directly affected women's well-being or emotional strain over dual roles. These factors were contributors, but they operated through their effects on perceived self-efficacy. Women who had a strong sense of coping efficacy (i.e., that they could manage the multiple demands of family and work, exert some influence over their work schedules, and get their husbands to help with various aspects of child care) experienced a low level of physical and emotional strain, good health, and a more positive sense of well-being. Neither theories nor empirical studies have given much attention to the positive spillover effects of women's satisfying work lives on their home lives.

Human stress is widely viewed as the emotional strain that arises when perceived task demands exceed perceived capability to manage them. Matsui and Onglatco (1992) showed that what is experienced as an occupational stressor depends partly on level of perceived self-efficacy. Women employees who have a low sense of efficacy are stressed by heavy work demands and role responsibilities. By contrast, those with a high sense of efficacy are frustrated and stressed by limited opportunities to make full use of their talents. A work life of blocked opportunities, thwarted aspirations, and personal nonfulfillment that takes up most of one's daily living can be a source of misery.

Interdependence of Gender-Socializing Subsystems

The research we have reviewed in this chapter documents the influential role played by each of the various societal subsystems in the differentiation of gender attributes and roles. In social cognitive theory (Bandura, 1986, 1999), human development and functioning are highly socially interdependent, richly contextualized, and conditionally manifested. In everyday life, these different subsystem sources of influence operate interdependently rather than in isolation. The multiple determination of behavior and reciprocity of influences adds greatly to the complexity of disentangling causal processes and their changing dynamics over the course of development. Further progress in understanding the sources, social functions, and personal and social effects of gender differentiation will require greater effort to clarify the complex interplay of the various subsystems of influence within the larger societal context. However, people are not simply the products of social forces acting on them. In the triadic reciprocity posited by social cognitive theory, people contribute to their self-development and social change through their agentic actions within the interrelated systems of influence.

ACKNOWLEDGMENT

This chapter was developed, in part, from material that originally appeared in Bussey and Bandura (1999).

REFERENCES

Ancis, J. R., & Phillips, S. D. (1996). Academic gender bias and women's behavioral agency self-efficacy. *Journal of Counseling and Development*, *75*, 131–137.

Astin, H. S. (1984). The meaning of work in women's lives: A sociopsychological model of career choice and work behavior. *Counseling Psychologist*, *12*, 117–126.

Bandura, A. (1969). Social-learning theory of identificatory processes. In D. A. Goslin (Ed.), *Handbook of socialization theory and research* (pp. 213–262). Chicago: Rand McNally.

Bandura, A. (1986). *Social foundations of thought and action: A social cognitive theory.* Englewood Cliffs, NJ: Prentice-Hall.

Bandura, A. (1991a). Self-regulation of motivation through anticipatory and self-regulatory mechanisms. In R. A. Dienstbier (Ed.), *Nebraska Symposium on Motivation: Vol. 38. Perspectives on motivation* (pp. 69–164). Lincoln: University of Nebraska Press.

Bandura, A. (1991b). Social cognitive theory of moral thought and action. In W. M. Kurtines & J. L. Gewirtz (Eds.), *Handbook of moral behavior and development* (Vol. 1, pp. 45–103). Hillsdale, NJ: Erlbaum.

Bandura, A. (1992). Social cognitive theory of social referencing. In S. Feinman (Ed.), *Social referencing and the social construction of reality in infancy* (pp. 175–208). New York: Plenum Press.

Bandura, A. (1995). *Self-efficacy in changing societies.* New York: Cambridge University Press.

Bandura, A. (1997). *Self-efficacy: The exercise of control.* New York: Freeman.

Bandura, A. (1999). Social cognitive theory of personality. In L. A. Pervin & O. P. John (Eds.), *Handbook of personality* (2nd ed., pp. 154–196). New York: Guilford Press.

Bandura, A. (2001). Social cognitive theory: An agentic perspective. *Annual Review of Psychology* (Vol. 52, pp. 1–26). Palo Alto, CA: Annual Reviews.

Bandura, A. (2002). Social cognitive theory in cultural context. *Journal of Applied Psychology: An International Review, 51,* 269–290.

Bandura, A., Barbaranelli, C., Caprara, C. V., & Pastorelli, C. (2001). Self-efficacy beliefs as shapers of children's aspirations and career trajectories. *Child Development, 72,* 187–206.

Bandura, A., Grusec, J. E., & Menlove, F. L. (1967). Some social determinants of self-monitoring reinforcement systems. *Journal of Personality and Social Psychology, 5,* 449–455.

Bandura, A., & Walters, R. H. (1959). *Adolescent aggression.* New York: Ronald Press.

Banerjee, R., & Lintern, V. (2000). Boys will be boys: The effect of social evaluation concerns on gender-typing. *Social Development, 9,* 397–408.

Bauer, P. J. (1993), Memory for gender-consistent and gender-inconsistent event sequences by twenty-five-month-old children. *Child Development, 64,* 285–297.

Beall, A. E., & Sternberg, R. J. (Eds.). (1993). *The psychology of gender.* New York: Guilford Press.

Berscheid, E. (1993). Foreword. In A. E. Beall & R. J. Sternberg (Eds.), *The psychology of gender* (pp. vii–xvii). New York: Guilford Press.

Betz, N. E., & Hackett, G. (1981). The relationship of career-related self-efficacy expectations to perceived career options in college women and men. *Journal of Counseling Psychology, 28,* 399–410.

Betz, N. E., & Hackett, G. (1983). The relationship of mathematics self-efficacy expectations to the selection of science-based college majors. *Journal of Vocational Behavior, 23,* 329–345.

Block, J. H. (1983). Differential premises arising from differential socialization of the sexes: Some conjectures. *Child Development*, *54*, 1335–1354.

Browne, B. A. (1998). Gender stereotypes in advertising on children's television in the 1990s: A cross-national analysis. *Journal of Advertising*, *XXVII*, 83–96.

Buss, D. M. (1995). Psychological sex differences: Origins through sexual selection. *American Psychologist*, *50*, 164–168.

Bussey, K., & Bandura, A. (1984). Influence of gender constancy and social power on sex-linked modeling. *Journal of Personality and Social Psychology*, *47*, 1292–1302.

Bussey, K., & Bandura, A. (1992). Self-regulatory mechanisms governing gender development. *Child Development*, *63*, 1236–1250.

Bussey, K., & Bandura, A. (1999). Social cognitive theory of gender development and differentiation. *Psychological Review*, *106*, 676–713.

Bussey, K., & Perry, D. G. (1982). Same-sex imitation: Lie avoidance of cross-sex models or the acceptance of same-sex models? *Sex Roles*, *8*, 773–794.

Caldera, Y. M., Huston, A. C., & O'Brien, M. (1989). Social interactions and play patterns of parents and toddlers with feminine, masculine and neutral toys. *Child Development*, *60*, 70–76.

Campenni, C. E. (1999). Gender stereotyping of children's toys: A comparison of parents and nonparents. *Sex Roles*, *40*, 121–138.

Collins, A. W., & Russell, G. (1991). Mother–child and father–child relationships in middle childhood and adolescence: A developmental analysis. *Developmental Review*, *11*, 99–136.

Collis, B. (1985). Psychosocial implications of sex differences in attitudes toward computers: Results of a survey. *International Journal of Women's Studies*, *8*, 207–213.

Coltrane, S., & Messineo, M. (2000). The perpetuation of subtle prejudice: Race and gender imagery in 1990s television advertising. *Sex Roles*, *42*, 363–389.

Deaux, K., & Major, B. (1987). Putting gender into context: An interactive model of gender related behavior. *Psychological Review*, *94*, 369–389.

Dietz, T. L. (1998). An examination of violence and gender role portrayals in video games: Implications for gender socialization and aggressive behavior. *Sex Roles*, *38*, 425–443.

Durkin, K. (1985). Television and sex-role acquisition: I. Content. *British Journal of Social Psychology*, *24*, 101–113.

Dweck, C. S., Davidson, W., Nelson, S., & Enna, B. (1978). Sex differences in learned helplessness: II. The contingencies of evaluative feedback in the classroom: III. An experimental analysis. *Developmental Psychology*, *14*, 268–276.

Eagly, A. H., Wood, W., & Diekman, A. (2000). Social role theory of sex differences and similarities: A current appraisal. In T. Eckes & H. M. Trautner (Eds.), *The developmental social psychology of gender* (pp. 123–174). Mahwah, NJ: Erlbaum.

Eccles, J. S. (1987). Gender roles and women's achievement-related decisions. *Psychology of Women Quarterly*, *11*, 135–172.

Eccles, J. S. (1989). Bringing young women to math and science. In M. Crawford & M. Gentry (Eds.), *Gender and thought* (pp. 36–58). New York: Springer-Verlag.

Elliott, J. (1977). The power and pathology of prejudice. In P. G. Zimbardo & F. L. Ruch (Eds.), *Psychology and life* (9th ed., pp. 589–590). Glenview, IL: Scott, Foresman.

Epstein, C. F. (1997). The multiple realities of sameness and difference: Ideology and practice. *Journal of Social Issues, 53*, 259–278.

Etaugh, C., & Liss, M. B. (1992). Home, school, and playroom: Training grounds for adult gender roles. *Sex Roles, 26*, 129–147.

Fagot, B. I. (1977). Consequences of moderate cross-gender behavior in preschool children. *Child Development, 48*, 902–907.

Fagot, B. I. (1985). Changes in thinking about early sex role development. *Developmental Review, 5*, 83–98.

Fagot, B. I., & Hagen, R. (1991). Observations of parent reactions to sex-stereotyped behaviors: Age and sex effects. *Child Development, 62*, 617–628.

Fagot, B. I., & Leinbach, M. D. (1991). Attractiveness in young children: Sex-differentiated reactions of adults. *Sex Roles, 25*, 269–284.

Feinman, S. (Ed.). (1992). *Social referencing and the social construction of reality in infancy.* New York: Plenum Press.

Freud, S. (1916). Introductory lectures on psychoanalysis. In J. Strachey (Ed. & Trans.), *Standard Edition, 18* (pp. 15–239). London: Hogarth Press, 1963.

Furnham, A., & Mak, T. (1999). Sex-role stereotyping in television commercials: A review and comparison of fourteen studies done on five continents over 25 years. *Sex Roles, 41*, 413–437.

Gould, S. J. (1987). *An urchin in the storm.* New York: Norton.

Hackett, G. (1995). Self-efficacy in career choice and development. In A. Bandura (Ed.), *Self-efficacy in changing societies* (pp. 232–258). New York: Cambridge University Press.

Hayden-Thomson, L., Rubin, K. H., & Hymel, S. (1987). Sex preferences in sociometric choices. *Developmental Psychology, 23*, 558–562.

Huston, A. C. (1983). Sex typing. In P. H. Mussen (Series Ed.) & E. M. Hetherington (Vol. Ed.), *Handbook of child psychology: Vol. 4. Socialization, personality, and social development* (4th ed., pp. 387–467). New York: Wiley.

Hyde, J. S., Fennema, E., & Lamon, S. J. (1990). Gender differences in mathematics performance: A meta-analysis. *Psychological Bulletin, 107*, 139–155.

Hyde, J. S., & Linn, M. C. (1988). Gender differences in verbal ability: A meta-analysis. *Psychological Bulletin, 104*, 53–69.

Idle, T., Wood, E., & Desmarais, S. (1993). Gender role socialization in toy play situations: Mothers and fathers with their sons and daughters. *Sex Roles, 28*, 679–691.

Jacobs, J. A. (1989). *Revolving doors: Sex segregation and women's careers.* Stanford, CA: Stanford University Press.

Junge, M. E., & Dretzke, B. J. (1995). Mathematical self-efficacy gender differences in gifted/talented adolescents. *Gifted Child Quarterly, 39*, 22–28.

Kohlberg, L. (1966). A cognitive-developmental analysis of children's sex-role concepts and attitudes. In E. E. Maccoby (Ed.), *The development of sex differences* (pp. 82–173). Stanford, CA: Stanford University Press.

Kuhn, D., Nash, S. C., & Brucken, L. (1978). Sex role concepts of two- and three-year-olds. *Child Development, 49*, 445–451.

Kujawski, J. H., & Bower, T. G. R. (1993). Same-sex preferential looking during infancy as a function of abstract representation. *British Journal of Developmental Psychology, 11*, 201–209.

Lamb, M. E., Easterbrooks, M. A., & Holden, G. W. (1980). Reinforcement and punishment among preschoolers: Characteristics, effects, and correlates. *Child Development, 51*, 1230–1236.

Leaper, C. (Ed.). (1994). *Childhood gender segregation: Causes and consequences.* San Francisco: Jossey-Bass.

Leaper, C., Leve, L., Strasser, T., & Schwartz, R. (1995). Mother–child communication sequences: Play activity, child gender, and marital status effects. *Merrill–Palmer Quarterly, 41*, 307–327.

Leinbach, M. D. (1990, April). *Infants' use of hair and clothing cues to discriminate pictures of men and women.* Paper presented at the International Conference on Infant Studies, Montreal, Quebec, Canada.

Lent, R. W., Brown, S. D., & Hackett, G. (1994). Toward a unifying social cognitive theory of career and academic interest, choice, and performance. *Journal of Vocational Behavior, 45*, 79–122.

Lewis, M., & Brooks-Gunn, J. (1979). *Social cognition and the acquisition of self.* New York: Plenum Press.

Lytton, H., & Romney, D. M. (1991). Parents' differential socialization of boys and girls: A meta-analysis. *Psychological Bulletin, 109*, 267–296.

Maccoby, E. E. (1990). Gender and relationships: A developmental account. *American Psychologist, 45*, 513–520.

Maccoby, E. E. (1998). *The two sexes: Growing up apart, coming together.* Cambridge, MA: Belknap Press.

Maccoby, E. E., & Jacklin, C. N. (1974). *The psychology of sex differences.* Stanford, CA: Stanford University Press.

Maddux, J. E. (1995). *Self-efficacy, adaptation, and adjustment: Theory, research and application.* New York: Plenum Press.

Martin, C. L. (2000). Cognitive theories gender development. In T. Eckes & H. M. Trautner (Eds.), *The developmental social psychology of gender* (pp. 91–121). Mahwah, NJ: Erlbaum.

Martin, C. L., & Halverson, C. F. (1981). A schematic processing model of sex typing and stereotyping in children. *Child Development, 52*, 1119–1134.

Matsui, T., Ikeda, H., & Ohnishi, R. (1989). Relations of sex-typed socializations to career self-efficacy expectations of college students. *Journal of Vocational Behavior, 35*, 1–16.

Matsui, T., & Onglatco, M. L. (1992). Career self-efficacy as a moderator of the relation between occupational stress and strain. *Journal of Vocational Behavior, 41*, 79–88.

Matsui, T., & Tsukamoto, S. (1991). Relation between career self-efficacy measures based on occupational titles and Holland codes and model environments: A methodological contribution. *Journal of Vocational Behavior, 38*, 78–91.

Mazzella, C., Durkin, K., Cerini, E., & Buralli, P. (1992). Sex role stereotyping in Australian television advertisements. *Sex Roles, 26*, 243–259.

McGhee, P. E., & Frueh, T. (1980). Television viewing and the learning of sex-role stereotypes. *Sex Roles, 6*, 179–188.

Meyer, B. (1980). The development of girls' sex-role attitudes. *Child Development, 51*, 508–514.

Mischel, W. (1970). A social learning view of sex differences in behavior. In P. H. Mussen (Ed.), *Carmichael's manual of child psychology* (Vol. 2, pp. 3–72). New York: Wiley.

Morse, L. W., & Handley, H. M. (1985). Listening to adolescents: Gender differences in science classroom interaction. In L. C. Wilkinson & C. B. Marrett (Eds.), *Gender influences in classroom interaction* (pp. 37–56). New York: Academic Press.

Ochman, J. M. (1996). The effects of nongender-role stereotyped, same-sex role models in storybooks on the self-esteem of children in grade three. *Sex Roles, 35*, 711–735.

Ozer, E. M. (1995). The impact of childcare responsibility and self-efficacy on the psychological health of working mothers. *Psychology of Women Quarterly, 19*, 315–336.

Perry, D. G., & Bussey, K. (1979). The social learning theory of sex differences: Imitation is alive and well. *Journal of Personality and Social Psychology, 37*, 1699–1712.

Peters, W. (1971). *A class divided.* New York: Doubleday.

Pomerleau, A., Bolduc, D., Malcuit, G., & Cossette, L. (1990). Pink or blue: Environmental gender stereotypes in the first two years of life. *Sex Roles, 22*, 359–367.

Poulin-Dubois, D. Serbin, L. A., & Derbyshire, A. (1998). Toddlers' intermodal and verbal knowledge about gender. *Merrill–Palmer Quarterly, 44*, 338–354.

Poulin-Dubois, D., Serbin, L. A., Kenyon, B., & Derbyshire, A. (1994). Infants' intermodal knowledge about gender. *Developmental Psychology, 30*, 436–442.

Raag, T., & Rackliff, C. L. (1998). Preschoolers' awareness of social expectations of gender: Relationships to toy choices. *Sex Roles, 38*, 685–700.

Rheingold, H. L., & Cook, K. V. (1975). The content of boys' and girls' rooms as an index of parents' behavior. *Child Development, 46*, 459–463.

Riley, M. W., Kahn, R. L., & Foner, A. (Eds.). (1994). *Age and structural lag.* New York: Wiley.

Rosenhan, D., Frederick, F., & Burrowes, A. (1968). Preaching and practicing: Effects of channel discrepancy on norm internalization. *Child Development, 39*, 291–301.

Rosenthal, T. L., & Zimmerman, B. J. (1978). *Social learning and cognition.* New York: Academic Press.

Sandnabba, N. K., & Ahlberg, C. (1999). Parents' attitudes and expectations about children's cross-gender behavior. *Sex Roles, 40*, 249–264.

Schunk, D. H. (1987). Peer models and children's behavioral change. *Review of Educational Research, 57*, 149–174.

Schwarzer, R. (Ed.). (1992). *Self-efficacy: Thought control of action.* Washington, DC: Hemisphere.

Sells, L. (1982). Leverage for equal opportunity through mastery of mathematics. In S. M. Humphreys (Ed.), *Women and minorities in science* (pp. 7–26). Boulder, CO: Westview Press.

Serbin, L. A., Poulin-Dubois, D., Colburne, K. A., Sen, M. G., & Eichstedt, J. A. (2001). Gender stereotyping in infancy: Visual preferences for and knowledge of gender-stereotyped toys in the second year. *International Journal of Behavioral Development, 25*, 7–15.

Shakin, M., Shakin, D., & Sternglanz, S. H. (1985). Infant clothing: Sex labeling for strangers. *Sex Roles, 12*, 955–963.

Siegal, M. (1987). Are sons and daughters treated more differently by fathers than by mothers? *Developmental Review, 7*, 183–209.

Simpson, A. W., & Erickson, M. T. (1983). Teachers' verbal and nonverbal communication patterns as a function of teacher race, student gender and student race. *American Educational Research Journal, 20*, 183–198.

Simpson, J. A., & Kenrick, D. T. (Eds.). (1997). *Evolutionary social psychology.* Mahwah, NJ: Erlbaum.

Stockard, J., & Johnson, M. M. (1992). *Sex and gender in society.* Englewood Cliffs, NJ: Prentice-Hall.

Thompson, T. L., & Zerbinos, E. (1995). Gender roles in animated cartoons: Has the picture changed in 20 years? *Sex Roles, 32*, 651–673.

Thompson, T. L., & Zerbinos, E. (1997). Television cartoons: Do children notice it's a boy's world? *Sex Roles, 37*, 415–432.

Thorne, B. (1986). Girls and boys together, but mostly apart. In W. W. Hartup & Z. Rubin (Eds.), *Relationships and development* (pp. 167–184). Hillsdale, NJ: Erlbaum.

Turner-Bowker, D. M. (1996). Gender stereotyped descriptors in children's picture books: Does "Curious Jane" exist in the literature? *Sex Roles, 35*, 461–488.

Walkerdine, V. (1989). *Counting girls out.* London: Virago Press.

West, C., & Zimmerman, D.H. (1991). Doing gender. In J. Lorber & S. A. Farrell (Eds.), *The social construction of gender* (pp. 13–37). Newbury Park, CA: Sage.

Wright, J. C., & Huston, A. C. (1983). A matter of form: Potentials of television for young viewers. *American Psychologist, 38*, 835–843.

Zahn-Waxler, C., Cole, P. M., & Barren, K. C. (1991). Guilt and empathy: Sex differences and implications for the development of depression. In J. Garber & K. A. Dodge (Eds.), *The development of emotion regulation and dysregulation* (pp. 243–272). New York: Cambridge University Press.

Zucker, K. S., Wilson-Smith, D. N., Kurita, J. A., & Stem, A. (1995). Children's appraisals of sex-typed behavior in their peers. *Sex Roles, 33*, 703–725.

6

Gender Socialization

A Parent × Child Model

EVA M. POMERANTZ
FLORRIE FEI-YIN NG
QIAN WANG

A wealth of evidence now indicates a number of significant psychological differences between females and males (for a review of the literature, see Feingold, 1994). A fundamental question is that of how these differences develop. The large body of work that indicates parents are a central influence in children's psychological development (for a review, see Parke & Buriel, 1998) suggests that parents play a major role in the development of these differences. However, given the increasing evidence for Parent × Child models of socialization in which parents and children influence children's psychological development (for a review, see Collins, Maccoby, Steinberg, Hetherington, & Bornstein, 2000), parents' role may depend on children's characteristics. Unfortunately, the application of Parent × Child models to the development of psychological sex differences has been rare (for some exceptions, see Keenan & Shaw, 1997; Kohlberg, 1966).[1] Our central goal in this chapter is to introduce a model in which parents and children contribute *jointly* to the develop-

[1] In this chapter, the term *sex* is used to refer to females and males. The term *gender* is used to refer to the social meanings attached to females and males.

ment of psychological sex differences. The key proposal underlying the model is that gender socialization arises from societal constructions of gender and from the distinct biological predispositions of girls and boys. Gender socialization is viewed as a dynamic process in which parents and children continually influence one another across the course of children's development.

MODELS OF SOCIALIZATION

Much of the theory and research on parents' role in the development of psychological sex differences has relied on unidirectional models of socialization in which parents differentially treat girls and boys, thereby fostering sex differences that were not already in place (e.g., Eccles, 1984; Pomerantz & Ruble, 1998). However, among investigators concerned with socialization more generally, such unidirectional models are increasingly being replaced with bidirectional models in which both parents and children are influential (e.g., Collins et al., 2000). Two general types of such models are applicable to understanding the development of sex differences. *Transactional models,* in which children's characteristics influence how parents treat them, are important to understanding the development of sex differences, because they can contribute to identifying the conditions under which parents *treat* girls and boys differently. *Interactional models,* in which children's characteristics influence the *effects* of parents' treatment on children, are informative about the conditions under which parents' differential treatment of girls and boys foster sex differences. Moreover, such models can provide insight into how sex differences develop even when differential treatment does not occur. The use of both models is important, because it can account for the substantial variability in the extent to which females and males differ (e.g., Feingold, 1994).

Parents' Differential Treatment: Transactional Models of Socialization

The question of whether parents treat girls and boys differently has been a subject of much controversy for many years (e.g., Lytton & Romney, 1991; Maccoby & Jacklin, 1974).[2] The large degree of variability in par-

[2] Differential treatment of girls and boys is most often studied by comparing parents' practices with girls and boys *between* families (e.g., Pomerantz & Ruble, 1998). Much rarer are comparisons of parents' practices with girls and boys *within* the same family (e.g., Crouter, Helms-Erikson, Updegraff, & McHale, 1999).

ents' differential treatment of girls and boys (Leaper, Anderson, & Sanders, 1998; Lytton & Romney, 1991) has led to a focus on the conditions under which differential treatment occurs. For example, investigators have examined the types of situations in which parents are most likely to treat girls and boys differently, as well as the types of parents most likely to do so (e.g., Bumpus, Crouter, & McHale, 1999; Leaper et al., 1998). Transactional models provide a useful framework for identifying such conditions. These models grew out of the argument that development has biological origins (e.g., Scarr, 1992). However, they have fostered an integrated account of development because of concern about the processes by which children's characteristics contribute to development. In fact, transactional models have been used even when a biological basis for children's characteristics is not assumed (e.g., Pomerantz & Eaton, 2001). A key tenet of such models is that children's characteristics evoke particular reactions from others that then play a role in children's subsequent development (e.g., Scarr, 1992), although evidence suggests that parents' reactions can also foster change in children (Maccoby, Snow, & Jacklin, 1984). For example, using a transactional model, Pomerantz and Eaton (2001) found that when children do poorly in school, mothers respond by supervising their homework, which appears to enhance children's performance over time.

In terms of understanding the development of sex differences, children's sex may be thought of as a characteristic indirectly influencing how parents treat them. It may shape parents' practices through two central pathways. The first arises from societal constructions of gender. As shown in Panel A of Figure 6.1 (see boxes A and B), parents' beliefs about gender and cues in the proximal environment that trigger such beliefs may lead parents to have both distinct perceptions of girls and boys and distinct goals for them (see box C), thereby causing parents to treat girls and boys differently. The second pathway arises from actual differences between girls and boys (see box D, Panel A, in Figure 6.1) resulting from prior socialization and biological predispositions. These distinct characteristics of girls and boys may lead parents to treat them differently. These two pathways suggest a set of key factors that influence whether parents treat girls and boys differently (see Table 6.1).

Societal Constructions of Gender

Despite efforts over the past three decades to eradicate gender stereotypes, there is much evidence for their existence (for a review, see Deaux & LaFrance, 1998). Many parents have different beliefs about the abilities of girls and boys (e.g., Jacobs & Eccles, 1992). For example, parents tend to see girls as more skilled than boys in language arts, but to see

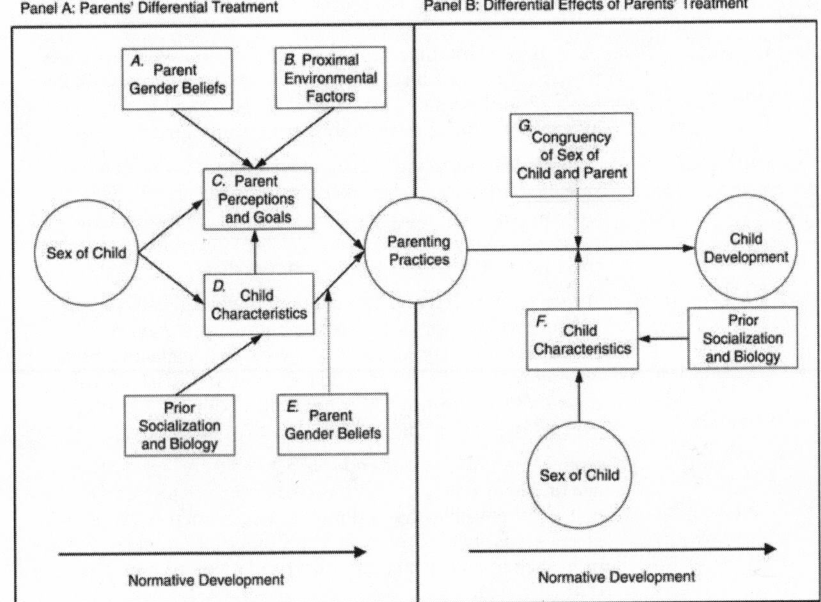

FIGURE 6.1. A transactional, interactional model of the role of parents and children in gender socialization. Dashed arrows represent moderating effects.

boys as more skilled in math and science. Moreover, college students tend to view females as highly communal (e.g., dependent, kind, sensitive, and sympathetic), but to view males as highly agentic (e.g., dominant, decisive, independent, and rational; Bergen & Williams, 1991; Eagly & Mladinic, 1989). Similar trends are evident in people's beliefs about the roles that females and males should fill within society, in large part as a result of the actual distribution of roles (see Eagly, Wood, & Johannesen-Schmidt, Chapter 12, this volume). For example, females are often viewed as fit for the role of caretaker, whereas males are viewed as fit for the role of breadwinner.

Such beliefs about gender may cause parents to perceive their children as possessing gender-stereotypical characteristics (e.g., girls are seen as dependent and boys are seen as independent) and to hold gender-stereotypical socialization goals for their children (e.g., girls should be sensitive and boys should be assertive). This may influence parents' interactions with their children, leading them to treat girls and boys differently (see Pomerantz, Saxon, & Kenney, 2001). For example, when parents view their daughters as possessing the stereotypically feminine

TABLE 6.1. Factors Influencing Parents' Differential Treatment

Parents' gender beliefs	Parents who endorse gender stereotypes may be most likely to treat girls and boys differently (e.g., parents who believe boys should be more assertive than girls may encourage autonomy among boys more than among girls).
Environmental gender-related cues	When cues in the immediate environment make gender salient, parents may be most likely to act on gender stereotypes (e.g., after reading a fairy tale in which the princess is saved by the prince, parents may treat girls, more than boys, as if they were dependent).
Parents' motivation	When parents have goals other than ensuring that gender stereotypes do not influence their interactions with their children, they may be most likely to treat girls and boys differentially (e.g., parents concerned with ensuring that their children do not fight may talk about the emotional aspects of conflict more with girls than with boys).
Parents' ability	Even if parents do not endorse gender stereotypes, they may act on them when they do not have the cognitive resources to stop themselves from doing so (e.g., when parents' attention is focused on preparing dinner, they may respond more negatively to the aggressive behavior of girls than to that of boys).
Relevant areas of socialization	Parents may only treat girls and boys differently in areas related to gender stereotypes or to children's characteristics that vary by sex (e.g., parents will help girls more than they do boys with math because of gender stereotypes about math, but such a difference will not be evident for history).
Relevant types of parenting practices	Parents may only use practices differentially with girls and boys that are related to gender stereotypes or to children's characteristics that vary by sex (e.g., parents may monitor the progress of girls more than that of boys, because of their stereotypical perceptions that girls are more in need of such supervision, but such a difference may not be evident in parents' use of rule enforcement).
Children's characteristics	Parents may be most likely to engage in differential treatment when children have gender-related characteristics that elicit such treatment (e.g., parents may use gentle discipline with girls more than with boys when girls internalize parents' agenda more than boys do).
Children's normative development	At times of children's lives when gender is particularly salient to parents, or when children are particularly likely to adopt gender-related characteristics, parents' differential treatment of girls and boys may be highest (e.g., parents may be particularly likely to make decisions for girls more than for boys during adolescence, because parents may be particularly likely to see gender stereotypes as relevant at this time).

characteristic of dependence, they may be particularly likely to aid their daughters in solving challenges. Beliefs about what is normative for girls and boys may also lead parents to see the same behavior in girls and boys differently and react differently to it (see Keenan & Shaw, 1997). For example, because of gender stereotypes about emotional expression, when girls are feeling anxious, parents may not make much of it, because such a state is often assumed to be normal for girls; in contrast, anxiety in boys may lead parents to see them as having problems.

Several lines of research support the idea that parents' beliefs about gender influence their perceptions and goals, thereby influencing their treatment of girls and boys. Research indicates that parents' differential expectations for their daughters' and sons' mathematical, athletic, and social performance are accounted for by parents' beliefs about the talents of females and males in these areas (e.g., Jacobs & Eccles, 1992). For example, parents who endorse the stereotype that females do more poorly than males at math have relatively low expectations for their daughters' performance in math, but relatively high expectations for their sons' performance. Evidence also suggests that parents who divide household work along traditional gender lines are more likely to treat their daughters and sons differently than are parents from egalitarian households (e.g., Crouter, Manke, & McHale, 1995). For example, parents from traditional households are particularly more likely to make decisions for their daughters than for their sons (Bumpus et al., 1999).

A major strength of the gender stereotype proposal is that it suggests several factors that influence whether parents treat girls and boys differentially, thereby providing an account of the variability in parents' differential treatment. Perhaps most obviously, to the extent that there is variability in parents' beliefs about gender, there will be variability in their differential treatment of girls and boys, with parents who endorse gender stereotypes being most likely to treat their daughters and sons differently. However, even parents who do not endorse gender stereotypes may act on such stereotypes when cues (e.g., toys or television) in the proximal environment make them salient. Although parents may sometimes be able to keep such cues from influencing their behavior, often they may have other goals (e.g., being sensitive to children's needs or ensuring that children do not fight with their siblings) that decrease their motivation to do so. Moreover, parents may not always have the ability to avoid the influence of gender stereotypes, because their cognitive resources (e.g., attention or memory) are taxed (see Deaux & Major, 1987). In line with the idea that parents may not always be able to engage in practices in which they believe, correlations between parents' socialization beliefs and behaviors are quite low (Holden & Edwards, 1989). Leaper et al.'s (1998) meta-analysis also indicates that parents are more likely to treat girls and boys differently when behavioral observations, rather than self-report methods, are used. Indeed, although mothers use controlling and autonomy-supportive practices with girls and boys differently in their everyday interactions (Pomerantz & Ruble, 1998), this does not manifest itself in mothers' beliefs (Pomerantz, 1995).

The proposal that gender stereotypes underlie parents' differential treatment of girls and boys also suggests that parents do not engage in such treatment pervasively. Instead, they may treat girls and boys differently only in areas in which gender-linked perceptions of children or gender socialization goals for children are relevant. As Jacobs and Eccles (1992) have shown, parents are likely to have differential expectations for girls and boys in areas in which there are culturally held stereotypes about the abilities of females and males—for example, in mathematics and social interactions. However, as these investigators highlight, differences would not be expected in areas for which there are no gender stereotypes—for example, history and geography. Research conducted by Crouter et al. (1995) makes a similar point by suggesting that only household chores that fall along gendered lines (e.g., cleaning the bathroom and taking out the garbage) may be distributed differently to girls and boys by parents.

Along comparable lines, the types of different practices that parents use with girls and boys may only be those for which gender-linked perceptions of children or gender socialization goals are relevant. For example, Pomerantz et al. (2001) have speculated that perceptions of girls as more helpless than boys lead parents to monitor the progress of girls more often than that of boys. However, such gender-stereotypical perceptions may not be relevant to parents' other socialization practices, such as their enforcement of rules. Thus, grouping together multiple forms of parenting practices may obscure parents' differential treatment of girls and boys (Block, 1983). Indeed, most prior work that has not found evidence for parents' differential treatment has examined parents' practices globally (e.g., Lytton & Romney, 1991). However, in their meta-analysis, which focused only on parents' use of directive speech, Leaper et al. (1998) found that parents were more directive when talking to girls than to boys. Along similar lines, Pomerantz and Ruble (1998) found that mothers were more controlling and less supportive of autonomy in terms of their involvement in tasks such as homework, decision making, and responses to their children's success, but not in terms of how they disciplined their children.

Actual Differences between Girls and Boys

Although gender stereotypes, and the environmental cues that make them salient, are important in parents' treatment of girls and boys, actual differences between girls and boys are also important (see Deaux & Major, 1987). Indeed, one critical reason that parents may perceive girls and boys differently, as well as have different goals for them, is because of differences in the characteristics of girls and boys. Such differences may also directly influence parents' practices. Although differences in the characteristics of girls and boys may be a consequence of prior socialization by parents, as well as peers, teachers, and the media, they may also be due to biological influences. There is now evidence that many psychological characteristics are at least partially biologically based (for a review, see Plomin & Caspi, 1999). Moreover, research suggests that biology plays a role in some sex differences in children's psychological characteristics (see Hampson & Moffat, Chapter 3, this volume; Hines, Chapter 2, this volume). For example, gonadal hormones present during prenatal and neonatal development contribute to children's sex differences in characteristics such as activity level, toy preference, and cognitive abilities (for a review, see Collaer & Hines, 1995), and may contribute to other sex differences as well.

Regardless of the origins of the sex differences in children's characteristics, over time, parents may respond to these differences in interactions with their children. Thus, one reason that parents may treat girls and boys differently is because they are reacting to girls and boys' distinct characteristics. Notably, work by Jussim (1991) on teachers' initial expectancies for children's performance indicates that although these expectancies account for a portion of the variance in teachers' later perceptions, children's actual ability is also a strong predictor. Parents and children have an established interaction history in which children's actual characteristics may assume at least equal weight with the ideas parents have formed about them as a consequence of gender stereotypes.

A number of well-documented sex differences among children may influence the practices parents use with them. We highlight three differences that may be particularly important. First, in the early years of children's development, girls are more cognitively advanced than are boys (e.g., Maccoby & Jacklin, 1974; Plomin, 1989). For example, as early as 8 months of age, girls have better word comprehension than do boys (e.g., Fenson et al., 1994). Moreover, as soon as children enter school, girls earn better grades than do boys (for a review, see American Association of University Women, 1992), perhaps in part as a result of differences in physical activity levels evident at birth (Campbell & Eaton, 1999) that may make it difficult for boys to remain focused in school. These sex differences may cause parents to engage in more structured instruction with boys than with girls. Indeed, Crowley, Callanan, Tennenbaum, and Allen (2001) found that parents explained museum science displays to boys more often than to girls. When parents do explain things to girls, they may do so at a more advanced cognitive level than they do with boys.

Second, girls appear to be more responsive than are boys to their parents' socialization attempts. As early as the second year of life, girls embrace their mothers' agenda more often than do boys, complying with their mothers' requests eagerly, even when their mothers are not around (e.g., Kochanska, 2002; Kochanska, Coy, & Murray, 2001). Before they are 2 years of age, girls are also better than boys at imitating their mothers in the context of instruction (Forman & Kochanska, 2001). This may alleviate the need for parents, or at least mothers, to use heavy-handed socialization practices with girls (see Leaper, 2002). Supportive of this proposal, Kochanska (1997) has found that when children do not follow their mothers' instructions, mothers use more gentle discipline with girls than with boys, psychologically guiding them rather than using power.

Third, as early as the second year of life, children tend to prefer gender-stereotypical activities (for a review, see Ruble & Martin, 1998). Such preferences, accompanied by the tendency for boys, from birth, to be more physically active than girls (see Campbell & Eaton, 1999), may play a role in parents' well-documented provision of gender-stereotypical activities (e.g., rough-and-tumble play or pretend tea parties; Lytton & Romney, 1991).

The sex differences in children's characteristics may contribute to the variability in parents' differential treatment and, consequently, the variability in the development of subsequent sex differences for several reasons. For one, the size of the sex differences in children's characteristics is quite small, suggesting that not all girls and boys possess gendered qualities to the same extent, presumably due to variability in their their socialization experiences and biological makeup. Thus, one reason for the variability in parents' differential treatment may be the variability among children's characteristics that elicit such treatment. In addition, similar to gender stereotypes, children's characteristics must be relevant to the area of socialization, as well as to the type of practice to be used, if they are to lead to differential treatment by parents. For example, girls' cognitive edge over boys may elicit only the types of parents' practices (e.g., instruction) that are influenced by children's cognitive abilities.

The characteristics that children bring to interactions with their parents may also contribute to variability in parents' differential treatment, because parents may not respond uniformly to such characteristics. Indeed, there is much variability in how parents respond when children engage in behavior inconsistent with gender stereotypes (e.g., Caldera, Huston, & O'Brien, 1989). A key influence on parents' responses may be their endorsement of gender stereotypes (see box E, Panel A in Figure 6.1). Parents who endorse such stereotypes may act to maintain characteristics in their children that are consistent with stereotypes but act to change characteristics that are inconsistent. Other factors besides parents' beliefs about gender may also be important. For example, parents who are particularly responsive to their children may react to children's individual characteristics, regardless of gender stereotypes; in contrast, parents who are not responsive may allow gender stereotypes to guide interactions with their children.

Normative Development

Parents' interaction with their children takes place over the course of children's development. With movement from one phase of development to the next, most children typically experience a number of significant changes. As highlighted at the bottom of Panel A in Figure 6.1, these normative developmental changes may influence parents' differential treatment of girls and boys. For example, the salience of gender stereotypes may wax and wane as children progress through life. On the one hand, as parents get to know their children over time, gender stereotypes may be less relevant. In line with this idea, parents' differential treatment appears to decrease as children get older (Lytton & Romney, 1991), although this trend could be a result of investigators' heightened reliance on children's reports as children get older. On the other hand, gender stereotypes may become more relevant as children enter adolescence, which has been characterized as a time when issues of gender become particularly important (see Hill & Lynch, 1983). Relatedly, children's own characteristics may change as they make their way through life. Children's adoption of gendered characteristics changes with age, hitting its peak at the beginning of adolescence (for a review, see Ruble & Martin, 1998). Thus, early adolescence may be a time of heightened differential treatment both because parents are particularly likely to see their children through the lens of gender stereotypes, and because children are particularly likely to adopt gendered characteristics.

Summary and Future Directions

Transactional models of socialization provide an important framework for understanding parents' differential treatment of girls and boys. The guiding idea, illustrated in Panel A, Figure 6.1, is that children's sex indirectly influences how parents treat them. First, societal constructions of gender may lead parents to perceive their children in a gender-stereotypical manner, as well as to hold gender-stereotypical goals, which may cause parents to treat girls and boys differently under some conditions. Second, a number of actual differences between girls and boys may lead parents to use different practices with them. Given that there may be changes in the salience of gender stereotypes, as well as children's actual characteristics, as children move from one phase of development to the next, children's normative development may also play a moderating role.

Fully understanding parents' differential treatment will involve research that examines characteristics of both parents and children in the differential treatment of girls and boys. Several paradigms may provide insight into such treatment. First, the correlational research examining parents' daily interactions with their children (e.g., Bumpus et al., 1999; Pomerantz & Ruble, 1998) needs to be extended to examine the eliciting role of *both* parents' beliefs about gender and sex differences in children's characteristics. Second, experimental paradigms in which fictional children's characteristics are manipulated and parents' responses are then assessed (e.g., Bugental, Caporael, & Shennum, 1980) might be extended to manipulate children's sex (see Kronsberg, Schmaling, & Fagot, 1985). Third, designs examining between- and within-family variance in parenting (e.g., Plomin, Reiss, Hetherington, & Howe, 1994) that incorporate children's sex might be useful in understanding the role of parents and children in parents' differential treatment of girls and boys (see Crouter, Helms-Erikson, Updegraff, & McHale, 1999).

Effects of Parents' Treatment: Interactional Models of Socialization

Questions about whether parents treat girls and boys differently often become so embroiled that important questions about the effects of differential treatment are rarely asked. Interactional models of socialization are essential to answering such questions. The essence of these models is that the effects of parents' practices are dependent on children's preexisting characteristics—presumed to be a consequence of prior socialization experiences or biological predispositions. For example, Caspi et al. (2002) found that boys abused by their parents grow up to engage in heightened delinquency, *unless* they possess a gene affecting the synthesis of neurotransmitters. Interactional models have two major implications for understanding the socialization of sex differences in children. First, these models suggest that when parents treat girls and boys differently, these practices may not affect all children similarly. Instead, the effects of parents' differential treatment may be limited to children possessing characteristics that make them responsive to such treatment (see box F, Panel B in Figure 6.1). Because girls and boys may differ in terms of responsiveness to their parents' practices, even when parents do not engage in differential treatment, parents' socialization attempts may have differential effects on girls and boys. Second, following from prior work (see Bell, Chapter 7, and Bussey & Bandura, Chapter 5, this volume), children's sex, in conjunction with the parent's own sex, may moderate the effect of parental practices (see box G, Panel B in Figure 6.1) such that children are more responsive to the practices of parents of the same sex. Thus, even when parents do not treat girls and boys differentially, their practices may foster distinct developmental trajectories for both. As highlighted in Table 6.2, application of interactional models of socialization to the development of sex differences suggests several important factors that may influence parents' contribution to the development of sex differences.

Children's Characteristics

Increasingly, research has documented that children are differentially influenced by their parents' socialization practices (for a review, see Collins et al., 2000). This has important implications for understanding the role of parents in children's gender socialization, because it suggests that parents' differential treatment of girls and boys may affect only some children. Consequently, many children's psychological development may not take place along gendered lines, thereby leading to variability in the sex differences. A number of characteristics of children may influence their responsiveness to parents' socialization attempts. We highlight three characteristics that may be particularly influential in gender socialization. As we subsequently discuss, there are also sex differences in these characteristics.

Children's responsiveness to parents' socialization attempts depends in part on their ability to follow through on these attempts. On a simple, cognitive level, children need to have the ability to attend to their parents' requests, then to understand them, and subsequently to carry them out. Moreover, because parents often ask children to engage in activities that conflict with children's own desires (e.g., cleaning up a mess or sharing a prized toy), children also need to be able to postpone their own desires to fulfill those of their parents, which requires effortful control (e.g., Kochanska, Murray, & Harlan, 2000). When the success of parents' socialization attempts depends on children having the ability to respond to these attempts, parents' differential attempts with girls and boys may only affect children who possess such ability. For example, parents are more likely to monitor the academic progress of girls than that of boys (Pomerantz & Ruble, 1998); this may lead to sex differences in performance only among children who can follow through on the suggestions their parents offer in the course of monitoring.

TABLE 6.2. Factors Influencing the Effects of Parents' Treatment

Children's ability	Among children who have the ability to follow through on their parents' requests (e.g., because they are able to exert effortful control), parents' differential treatment may be most likely to foster sex differences. Because, early, on girls' abilities are apt to be more advanced than are those of boys, even when parents do not engage in differential treatment, sex differences may develop because parents will be more successful in their socialization attempts with girls than with boys.
Children's sensitivity	Among children who are sensitive to their parents' socialization practices (e.g., because they are easily induced to feel guilty), parents' differential treatment may be most likely to foster sex differences. Because girls tend to be more sensitive than boys, even when parents do not engage in differential treatment, sex differences may develop, because parents may be more successful in their socialization attempts with girls than with boys.
Children's motivation	Among children who are motivated to follow through on their parents' requests (e.g., because they see their relationships with their parents as self-defining), parents' differential treatment may be most likely to foster sex differences. Given that girls are more likely than boys to be motivated, even when parents do not engage in differential treatment, sex differences may develop, because parents may be more successful in their socialization attempts with girls than with boys.
Relevant types of parenting practices	The effects of children's ability, sensitivity, and motivation may be limited to types of parenting practices (e.g., gentle discipline) that depend on such characteristics for success.
Congruency of sex of child and parent	Because of sex differences in status, girls may be more likely than boys to be amenable to their mothers' socialization attempts. Moreover, children may mainly imitate the behavior of their same-sex parent.
Children's normative development	At times in children's lives when gender is particularly salient (e.g., early adolescence), the effects of parents' differential treatment may be the strongest, unless children have a strong desire not to conform with gender norms.

Children's sensitivity to their parents' socialization attempts may also play a role in their responsiveness to these attempts. Fearful children are particularly likely to internalize rules when their mothers use gentle discipline with them, but such a subtle approach is ineffective with children who are not fearful (e.g., Kochanska, 1995, 1997). This may be because fearful children are more sensitive to parents' disciplinary attempts, with even subtle hints from parents eliciting guilt when children have violated a rule. Thus, when the effects of parents' practices depend on children's sensitivity, parents' differential use of such practices with girls and boys may contribute to the development of sex differences only among children prone to guilt. For example, mothers' tendency to use more gentle discipline with girls than with boys (Kochanska, 1997) may foster sex differences in the internalization of rules only among children prone to guilt.

Motivation to comply with parental requests is another characteristic of children that may influence the effectiveness of parents' socialization attempts. When children define themselves in terms of their relationships with their parents, they may strive to maintain harmonious relationships (see Markus & Kitayama, 1991). As a consequence, children's inclusion of their relationships with their parents in their views of themselves may make them particularly motivated to take on their parents' goals for them as their own. Iyengar and Lepper (1999) found that children of Asian descent are more intrinsically motivated than are children of European descent when their mothers make decisions for them, presumably because they transform their mothers' decisions into their own. As Iyengar and Lepper suggest, this may be due to cultural differences in children's tendency to include their relationships with their parents in their views of themselves. Children who hold such views of themselves are also particularly likely to internalize goals valued by their parents, in that they are intrinsically motivated to meet academic goals (Wang & Pomerantz, 2003). Thus, when the success of parental practices is contingent on children's motivation to comply with parents' requests, differential use of such practices with girls and boys may most strongly affect children who view their relationships with their parents as self-defining. For example, parents who expect their sons to do better in math than their daughters (e.g., Jacobs & Eccles, 1992) may foster sex differences in performance in math most among children who include the relationships with parents in their views of themselves given that such children may be the most motivated to adopt their parents' goals for them.

Girls are more likely than boys to possess a number of the characteristics that heighten responsiveness to parents' socialization attempts. First, girls may be more able than boys to respond to parental socialization attempts. As we highlighted earlier, girls' cognitive abilities early in life are more advanced than are those of boys (e.g., Maccoby & Jacklin, 1974; Plomin, 1989). Moreover, before the age of 2 years, girls are more advanced than boys in terms of effortful control (e.g., Kochanska, Murray, & Coy, 1997; Kochanska et al., 2000). Second, girls, more than boys, may be sensitive to parents' socialization attempts. At least as early as the third year of life, girls are more prone than boys to experiencing guilt (e.g., Kochanska, 2002; Kochanska, Gross, Lin, & Nichols, 2002). Third, girls may be more motivated than are boys to internalize parents' socialization attempts. For example, research on adults indicates that females are more likely than males to include their relationships with close others in their views of themselves (for a review, see Gardner & Gabriel, Chapter 8, this volume).

Several lines of research support the idea that these characteristics lead girls to be particularly responsive to their parents' socialization attempts. First, as noted earlier, girls embrace their mothers' agenda more than do boys, complying with requests even when their mothers are not around (e.g., Kochanska, Askan, & Koenig, 1995; Kochanska et al., 2001). They are also better at imitating their mothers in the context of instruction (Forman & Kochanska, 2001). Second, Tenenbaum and Leaper's (2002) meta-analysis indicates that mothers' beliefs about gender are more strongly linked to girls' than to boys' beliefs about gender. Third, research suggests that girls take parents' praise to heart more than do boys (Kempner, Pomerantz, Ng, & Wang, 2003). For example, when mothers react to children's successes in school with person-oriented praise (e.g., "You're a good girl"), girls are more likely than boys to feel that their worth as a person is contingent on doing well in school.

The sex difference in children's responsiveness to their parents' socialization attempts suggests that even when parents do not treat girls and boys differently, they may contribute to the development of subsequent sex differences in children. However, there may be a great deal of variability in this. First, because the size of the sex differences in the characteristics that influence children's responsiveness to parents' socialization attempts is small, not all girls may be more responsive than all boys. Second, girls may not be more responsive than boys to all of parents' socialization attempts. Instead, their heightened amenability may be limited to those parental practices that are contingent on the characteristics that girls possess to a greater extent than do boys. Third, other factors may influence gender socialization that counteract girls' heightened responsiveness, especially to parents' gender-stereotypical practices. For example, because stereotypical masculine characteristics are often valued more than stereotypical feminine characteristics, girls may be more resistant than boys to attempts by parents to cultivate gender-consistent behavior.

Congruency of Sex of Child and Parent

The match between children and parents' sex may play an important role in the gender socialization process. There are differences in the status and power of women and men (see Pratto & Walker, Chapter 11, and Ridgeway & Bourg, Chapter 10, this volume). It is possible that one reason girls have been found to be more amenable than boys to their parents' socialization attempts is because mothers, rather than fathers, are studied so often. Perhaps sons feel that they have higher status than their mothers. As a consequence, they may be less likely to follow their mothers' lead than to follow that of their fathers. In line with this perspective, Leaper (2000) found that boys give in to their mothers less often than to their fathers. Girls may be highly amenable to both their mothers' and fathers' socialization attempts, whereas boys may be amenable only to those of their fathers.

The match between children's and parents' sex may also play an important role in the extent to which children model their parents' behavior. Children may often observe and then take on the behavior of their same-sex parent, with whom they identify strongly (see Bell, Chapter 7, and Bussey & Bandura, Chapter 5, this volume). Because mothers more often than fathers do more of the child rearing (see Pleck, 1997), this may mean that girls are more easily socialized than are boys, because they have more time to observe and imitate their same-sex parent. For example, girls may be more likely to interact in a mature manner with others, because they frequently see their mothers doing so, and they spend time imitating them; boys, however, may not attend to such behavior on the part of their mothers, and may have only a limited opportunity to observe it in their fathers. Moreover, the communal behaviors typical of child rearing may be passed on to girls more often than to boys, because girls watch their mothers engage in such behaviors on a regular basis (see Bell, Chapter 7, this volume). Indeed, even parents whose purpose is to raise their daughters in a gender-neutral manner may foster a communal orientation in girls, if mothers do the bulk of the child rearing.

Normative Development

Children's phase of development may play a role in how parents influence them (see bottom of Panel B, Figure 6.1). Kohlberg (1966) has argued that children's attention to same-sex models intensifies once they have a sense of the permanence of categorical sex (e.g., "I am a girl, and I will be a girl no matter what"). This development—often referred to as *attainment of gender constancy*—emerges sometime between the ages of 3 and 7 (for a review, see Ruble & Martin, 1998). In line with Kohlberg's idea, children, particularly boys, spend more time looking at same-sex models after they have achieved gender constancy than prior to doing so (Slaby & Frey, 1976). A similar trend may be evident for many forms of parents' differential treatment. For example, when children have a sense of the permanence of categorical sex, they may be more responsive to their parents' encouragement of gender-stereotypical activities. In addition, as noted earlier, with entry into adolescence, children are particularly likely to adopt gendered characteristics (see Ruble & Martin, 1998). Thus, differences between girls and boys' responsiveness to parents may also be heightened at this time. However, although the evidence is not entirely consistent, adolescence is also a time of heightened flexibility among children in their beliefs about females and males (Ruble & Martin, 1998). Consequently, it is also possible that children may be particularly likely to reject attempts by their parents to treat them in a gender-stereotypical manner at this time, and that they spend little time modeling the behavior of their same-sex parent.

Summary and Future Directions

Interactional models of socialization in which the effects of parents' practices are dependent on children's characteristics provide a useful framework for understanding the role of parents' practices in the development of psychological sex differences (see Panel B, Figure 6.1). Several key proposals emerge from this framework. First, parents' differential treatment of girls and boys may be most influential among children who have characteristics that heighten their responsiveness to parental practices. Second, even when parents do not treat girls and boys differently, sex differences may develop, because girls and boys may differ in the characteristics that heighten their responsiveness to parental practices. Third, the match between children's sex and that of their parents may play an important moderating role. The normative developmental changes that children experience may also influence their responsiveness to parental practices, thereby causing the role of parents in the development of sex differences to wax and wane as children progress through life.

Much progress has been made in understanding the characteristics of children that heighten responsiveness to parents' socialization attempts. Moreover, sex differences in these characteristics have been well documented. Unfortunately, there has been little attempt to integrate these two lines of work. Three endeavors are important in this vein. First, with only a few exceptions (e.g., Frome & Eccles, 1998; Kuebli, Butler, & Fivush, 1995), research exploring parents' differential treatment of girls and boys rarely examines what ensues over time for children. Given the evidence for interactional models of socialization, studies need to look at characteristics of children that influence over time the effects of parents' differential treatment. Second, more research examining the issue of sex differences in children's responsiveness to parents' practices is needed. It will be important to identify the role of prior socialization and biological predispositions in the early sex differences related to responsiveness. Third, although some attention has been directed to the role of fathers in understanding parents' differential treatment of girls and boys (see Siegal, 1987), the effects of fathers' practices on children have received relatively little attention, particularly in the context of understanding the development of sex differences. This will be particularly valuable in understanding whether girls are more responsive than boys to fathers', as well as to mothers' socialization attempts.

CONCLUDING REMARKS

Our goal in this chapter has been to propose a general framework from which to generate hypotheses about the conditions under which parents contribute to the development of sex differences. We have used a number of lines of work to elaborate on the simple notion that parents treat girls and boys differently, which, in turn, sets girls and boys on diverse developmental trajectories. As shown in Panel A, Figure 6.1, using transactional models of socialization, we have suggested two pathways by which children's sex influences how parents treat them. First, parents' endorsement of gender stereotypes (box A), as well as cues in the proximal environment triggering such stereotypes (box B), influence how parents perceive both girls and boys, and the goals they have for them (box C). Second, a number of actual differences between girls' and boys' characteristics (box D), due most likely to prior socialization experiences and to biological influences, may elicit parents' differential treatment. Together, these two mechanisms portray a picture of parents' differential treatment as originating from societal constructions of gender and girls' and boys' distinct biological predispositions. As children move from one phase of life to the next, parents' beliefs about gender and children's gendered characteristics may change, thereby leading parents' differential treatment to vary over the course of children's development.

As shown in Panel B, Figure 6.1, we have attempted to move beyond issues of parents' differential treatment of girls and boys, to the role of such treatment in the development of children's sex differences. In this vein, we have drawn on interactional models of socialization in which the effects of parents' practices are dependent on children's own characteristics. First, children's characteristics may moderate the effects of parents' differential treatment of children (see box F), so that it leads to sex differences only among some children. Even when parents do not treat girls and boys differentially, their practices may lead to sex differences, because of differences in the characteristics of girls and boys that influence their amenability to parental practices. Second, the congruency of child and parental sex is important (see box G). Notably, these effects may wax and wane with changes in children's adoption of gendered-characteristics as they move from one developmental phase to the next.

At each point in the model, there is room for variability in the socialization process that may foster variability in the development of sex differences. As highlighted in Table 6.1, whether parents treat girls and boys differently is dependent on the extent to which they hold gender-stereotypical beliefs, cues in the environment that elicit gender stereotypes, and their motivation and ability to disregard such cues. Similarly, not all children have gendered characteristics that may elicit differential treatment from parents. A focus on these mechanisms suggests that the areas in which differential treatment occurs, as well as the types of practices in which it manifests itself, will be related to gender stereotypes and children's gendered characteristics. Additional variability is introduced when the effects of parenting practices are taken into account. As highlighted in Table 6.2, not all children are similarly responsive to parents' differential treatment. Moreover, although girls and boys may react differently to parents' socialization attempts, variability in the sex differences in characteristics that cause such distinct reactions may lead to variability in the development of sex differences. Finally, because socialization processes may change as children progress through life, further variability is introduced into the equation.

Although we have focused on the role of parents in gender socialization, we believe the model we have introduced is applicable to other forces that contribute to gender socialization. Much of the early work attempting to elucidate sex differences, particularly those in achievement-related processes, focused on teachers. This work was guided by the idea that teachers treat girls and boys differently, thereby fostering sex differences (e.g., Dweck, Davidson, Nelson, & Enna, 1978). However, the factors we have proposed that influence parents' socialization of sex differences may also be important in teacher socialization. Indeed, in a landmark study on teacher socialization, Parsons, Kaczala, and Meece (1982) showed that both teachers' beliefs about the abilities of girls and boys and children's characteristics play important roles in teachers' contributions to the development of sex differences in children. Our model is also relevant to the burgeoning work on the role played by peers in the development of sex differences (see Maccoby, 1998).

The focus of this chapter represents a microanalytical approach to understanding how psychological sex differences develop. Placing such a model in the context of the larger culture is important. Gender-related beliefs may differ from culture to culture. For example, as Eagly and colleagues (Chapter 12, this volume) emphasize, the distribution of women and men into social roles is a product of social, economic, technological, and ecological forces present in a society; such distribution may influence the gender stereotypes that members of a society hold, as well as the characteristics that females and males develop. Thus, parents' differential treatment of girls and boys, as well as children's reactions to such treatment, may vary from culture to culture, with increased gender socialization taking place in cultures in which the division of social roles is strongly based on gender (see Leaper, 2002). Such cultures may include patriarchal societies in which males have more power, status, and control of resources than do females, as well as agrarian societies in which men are mainly responsible for agricultural labor, and women for child rearing and household chores (see Wood & Eagly, 2002). Moreover, the pressure to abide by societal norms varies from culture to culture (Triandis, 1994). As a consequence, parents' adherence to gender stereotypes may vary from society to society. Thus, in cultures in which adherence to norms is strong, gender socialization would be expected to be strong. Finally, the processes by which socialization occurs appear to differ across cultures (for a review, see Chao & Tseng, 2002). This may be true for gender socialization as well.

The question of how females and males come to differ psychologically is important, and it has intrigued investigators for decades in a variety of fields. There is often a tendency to attribute the development of psychological sex differences mainly to social factors or primarily to biological factors. However, the application of theory and research implicating both parents and children as important in the socialization process suggests that the two jointly contribute to the development of psychological sex differences.

ACKNOWLEDGMENTS

This chapter benefited from the helpful comments of Missa Murry Eaton, Gwen Kenney, Sungok Shim, Karen Rudoph, and Allison Ryan. Work on this chapter was supported by National Science Foundation Grant No. BCS-9809292 and National Institute of Mental Health and Office for Research on Women's Health Grant No. R01 MH57505 to Eva M. Pomerantz.

REFERENCES

American Association of University Women. (1992). *AAUW report: How schools shortchange girls*. Washington, DC: American Association of University Women Educational Foundation.

Bergen, D. J., & Williams, J. E. (1991). Sex stereotypes in the United States: 1972–1988. *Sex Roles, 24*, 413–424.

Block, J. H. (1983). Differential premises arising from differential socialization of the sexes: Some conjectures. *Child Development, 54*, 1335–1354.

Bugental, D. B., Caporael, L., & Shennum, W. A. (1980). Experimentally produced child uncontrollability: Effects on the potency of adult communication patterns. *Child Development, 51*, 520–528.

Bumpus, M. F., Crouter, A. C., & McHale, S. M. (1999). Parental autonomy granting during adolescence: Exploring gender differences in context. *Developmental Psychology, 37*, 163–173.

Caldera, Y. M., Huston, A. C., & O'Brien, M. (1989). Social interactions and play patterns of parents and toddlers with feminine, masculine, and neutral toys. *Child Development, 60*, 70–76.

Campbell, D. W., & Eaton, W. O. (1999). Sex differences in the activity level of infants. *Infant and Child Development, 8*, 1–17.

Caspi, A., McClay, J., Moffitt, T., Mill, J., Martin, J., Craig, I. W., et al. (2002). Role of genotype in the cycle of violence in maltreated children. *Science, 297*, 851–854.

Chao, R., & Tseng, V. (2002). Parenting of Asians. In M. H. Bornstein (Ed.), *Handbook of parenting: Vol. 4. Social conditions and applied parenting* (2nd ed., pp. 59–93). Mahwah, NJ: Erlbaum.

Collaer, M. L., & Hines, M. (1995). Human behavioral sex differences: A role for gonadal hormones during early development? *Psychological Bulletin, 118*, 55–107.

Collins, W. A., Maccoby, E. E., Steinberg, L., Hetherington, E. M., & Bornstein, M. (2000). Contemporary research on parenting: The case for nature and nurture. *American Psychologist, 55*, 218–232.

Crouter, A. C., Helms-Erikson, H., Updegraff, K., & McHale, S. M. (1999). Conditions underlying parents' knowledge about children's daily lives in middle childhood: Between- and within-family comparisons. *Child Development, 70,* 246–259.

Crouter, A. C., Manke, B. A., & McHale, S. M. (1995). The family context of gender intensification in early adolescence. *Child Development, 66,* 317–329.

Crowley, K., Callanan, M. A., Tenenbaum, H. R., & Allen, E. (2001). Parents explain more often to boys than to girls during shared scientific thinking. *Psychological Science, 12,* 258–261.

Deaux, K., & LaFrance, M. (1998). Gender. In D. T. Gilbert & S. T. Fiske (Eds.), *The handbook of social psychology* (4th ed., Vol. 1, pp. 788–827). New York: McGraw-Hill.

Deaux, K., & Major, B. (1987). Putting gender into context: An interactive model of gender-related behavior. *Psychological Review, 94,* 369–389.

Dweck, C. S., Davidson, W., Nelson, S., & Enna, B. (1978). Sex differences in learned helplessness: II. Contingencies of evaluative feedback in the classroom. III. An experimental analysis. *Developmental Psychology, 14,* 268–276.

Eagly, A. H., & Mladinic, A. (1989). Gender stereotypes and attitudes toward women and men. *Personality and Social Psychology Bulletin, 15,* 543–558.

Eccles, J. S. (1984). Sex differences in achievement patterns. In T. Sonderegger (Ed.), *Nebraska Symposium on Motivation* (Vol. 32, pp. 98–132). Lincoln: University of Nebraska Press.

Feingold, A. (1994). Gender differences in personality: A meta-analysis. *Psychological Bulletin, 116,* 429–456.

Fenson, L., Dale, P. S., Reznick, J. S., Bates, E., Thal, D. J., & Pethick, S. J. (1994). Variaibility in early communicative development. *Monographs of the Society for Research on Child Development, 59* (Serial No. 242).

Forman, D. R., & Kochanska, G. (2001). Viewing imitation as child responsiveness: A link between teaching and discipline domains of socialization. *Developmental Psychology, 37,* 198–206.

Frome, P. M., & Eccles, J. S. (1998). Parents' influence on children's achievement-related perceptions. *Journal of Personality and Social Psychology, 74,* 435–452.

Hill, J. P., & Lynch, J. H. (1983). The intensification of gender-related role expectations during early adolescence. In J. Brooks-Gunn & A. C. Perersen (Eds.), *Girls at puberty: Biological and psychosocial perspectives* (pp. 201–228). New York: Plenum Press.

Holden, G. W., & Edwards, L. A. (1989). Parental attitudes toward child rearing: Instruments, issues, and implications. *Psychological Bulletin, 106,* 29–58.

Iyengar, S. S., & Lepper, M. R. (1999). Rethinking the value of choice: A cultural perspective on intrinsic motivation. *Journal of Personality and Social Psychology, 76,* 349–366.

Jacobs, J., & Eccles, J. (1992). The impact of mothers' gender-role steroetypic beliefs on mothers' and children's ability perceptions. *Journal of Personality and Social Psychology, 63,* 932–944.

Jussim, L. (1991). Social perception and social reality: A reflection-construction model. *Psychological Review, 98,* 54–73.

Keenan, K., & Shaw, D. (1997). Developmental and social influences on young girls' early problem behavior. *Psychological Bulletin, 121,* 95–113.

Kempner, S., Pomerantz, E. M., Ng, F. F., & Wang, Q. (2003). Mothers' everyday reactions to children's academic success: Sex differences in children's responses. Manuscript in preparation.

Kochanska, G. (1995). Children's temperament, mother's discipline, and security of attachment: Multiple pathways to emerging internalization. *Child Development, 66,* 597–615.

Kochanska, G. (1997). Multiple pathways to conscience for children with different temperaments: From toddlerhood to age 5. *Developmental Psychology, 33,* 228–240.

Kochanska, G. (2002). Committed compliance, moral self, and internalization: A mediational model. *Developmental Psychology, 38,* 339–351.

Kochanska, G., Askan, N., & Koenig, A. L. (1995). A longitudinal study of the roots of preschoolers' conscience: Committed compliance and emerging internalization. *Child Development, 66,* 1752–1769.

Kochanska, G., Coy, K. C., & Murray, K. T. (2001). The development of self-regulation in the first four years of life. *Child Development, 72,* 1091–1011.

Kochanska, G., Gross, J. N., Lin, M., & Nichols, K. E. (2002). Guilt in young children: Development, determinants, and relations with a broader system of standards. *Child Development, 73,* 461–482.

Kochanska, G., Murray, K. T., & Coy, K. C. (1997). Inhibitory control as a contributor to conscience in childhood: From toddler to early school age. *Child Development, 68,* 263–277.

Kochanska, G., Murray, K. T., & Harlan, E. T. (2000). Effortful control in early childhood: Continuity and change, antecedents, and implications for social development. *Developmental Psychology, 36,* 220–232.

Kohlberg, L. (1966). A cognitive-developmental analysis of children's sex-role concepts and attitudes. In E. E. Maccoby (Ed.), *The development of sex differences* (pp. 82–173). Stanford, CA: Stanford University Press.

Kronsberg, S., Schmaling, K., & Fagot, B. I. (1985). Risk in a parent's eyes: Effects of gender and parenting experience. *Sex Roles, 13,* 329–341.

Kuebli, J., Butler, S., & Fivush, R. (1995). Mother–child talk about past emotions: Relations of maternal language and child gender over time. *Cognition and Emotion, 9,* 265–283.

Leaper, C. (2000). Gender, affiliation, assertion, and the interactive context of parent–child play. *Developmental Psychology, 34,* 3–27.

Leaper, C. (2002). Parenting girls and boys. In M. H. Bornstein (Ed.), *Handbook of parenting: Vol. 1. Children and parenting* (2nd ed., pp. 189–225). Mahwah, NJ: Erlbaum.

Leaper, C., Anderson, K. J., & Sanders, P. (1998). Moderators of gender effects on parents' talk to their children: A meta-analysis. *Developmental Psychology, 34,* 3–27.

Lytton, H., & Romney, D. M. (1991). Parents' differential socialization of boys and girls: A meta-analysis. *Psychological Bulletin, 109,* 267–296.

Maccoby, E. E. (1998). *The two sexes: Growing up apart, coming together.* Cambridge, MA: Harvard University Press.

Maccoby, E. E., & Jacklin, C. N. (1974). *The psychology of sex differences.* Stanford, CA: Stanford University Press.

Maccoby, E. E., Snow, M. E., & Jacklin, C. N. (1984). Children's dispositions and mother–child interaction at 12 and 18 months: A short term longitudinal study. *Developmental Psychology, 20,* 459–472.

Markus, H. R., & Kitayama, S. (1991). Culture and the self: Implications for cognition, emotion, and motivation. *Psychological Review, 98,* 224–253.

Parke, R. D., & Buriel, R. (1998). Socialization in the family: Ethnic and ecological perspectives. In N. Eisenberg (Ed.), *Handbook of child psychology: Vol. 3. Social, emotional, and personality development* (5th ed., pp. 463–552). New York: Wiley.

Parsons, J. E., Kaczala, C. M., & Meece, J. L. (1982). Socialization of achievement attitudes and beliefs: Classroom influences. *Child Development, 53,* 322–339.

Pleck, J. H. (1997). Paternal involvement: Levels, sources, and consequences. In M. E. Lamb (Ed.), *The role of the father in child development* (pp. 66–103). New York: Wiley.

Plomin, R. (1989). Environment and genes: Determinants of behavior. *American Psychologist, 44,* 105–111.

Plomin, R., & Caspi, A. (1999). Behavioral gentics. In L. A. Pervin & O. P. John (Eds.), *Handbook of personality: Theory and research* (2nd ed., pp. 251–276). New York: Guilford Press.

Plomin, R., Reiss, D., Hetherington, E. M., & Howe, G. W. (1994). Nature and nurture: Genetic contributions to measures of the family environment. *Developmental Psychology, 30,* 32–43.

Pomerantz, E. M. (1995). *The role of parental autonomy granting and control in the development of sex differences in self-evaluative processes.* Unpublished dissertation, New York University, New York.

Pomerantz, E. M., & Eaton, M. M. (2001). Maternal intrusive support in the academic context: Transactional socialization processes. *Developmental Psychology, 37,* 174–186.

Pomerantz, E. M., & Ruble, D. N. (1998). The role of maternal control in the development of sex differences in child self-evaluative factors. *Child Development, 69,* 458–478.

Pomerantz, E. M., Saxon, J. L., & Kenney, G. A. (2001). Self-evaluation: The development of sex differences. In G. B. Moskowitz (Ed.), *Cognitive social psychology: On the tenure and future of social cognition* (pp. 59–74). Mahwah, NJ: Erlbaum.

Ruble, D. N., & Martin, C. L. (1998). Gender development. In N. Eisenberg (Ed.), *Handbook of child development: Vol. 3. Social, emotional, and personality development* (5th ed., pp. 933–1016). New York: Wiley.

Scarr, S. (1992). Developmental theories for the 1990s: Development and individual differences. *Child Development, 63,* 1–19.

Siegal, M. (1987). Are sons and daughters treated more differently by fathers than by mothers? *Developmental Review, 7,* 182–209.

Slaby, R. G., & Frey, K. S. (1976). Development of gender constancy and selective attention to same-sex models. *Child Development, 46,* 849–856.

Tenenbaum, H. R., & Leaper, C. (2002). Are parents' gender schemas related to their children's gender-related cognitions?: A meta-analysis. *Developmental Psychology, 38,* 615–630.

Triandis, H. C. (1994). *Culture and social behavior.* New York: McGraw-Hill.

Wang, Q., & Pomerantz, E. M. (2003). *Children's inclusion of their relationships with their parents in their self-construals: Implications for children's well-being.* Manuscript under review.

Wood, W., & Eagly, A. H. (2002). A cross-cultural analysis of the behavior of women and men: Implications for the origins of sex differences. *Psychological Bulletin, 128,* 699–727.

7

Psychoanalytic Theories of Gender

LESLIE C. BELL

A man has long hair that he hides behind and is loath to cut lest he appear to be "giving in" to his wife. He wears loose clothing and sandals, and is fearful of being controlled by women, yet has trouble standing up to his wife to state any of his needs. He alternates between experiencing himself as in control and powerful in anonymous sexual encounters, and as weak and ineffectual at home and at work. Responsible for the bulk of expenses and domestic tasks in his household, he likes it that way, because it keeps him in charge.

A woman has cropped, short hair, and multiple piercings and tattoos. She wears baggy boys' clothes and sneakers, and has primarily been in serially monogamous relationships in which she has trouble asking for and getting what she wants from girlfriends. She also has trouble setting limits with people to whom she is close, but in her public life is able to go after what she wants and get it. She has a gentle manner and is soft-spoken. Because she supports her girlfriend financially and is responsible for most domestic tasks, she resents her girlfriend.

These two individuals occupy their genders in both expected and unexpected ways. This man and this woman also feel, think, and act in ways that they wish they did not. We might also consider a woman who holds strong feminist ideals, yet finds herself wishing to be financially taken care of by a man and feels that she is deserving of such care. Or a man who seems radically independent in most of the public world, yet finds himself feeling like a dependent child in relation to his female boss, wishes to please her, and feels easily scorned by her.

How do we account for these seemingly inconsistent and conflicted representations of gender in which we find ourselves acting, feeling, and thinking in ways that we wish we did not? At the same time, how do we account for individuals who occupy their gender in more conventional ways? A useful psychology of gender needs to make sense of both the seemingly fixed and universal, and the seemingly fluid and individual aspects of gender. It should provide an explanation of gender's seeming intractability and universality, and of individuals' ability to manifest and experience gender in endlessly multiple ways. At the same time, a psychology of gender should make sense of the conflicted nature of gender, of the ways in which it is not always an easy fit and sometimes feels uncomfortable, and of the ways in which gender sometimes feels just right, extremely enjoyable, as though it fits us perfectly.

This chapter demonstrates the particular utility of psychoanalytic theory in understanding gender. Psychoanalytic theory has been concerned from its beginnings with questions of gender, starting with Freud's *Studies on Hysteria*, in which he examined the ways that psychological symptoms manifest themselves in women, often in response to gender-specific experiences and limitations in their family and social lives (Breuer & Freud, 1895). I first describe what distinguishes psychoanalytic theory from other theories of development and gender, and outline Freud's initial contributions to the understanding of gender. I then describe the particular contributions and revisions to Freud's theory provided by second-wave feminist psychoanalytic theorists, who not only redress some of the sexism in Freud's initial theories but also provide a way to understand gender's seeming universality and intractability. Finally, I discuss contemporary feminist psychoanalytic theorists influenced by postmodernism, who argue for gender's particularity and fluidity, as well as for its universality and intractability.[1]

---

[1]Because psychoanalytic theory is generally generated by clinicians principally interested in the treatment of their particular patients, the evidence presented is clinical; that is, clinicians describe the dilemmas, sufferings, and difficulties of their particular patients as evidence of the theory they propound, and use their patients' cure as evidence of the theory's utility. Historically, psychoanalytic theory has been isolated from mainstream psychology because of its reliance on concepts that are difficult to study with traditional, empirical techniques, and that seemingly rely on subjective rather than objective knowledge. In this chapter, I present primarily clinical evidence in support of psychoanalytic theory, but empirical psychology has certainly been interested since the mid-1940s in determining the empirical validity of various psychoanalytic concepts (Hornstein, 1992). These experiments have, however, chiefly confirmed or denied the validity of concepts and have not focused on advancing theory. For an interesting discussion of these issues, see Hornstein (1992).

TRADITIONAL PSYCHOANALYTIC THEORY

Psychoanalysis occupies a curious position in that it is a treatment providing a cure for the troubles that ail individuals and a process of discovering meaning that may be true for particular individuals, and that may also generate findings characteristic of groups of individuals. Because many of Freud's patients were women and he was a man, because his work occurred during the Victorian era, during which gender prescriptions were quite rigid, and perhaps because of his own personal experiences of gender, Freud focused on the differences between male and female development in general and the development of gender in particular (1905, 1925, 1931, 1932, 1937). Other theorists at the time generally did not concern themselves with differences in male and female development but instead assumed male development to be the norm (e.g., Hall, 1904; Piaget, 1929). Freud was perhaps the first gender theorist in his insistence that biological sex is not the same as acquired gender, that biology is not destiny, and that gender is made and not inborn. He did not go quite as far as subsequent theorists in making these claims, and at times he can sound deterministic, as though biology is in fact destiny. But the tools and insights he provided us are invaluable in understanding gender in its universal and particular aspects.

Two of Freud's early findings that have endured and are particularly important in the psychology of gender include the notion of internal conflict and the idea that we have an unconscious part of ourselves that motivates us, but of which we remain unaware. These two findings are related and have important implications for our experiences of gender as contradictory and unexplained by our conscious desires and feelings.

Freud became intrigued by female patients who at the time were diagnosed with hysteria; that is, they exhibited physical symptoms such as paralysis, shortness of breath, tics, and loss of sense of smell, when there was nothing physically wrong with them (Breuer & Freud, 1895). They were generally assumed to be incurable or if curable, then by medical science. Freud believed there to be meaning in the symptoms the young women manifested. Along with his colleague Breuer and one of Breuer's patients, Bertha Pappenheim (otherwise known as Anna O), Freud came upon the talking cure. After trying hypnosis and other techniques, Freud, Breuer, and their patients used talking to trace symptoms back to their origins, which sometimes led to the elimination of the symptom, when it was accounted for and fully understood. They found that, from the point of view of a person's unconscious fantasies or beliefs, there is meaning in symptoms that may appear to be crazy and irrational. An unconscious part of the mind reflects desires, wishes, and fantasies that are not conscious to us in our waking lives but inform the ways that we think, act, and feel. Symptoms were traced to meaningful experiences that caused such profound inner conflict that women developed physical symptoms to manage the conflict. For example, one patient could not tolerate the anger and resentment that she felt over having to tend her dying father. Another patient could not tolerate the shame and anger she felt at having been sexually abused by her father's friend. Both women developed physical symptoms rather than consciously experiencing personally and socially unacceptable feelings. The notion of internal conflict helps to explain why the man with long hair, mentioned earlier, may have anonymous sex despite not wanting to. He cannot tolerate the feelings of dependence and helplessness that he feels in relation to his wife, so he has sex with women on whom he is not dependent, so as not to feel his neediness. The existence of an unconscious part of ourselves explains some of the contradictions that we feel in relation to our experiences of gender, such as why the woman with feminist ideals, mentioned earlier, may long for a sugar daddy.

Psychoanalysis, in its attempt to provide a cure to patients, makes somewhat universal claims about healthy development and gender. Many early psychoanalysts interpreted Freud as arguing that mature sexuality and gender development involved heterosexuality and a rigid adherence to one's prescribed gender role. One sees evidence of this in the historical (and recent) treatment of gays and lesbians, whom some psychoanalysts attempted to "cure" of their homosexuality (Isay, 1990; Mitchell, 1981). Yet in *Three Essays on the Theory of Sexuality* (1905) and "The Psychogenesis of a Case of Homosexuality in a Woman" (1920), Freud himself appeared to be a sex radical who theorized about great variability in both gender and sexuality (Chodorow, 2000). More contemporary psychoanalytic theory returns to the radicalism of Freud and claims that mature gender involves the capacity for more fluidity, less splitting, and less rigidity in terms of gender, the body, and sexuality. It advocates as healthy the capacity to play with gender categories in relationships with others rather than to be limited and constrained by them (Aron, 1995; Benjamin, 1995; 1998; Dimen, 1991, 1995; Elise, 1998, 2000; Goldner, 1991; Harris, 1991, 1996; Sweetnam, 1996, 1999).

At the same time that it is making universal claims, however, psychoanalysis is always working to make meaning of patients' own very particular and individual experiences of development and gender. Psychoanalysis recognizes the tremendous diversity and variability in individual experiences of universal phenomena, for example, breast feeding and early tending by caregivers, attachment to and separation from caregivers, and bodily, social and psychological changes accompanying puberty. In psychoanalytic theory, there is never a one-to-one relationship between objective and observable circumstances in one's development and subjective experiences of it. For example, two different girls may have mothers who appear to respond with delight and pride in their daughters' menarche. One of the girls may experience this as affirming, and feel delighted and proud herself about her body's changes. The other girl may experience this response as intrusive and feel misunderstood in what she experiences as a shameful and unwelcome change in her body. These subjective differences in objectively similar relationships produce very different experiences of gender in these two girls. Psychoanalytic theory, through its conceptualization of the unconscious, allows us to understand how these two girls could have such vastly different experiences of the same observable interaction. The unconscious idiosyncratically influences the fantasied meanings that we attribute to such an experience. Psychoanalysis provides us with a theory that considers both fantasied meanings and materially observable phenomena to account fully for individuals' experiences of gender.

Although the methods of psychoanalysis are useful for understanding gender, it is also true that psychoanalysis has been substantively interested in gender and sexuality from its inception (Freud, 1905, 1920, 1925, 1931, 1932, 1937; Horney, 1926, 1932; Rivière, 1929). Freud located sexuality and the body at the center of development in general and gender development in particular. The earliest physical and sensual handling and tending of the infant are the first ways the baby comes to know him- or herself in relation to an other. This has implications for gender in that experiencing one's body in relation to an other contributes to one's sense of self and gender. So in very basic and fundamental ways, one's experience of gender, the body, and sexuality are linked.

Moreover, in particularly elastic moments in *Three Essays on the Theory of Sexuality*, Freud (1905) argued that whereas gender is always related to sexuality, neither fully causes the other. Instead, he argued that men and women are both masculine and feminine, passive and active, and inherently bisexual in orientation, and that one's gender experience is not predictive of whom one loves; that is, a man may be male and masculine in his erotic life, but may love men, and a woman may be masculine and also love men. Individuals may experience masculine and feminine aspects of themselves in relation to the same person, and may seek out love objects that correspond to both masculine and feminine ideals. Freud also discussed how the same experience or constitution can result in different sexualities—that one may grow up in a similar looking family and have similar experiences, or seem to have a similar temperament to another person and develop quite differently from him/her. Freud was revolutionary in arguing that individuals' experiences are more multiple and varied than would be predicted by their material circumstances.

Freud made the radical claim that men are made and not born, that boys' development into heterosexual men needs to be explained and is not just natural. Freud developed the theory of the Oedipus complex to account for how men are made from boys originally attached to their mothers. It explains how they become men who identify with their fathers and romantically love women other than their mothers. The theory of the Oedipus complex has been rightly critiqued over the years by feminists, gays, and lesbians, who argue that it is phallocentric, that it holds the penis in too high regard, and that it assumes that maturity entails heterosexuality (Benjamin, 1988; Chodorow, 1978, 1992; Isay, 1990, to name a few). Yet there are in fact puzzles to be solved in male development. How do boys manage not to stay identified with their mothers, who are more central figures in their early caretaking than are their fathers? How and why does masculinity develop given that it is women who are most centrally involved in child rearing? And how do heterosexual boys shift their love from their mothers to other women? Why would a boy ever give up a mother's love, and his love for her?

Freud chose the myth of Oedipus to illustrate his theory of male development. He argued that myths and fairy tales often reflect a collective unconscious, something that is fundamentally true about human life but remains generally hidden from conscious life, only to be told in story and fantasy form. Myths and fairy tales persist throughout time, argued Freud, because they reflect something essential in human experience. Freud proposed that boys face similar dilemmas, passions, and conflicts as did Oedipus. In a very simplified form, an oracle decreed that Oedipus would eventually kill his father and marry his mother, and to prevent this fate from befalling them and him, Oedipus's parents sent him to live elsewhere. As an adult, Oedipus unwittingly killed his father and married his mother. When he discovered this, he was so despairing and devastated that he gouged out both of his eyes and exiled himself. Freud took from the myth, and from evidence in his clinical work with patients, that boys generally unconsciously wish to marry their mothers and kill off their fathers, so that they have no competition for their mothers' affection. Oedipus lived out this wish, but most of us, Freud argued, merely unconsciously wish and do not act on these desires. But we do require a way out of this dilemma, which Freud described as the resolution of the Oedipus complex.

In Freud's theory, little boys desire to have their mother as their own love object. They are angry with their fathers for having their mother and wish to kill the father to be able to claim the mother as theirs. However, when boys are around 4–6 years old, they become aware of the differences between the sexes.[2] Prior to this age, children do not differentiate themselves or others by sex, claimed Freud. At this age, the boy notices the absence of a penis in women and imagines the he could also be deprived of his penis. He fears that the father will deprive him of his penis as punishment for desiring the mother and wanting to unseat the father. To preserve himself, the boy must give up his heterosexual attachment to his mother. What he gains is identification with his father and the capacity to love woman other than his mother later in life.

Freud (1925, 1931, 1932) argued that girls face similar developmental dilemmas, but also some that diverge from those of male development. The questions, as he saw them, were as follows: How does femininity develop, and why do women submit to its limitations? How do heterosexual girls shift their love from their mothers to their fathers, and then to other men? Why would a girl ever give up a mother's love, and her love for her mother? How and why do girls change the organ from which they derive pleasure from the clitoris to the vagina? Freud argued that girls, in complement to boys, desire to marry the father and kill the mother, who is a rival for the father's affection. Girls spend their early lives attached to the mother in the same ways as do boys. Between 4 and 6 years of age, however, girls recognize that they lack a penis and experience themselves as castrated and inferior to boys and men. They then feel contempt for their mothers and other women who also lack a penis, blaming the mother for their own lack. Contempt and anger at the mother fuel the girl's turning from her mother and toward her father as a love object. Upon realizing that she cannot have a penis, she gives up active sexuality based in the clitoris for passive sexuality based in the vagina, and wishes for a child from the father rather than a penis. She then has a rivalrous relationship with the mother that is similar to that of the boy with the father. However, the girl does not have to fear castration or retribution from the inferior mother, so she has a more difficult time giving up the father as a love object than boys have giving up the mother. Identification with the mother is also more complicated than a boy's identification with the father, because the girl has not resolved her contemptuous and angry feelings at the mother, and she holds her mother to be inferior.

Many feminists, gays, lesbians, and other critics have continued to rework rather than reject Freud's theory of the Oedipus complex, because the compelling questions that Freud originally asked still need to be an-

---

[2] This has since been empirically refuted. Evidence suggests that children recognize sex differences as early as 18–24 months of age (Fast, 1984).

swered. And the psychoanalytic method that he developed for answering them remains among the most useful that we have for understanding the passions and discomforts of gender. Contemporary psychologists and social scientists interested in gender and sexuality have found useful Freud's attention to the family, the body, the unconscious, internal conflict, and internalization in the development of gender. They have modified and built on Freud's theory to rid it of phallocentrism, to problematize its assumption of heterosexuality, to assert the subjectivity of the mother, and to rid the theory of its biological determinist bent (Benjamin, 1988; Chasseguet-Smirgel, 1970; Chodorow, 1978; Fast, 1984).

SECOND-WAVE FEMINIST PSYCHOANALYTIC THEORIES

Early feminist psychoanalytic theorists tended to be clinicians who sought to redress the phallocentric nature of early psychoanalytic theory (Horney, 1926; Jacobson, 1968; Jones, 1927; Klein, 1928; Thompson, 1943). They made claims about girls' early knowledge of the vagina (Freud claimed girls were only aware of the clitoris), suggested that womb envy may be equally powerful and as plausible as penis envy, and argued for a distinct line of female development that from early on differed from male development, not just with the onset of the oedipal stage. They based much of their thinking on clinical experiences with female patients who had lived experiences of their bodies and genders that diverged widely from Freud's theory.

Many second-wave feminists writing during the 1970s and 1980s turned to psychoanalytic theory because it addressed gender and sexuality, and because it seemed to account for the persistence of gender inequalities, both in individual psyches and in cultural and social institutions, despite U.S. society's political and social commitment to gender equality. They took from Freud the premise that gender is not self-evident, that particular personality characteristics, such as active and passive, independent and dependent, do not universally differentiate the sexes. They accounted for the nature of entrenched gender and gender inequality by focusing on how these become lodged in and actually constitute the psyche. They went further than Freud in their attention to societal and cultural forces but retained a focus on the individual unconscious. Second-wave feminist psychoanalytic theorists also surpassed Freud by arguing not only about how gender develops but also how it reproduces itself.

I have chosen to focus on those feminist psychoanalytic theorists whose work has been most grounded in clinical work but still retains a focus on and interest in the interplay of the social and the psychological. Chodorow (1974, 1978) and Benjamin (1988) have had particularly far-reaching influence not only in the field of psychology but also in the humanities and other social sciences. In their work, they used the important concepts provided by psychoanalysis—the unconscious, internal conflict, the link between sexuality and gender, the role of early childhood experiences—to link the psychology of gender to the persistence of gender inequality.[3] One of the central problems they addressed is that women, as the usual primary parent of children, occupy the difficult position of being all important to children at the same time that they are devalued by society, and often by themselves. And children, in the process of individuation, may also insist on devaluing all that is feminine and maternal within themselves, both to defend against the mother's power and to assert their individuality. Girl children, then, have great difficulty in developing a female sense of self that is subjective and agentic, and boy children have difficulty relating to women without devaluing them. Chodorow and Benjamin, who both have roots in Marxism and philosophy, saw "the psychology of men and women as an intertwined conflictual whole, as part of a totality of social and psychological relations" (Chodorow, 1989, p. 5).

At the time of Chodorow's early writings, much feminist thinking was concerned with the split between the public and private sphere, in which men occupy the valued public sphere of work, politics, and culture, and women, the devalued private sphere of home and children. This split seemed central to gender inequality, and Chodorow worked to explain both its origins and its perpetuation (1974, 1978). She did not, as did many feminists at the time, look solely at social institutions, such as the state and the economy, but examined the role of families and early childhood experiences in producing both individual and social gender. At the time of Benjamin's early writing (1988), much feminist thinking was focused on how and why it is that men dominate women sexually. Power differences between men and women seemed to be traceable to the sexual domination of women by men, with the original gender inequality being created and perpetuated in the most private of places, the bedroom.[4]

[3] Dorothy Dinnerstein (1976), *The Mermaid and the Minotaur*, also made related arguments about the relationship between the psychology of gender and gender inequality, but she is neither clinically grounded nor steeped in social theory, and the impact of her ideas is not so far-reaching as is that of Chodorow and Benjamin.

[4] Gayle Rubin (1975), in her classic essay "The Traffic in Women: Notes towards a 'Political Economy' of Sex," laid the groundwork for work such as Benjamin's in her focus on the role of heterosexual marriage in perpetuating gender inequality, but Rubin focuses exclusively on social theory rather than clinical work.

Chodorow posed the original question that made possible subsequent explorations and understandings of the role of mothering in perpetuating gender. How is it that women come to want to be mothers, over and over again? Previously, women's mothering had been described as natural, because women give birth and lactate, but Chodorow sought to understand the psychology of mothering, the desire to mother, and not just its physical logic based on women's possession of uteruses and mammary glands. Particularly, if mothering is often a fundamental basis of gender inequality, why would women desire it? Of central importance to the issue of women's desire to mother is the question of boys' and girls' connection to and separation from their mothers. Chodorow argued that parenting arrangements in contemporary society, in which women are primarily responsible for parenting and men go out to work in the public sphere and have limited parenting responsibilities, produce different personality structures in girls and boys. For both boys and girls, Chodorow argued that although mothers may be socially devalued, they are extremely powerful in children's eyes and experiences. The mother is the primary figure in their early lives, and is the person both boys and girls most profoundly need early on. The puzzle for Chodorow then became, how do boys and girls manage to connect to and separate from their own mothers, and how does this connection and separation look different in boys and girls? Freud also considered this question, but with somewhat phallocentric results. He answered that boys fear the deprivation of the penis, so they separate from the mother, and that girls are angry with the mother for depriving them of a penis, so they separate from her as well. Chodorow came to understand this process without relying so much on the importance of the penis.

Girls, in Chodorow's model, grow up with an experience of sameness and continuity with their mothers. The mother who is a girl's primary love object is also the person with whom she identifies in terms of gender. However, because of the sameness in gender between mothers and daughters, because mothers experience their daughters as extensions of themselves, and because women often rely on relationships with their children, especially daughters, to fulfill their needs for connection and intimacy, girls must struggle intensely to attain a sense of separateness and individuation from their mothers. Heterosexual relationships for women are unlikely to be satisfying because of conflicts over closeness and separateness (based on their relationships with their mothers), and because of men's unavailability for connection and intimacy (discussion follows). Women, then, have a need for attachment beyond heterosexual relations with men, even if they are heterosexual, and Chodorow argued that they therefore mother and develop close attachments to their children, and the cycle continues.

Boys, on the other hand, grow up with an early experience of continuity with their mothers and a later experience of difference from their mothers, once they recognize gender difference. Because of their experience of difference, boys are more easily able to separate and individuate from their mothers. They identify with their fathers, who occupy the public sphere, and turn toward material achievement in the outside world, both as a means of achieving gender identity and of freeing themselves from their mothers' power. Later in life, men will desire to love and be close to women, grounded in the safe position in the public sphere they have occupied. Heterosexual activity and relationships for men will likely be a satisfying return to the primary oneness they originally experienced with their mothers.

Benjamin borrowed Chodorow's premise that women's mothering is central in the development and perpetuation of gender, and used it to understand how gender domination is anchored in women as much as it involves male exercise of power. Other feminists had explored the roots of male domination but had not pursued the question of female submission to domination. Benjamin required psychoanalytic theory to answer such a question, because, consciously, women certainly do not want to be dominated (most of the time), and consciously, most men do not want women to be reduced to less valuable human beings. But Benjamin aruged, in a familial constellation in which women are primarily responsible for child care and men base their identities in the public sphere of work, boys and girls experience their parents differently and so develop into dominant men and submissive women. Children experience their fathers as exciting subjects and agents in the outside world, capable of action on their own behalf and in possession of desire. By contrast, they experience their mothers as passive and not capable in the outside world but able to nurture in the private sphere, as objects of their fathers' desire but not in possession of their own. The mother's nurturing features are important but are socially denigrated and split off from the excitement of the father. Both boys and girls feel the desire for excitement as their own inner desire, then look to the exciting other (the father) for recognition of their desires. Both boys and girls seek what Benjamin termed *identificatory love* with the exciting father, who has freedom, autonomy, and desire.

Boys, in this formulation, can be recognized as like the exciting father and so gain subjecthood and desire. Yet this comes at the price of their attachment to the mother, and the qualities she possesses and engenders. They have achieved a certain form of subjectivity, but one that denigrates the qualities of women. Girls left with mothers who are themselves objectified will find it impossible, according to Benjamin, to develop a sense of true subjectivity. Girls are generally not recognized as being like the exciting father. As long as the person similar to them in gender (the mother) experiences herself as an object in relation to a subject (a man), girls will either (1) identify with their fathers as subjects and denigrate their mothers, and part of themselves by implication; or (2) identify with their mothers as objects. In terms of sexuality, this provides women with two different positions—that of a subordinate object with no desire, or that of a dominant subject with desire, who denies her dependency needs.

Although it is apparent that the psychology of gender just described flows from particular social structures and parenting arrangements, Chodorow and Benjamin also outlined the ways that the described forms of gender get translated into gender inequality. Chodorow argued that fathers' absence in the rearing of young children makes it so that boys' identification with masculinity, necessary to attain the correct gender role, happens through rejecting what stands for femininity. Boys come to recognize that what they are supposed to be is what their mothers are not. This rejection does not happen in a vacuum, however, but in a world in which men control not only major social institutions but also the very definition and constitution of society and culture. Rejecting femininity is then consonant with denigrating femininity, so that tasks, traits, and qualities associated with being feminine are considered less socially valuable than are tasks, traits, and qualities associated with being masculine. As a result, men are motivated to avoid being primary caretakers, or being in any social terms "feminine," leaving the socially devalued work of mothering to women.

Benjamin later asked why it is that masculinity and femininity are so polarized, that society imagines that we cannot be one without being the other, and that the dichotomies of subject–object, autonomous–dependent continue to shape the relationship between the sexes despite our society's formal commitment to equality. Other feminists sought to account for this puzzle by looking at social institutions that perpetuate inequality. Benjamin, using psychoanalytic theories, endeavored to explain the psychological persistence of these dichotomies in individual psychology and social life. She argued that as long as parenting arrangements are such that parents are split into either subject or object, either autonomous or dependent, children will develop into adults who can only tolerate a split and polarization in gender, who cannot withstand ambiguity in terms of gender. And as long as society continues to rely on these dichotomous categories to organize social institutions and our thinking itself, the split will remain.

Whereas these theories have been influential in the psychology of gender, they have also been criticized for their presumption of a heterosexual, nuclear, and intact family formation, and for their assumption of heterosexuality as the natural developmental outcome of gender development. These theories presupposed a heterosexual family formation in which both parents are present and the mother is the primary caregiver. Given that only 56% of families today meet these criteria (U.S. Bureau of the Census, 2001), some have argued for the inapplicability of second-wave feminist psychoanalytic theory to children and caregivers in other family formations. Chodorow and Benjamin also assumed that heterosexuality is the natural outcome of the gender development they described, that women will romantically and sexually love men, and men will romantically and sexually love women. Because homosexuality and bisexuality are known to be other possible developmental outcomes, others have argued for the inapplicability of Chodorow's and Benjamin's theories to children and, later, to adults who are gay, lesbian, bisexual, or transgendered. Chodorow and Benjamin, and others, have countered that despite the proliferation of various family formations, it is still true that women are responsible for the bulk of caregiving to children. And even if the other parent is a woman, it is generally true that one parent is more a secondary parent who goes out into the world, who is not so affiliated with the domestic sphere and caregiving responsibilities (Benjamin, 1988). Furthermore, Benjamin and others have argued that it is not essential to have two parents, or two parents of different genders, to have these split experiences of autonomy and dependency (1995, 1998). Rather, one might experience a single parent as alternately autonomous or dependent, but be unable to experience the parent as both at the same time. Or one might have split experiences of parents of the same gender. Some of the dynamics and processes discussed by these authors may then hold true despite appearances to the contrary. Although Chodorow and Benjamin both originally assumed heterosexuality to be the normal developmental outcome for men and women, Chodorow (1992) later questioned this assumed heterosexuality and now argues that heterosexuality needs to be explained at least as much as does homosexuality.

Chodorow's and Benjamin's early theories provided us with powerful tools for understanding gender's seeming universality and intractability. They helped to describe gender's origins as well as its reproduction in social and individual life. And they showed the ways that its location in individual psyches makes it particularly difficult to change. It is constitutive of the self, and subjectivity more generally, so it does not respond to mere suggestion or teaching. By locating the development of gender not only in families but also in social structures that depend on particular representations of gender, they further bolstered their arguments for gender's seeming entrenchment. Also, their focus on preoedipal development in boys and girls highlighted the importance of the primary caregiver, and the primary caregiver's gender. However, their theories have been shown to be somewhat overgeneralized, because clinical evidence suggests that individuals' experiences of gender sometimes fit general categories but often also manifest themselves in highly idiosyncratic and personal ways. The seemingly universal experiences of gender they discussed are extremely important, but do not fully account for the range of gendered experience that we witness clinically. Nor did they theorize the body and its relationship to sexuality, out of concerns about biological determinism.

CONTEMPORARY FEMINIST PSYCHOANALYTIC THEORIES

Contemporary feminist psychoanalytic theorists, Chodorow and Benjamin among them, now argue for gender's particularity and multiplicity, and at the same time recognize its universality and intractability. They recognize gender to be both personal and cultural, subjective and objective, fluid and nominal. Furthermore, they conceptualize a postoedipal phase of development during which individuals neither rigidly experience gender in one objectively observable way nor only experience gender fluidly in a purely subjective way. These theorists argue for a different form of healthy gender, one in which individuals need not solely accept the limitations of their gender but may instead sometimes experience themselves as multiply gendered, and other times as only one gender. Finally, they return to a focus on the body and sexuality in understanding the psychology of gender and are able to do so without the biological determinism that second-wave feminists so strongly avoided. The unconscious is the mediating factor that makes possible our idiosyncratic and personal versions of gender, the body, and sexuality. The contemporary feminist psychoanalytic theorists I discuss here ground their thinking in clinical work at the same time that they are influenced by second-wave feminist theorizing, postmodernism, and queer theory. They currently write and are engaged in debates about gender's social and individual nature, about gender and the nature of the self, and about the relationship of the body and sexuality to gender. In the current social context in which they write and work with patients, women have increasingly entered traditional male spheres of work and politics, and men have slowly entered traditional female spheres of parenting and domestic work.[5] The current social context also includes increased

[5] See Arlie Hochschild's (1997) *The Second Shift* for a discussion of this "stalled revolution."

attention to issues of transgendered identities and to the struggle of gays, lesbians, and bisexuals for equal rights.

Beginning with Freud, psychoanalysis has struggled to separate sex from gender, to recognize the distinction between biological sex and socially assigned attributes of gender, and not to conflate the two (Freud, 1905, 1920; Stoller, 1968). Psychoanalysis has more recently worked to separate cultural gender from personal gender, objective gender from subjective gender. Contemporary psychoanalysis recognizes that not all individuals experience social and cultural constructions of gender, or even similar family configurations that influence gender, in the same ways. For example, two men may both be muscular, walk with a swagger, make a lot of money, and have many sexual partners. On the face of it, they appear to be similarly gendered. However, one man may have grown up playing and being successful in athletics his whole life, may be comfortable in his body, enjoy his work, and be part of a long-term, nonmonogamous relationship in which both he and his partner have other sexual partners but remain lovingly committed to one another. And the other man may have grown up being picked on for his nerdiness and slight build, so he now works out compulsively so as never to feel physically vulnerable as he did when younger. He may similarly work extremely hard to be professionally successful but may be personally unfulfilled. And he may have multiple partners out of a fear of being close to a committed partner and feeling vulnerable. These men seem to be similarly gendered on the outside, but on the inside experience their gender quite differently.

The distinctions between these two men may be exaggerated, but the examples illustrate Fast's (1984) point that there is a distinction between objective gender, observed differences in personality, character, or behavior, that tends to differentiate and characterize the sexes, and subjective gender, personal constructions of masculinity and femininity, that constitutes one's sense of self as gendered. This distinction is important, because it expands our understanding of gender and the ways individuals actually experience it. We understand gender to be both individual and social, but always both. Chodorow also moves us toward understanding gender in its complexity as both cultural and personal (1995, 1999a, 1999b). We may exist in similar cultural contexts with regard to gender, but we manifest myriad personal experiences of gender that are unaccounted for merely by the cultural forces impinging on and constituting us. Something else that contributes to each individual's experience of gender Chodorow (1995) locates in the personal unconscious. Referring to previous work, she points to mother–daughter relationships and argues that they are not the same for all women, and even when experiences are similar, they take on different meanings for different women.

Whereas there are certain cultural and social realities of gender inequalities, Chodorow argues: "The existence of cultural and social gender inequality does not explain the range of fantasy interpretations and varieties of emotional castings women (and men) bring to this inequality" (p. 539).

These accounts afford us with more ability to account for variation in gender, which allows us better to understand the relationship between gender and culture, race, and class. They do so through attention both to cultural forces and individual ways of making sense of those forces. Traditional clinical psychoanalytic theory has been notoriously remiss in addressing issues of culture, race, and class, in part perhaps because of the relatively homogeneous cultural, racial, and class backgrounds of both psychoanalytic clinicians and their patients. These contemporary theories help to redress psychoanalysis's inattention to broader cultural categories that shape individual meaning.

In addition to expanding our understanding of gender to include cultural, social, familial, and individual aspects, contemporary feminist psychoanalytic theory focuses on understanding how we can escape from the dichotomous categories of gender described and explained so convincingly by second-wave feminists. They do so by borrowing from postmodern (Foucault, 1978) and queer theorists[6] (Butler, 1990; de Lauretis, 1991; Sedgewick, 1990). Queer and postmodern theorists argue that the dichotomous categories of masculine–feminine, subject–object, active–passive, contained–container, autonomy–dependency constitute our selfhood at the same time that they severely limit it. These categories, and the splits they produce and inspire, require us to choose between being one thing or another, and so extremely circumscribe our capacity to be fully human.

Contemporary theorists discuss and elaborate a postoedipal developmental period during which gender is not solely an oedipal achievement, a final arrival at a solid and fixed gender identity that corresponds to one's sexual anatomy. Contemporary theorists recognize the value of oedipal-level thinking about gender, in which rigid categories and binary oppositions predominate, in children but not in adults. Here, the child develops categories of thinking that organize his or her experience—male and female, black and white, can and cannot, subject and object, active and passive, and so on. It is developmentally appropriate that children should think using such categories. It is not developmentally ap-

[6] The academic and activist usage of the term *queer* seeks to break down the binary *straight–gay* by naming a new sexual category, queer, which is a chosen and not imposed identity. Queer theory seeks to understand the impact of such binaries on the construction of the self.

propriate, however, that adults should remain at this developmental stage. Several theorists argue that consolidating a stable gender identity is a developmental "accomplishment" that requires the activation of pathological processes such as disavowal and splitting (Benjamin, 1995, 1998; Goldner, 1991). It requires that we disavow and cut off parts of ourselves that could otherwise be expressed and experienced were it not for our loyalty to rigid and dichotomous categories of gender. These theorists argue that if an individual remains in the oedipal position, with its rigid understanding of difference, he or she may begin to experience psychological pathology. The insistence on black-and-white thinking, splitting, and polarization is not characteristic of mental health but of pathology. There is some evidence that rigid sex typing leads to behavioral inflexibility and difficulty adapting to unfamiliar situations for both men and women (Bem & Lenney, 1976; Helson & Picano, 1990), certainly not a hallmark of mental health. There is also evidence that rigidly feminine women suffer more than do rigidly masculine men (Heilbrun, 1984; Heiser & Gannon, 1984). Given Chodorow's and Benjamin's earlier arguments about the privileging of masculinity over femininity, it follows that rigid femininity would be more harmful socially than would rigid masculinity. Men who occupy rigidly masculine categories of gender at least benefit socially, if not personally, from doing so. Contemporary psychoanalytic theorists, when discussing a postoedipal developmental period, recognize the cultural and social categories of gender that create very different conditions and motivations for men and women to enter the postoedipal position.

A postoedipal developmental period includes the ability to experience ourselves, at times, as being different genders that are sometimes determinate of our selves and sometimes immaterial to our selves. Dimen (1991) argues that occupying only one gender may not always adequately represent our experiences of ourselves. When we have access to one set of gendered experiences, we may feel stifled, constrained, and limited. Aron (1995) finds that clinicians witness this phenomenon in their treatment of patients quite frequently, because they may alternately be experienced by their patients as maternal or paternal, male or female, regardless of their sex and gender. If clinicians cannot tolerate being experienced as differently gendered at different moments, they will not be fully available and helpful to their patients. And all people may experience themselves as differently gendered, both physically and emotionally, depending on the situation. Men or women may experience themselves as open, nurturing, and receptive, attributes socially coded as feminine, and may at different points experience themselves as penetrating and withholding, attributes socially coded as masculine. Harris (1991) argues that gender is not always what it seems to be. Sometimes it may seem an essential part of ourselves that is very defining of our selfhood; other times, it may seem insubstantial and insignificant. As she writes, "Gender may in some contexts be as thick and reified, as plausibly real as anything in our character. At other moments, gender may seem porous and insubstantial" (p. 212). So gender's salience in constituting our sense of self may at some moments be minimal, whereas in others it may be markedly high. A postoedipal experience of gender involves the ability to experience gender, at different moments, as essential and then insignificant.

Postoedipal gender, in contemporary psychoanalytic theory, is a true achievement. It includes the capacity to tolerate ambiguity and instability, and to occupy multiple categories of gender. One version of this entails a return to the overinclusive thinking characteristic of the preoedipal period described by Fast (1984). During the preoedipal period, children have the narcissistic sense that all sex and gender possibilities are open to them, that they can be all things: male and female, big and small, weak and strong, inside and outside. In the postoedipal period, one can experience oneself as both male and female, active and passive, and penetrating and containing, but with an adult experience of oneself and others as whole objects, not a child's narcissistic experience of him- or herself and others as part objects (Benjamin, 1995, 1998; Dimen, 1991, 1995; Elise, 1998; Goldner, 1991; Harris, 1991, 1996). Another postoedipal achievement entails a capacity to move back and forth between the overinclusivity of the postoedipal period and the rigidity of the oedipal period. There might be some experiences of overinclusivity in terms of gender, and other experiences of firm occupation of one gender or the other; that is, a man may at times experience himself to be both masculine and feminine, and at other moments to be exclusively masculine. Health would be signaled by the capacity to move between these different experiences of gender to experience most fully one's self (Aron, 1995; Sweetnam, 1996, 1999). In either case, we find a very different picture of "healthy" gender than in previous psychoanalytic accounts, in which men and women achieved a singular and unified gender that was true for them across time and space. For contemporary theorists, the development and experience of gender continues throughout life and is not finished following the oedipal period.

Whereas second-wave feminists shied away from using the body to understand the psychology of gender, in an effort to avoid the determinism characteristic of other bodily and biologically based theories, contemporary feminist psychoanalytic theorists now have at their disposal the ideas of postmodernism and queer theory, which situate the body within a social context. Postmodern theories understand the body to have different meanings and to evince different experiences, depending on the social forces that not only influence but also create a particular experience of the body. For example, some have argued that in contemporary U.S. society, with its focus on toned and fit female bodies, women may experience their bodies as disciplined or as out of control, whereas several years ago, with more focus on skinny bodies and less emphasis on tone, women may have experienced their bodies as deprived or as too indulged (Bordo, 1993). Queer theorists argue that bodies and what we do with them during sex certainly matter, or deviations from normative sexuality would not engender such hostility, fear, and discrimination (Butler, 1990; Foucault, 1978; Sedgewick, 1990). To discuss gender and sexuality without considering the body is, they argue, to be blind to the social significance of the body and what it does and does not do.

Contemporary feminist psychoanalytic theory is able to return to Freud's original insights about the fundamental importance of the body in the development of a gendered self, but theorists are now able to understand the body as both given and as constructed; that is, the body exists materially prior to the self but is brought into being and given meaning through its relationship to others. The body has some a priori material demands and desires, such as hunger, fatigue, comfort, and touch, but many of its demands, desires, and passions are brought into being through being tended to and related to by an other. McDougall (1985, 1995), a French feminist psychoanalyst, discusses female and male bodies as both given and constructed. She argues that the interiority of female sexual parts creates a different experience of the gendered self than does the exteriority of male sexual parts. There is more unknown to women about their bodies than there is to men, and this impacts both women's and men's experience of gender. Yet she also proposes that we understand female bodies and femininity to be mysterious and unknown, in an effort to defend against recognizing the uncertainties of male bodies and masculinity. Dimen (1999), like McDougall, argues that the body both predates construction and is constructed. Whereas the body is socially created, it may also be the site of deeply personal and subjective desire that has escaped construction. This desire may make possible the reclamation of the body and a unique experience of gender based in the personal, not the universal, body.

Contemporary feminist psychoanalytic theories account for a range of experiences of gender and for the diverse ways in which individuals experience and express their gender. At the same time, they do not lose sight of the powerful ways in which gender is a social category based in difference and inequality. Chodorow and Fast developed theories that allow for gender's particularity, its unique and subjective expression in each individual, and its social and objective nature. Benjamin, Dimen, Elise, Goldner, and Harris posit a postoedipal developmental period that follows a preoedipal period characterized by undifferentiation and multiplicity, and an oedipal period characterized by rigidity and stasis. The postoedipal period includes the capacity for overinclusivity and for experiencing one's gender multiply and fluidly. Also, as articulated by Aron and Sweetnam, it includes the capacity to move between fluid and rigid experiences of gender. Finally, McDougall, Dimen, and others have returned to the body, after second wave feminists eschewed it for years, to understand more fully the development of gender and the self. Present in each of these theories is a recognition of the ongoing development of gender. By conceiving of a postoedipal period, gender development is no longer relegated to oedipal notions of mature gender that are more rigid and restrictive than are most individuals' lived experiences of gender.

CONCLUSIONS

Psychoanalytic theories offer us a unique lens through which to understand the psychology of gender. They do so by focusing attention on outside forces that broadly impact experiences of gender and internal forces that make meaning of gender in very particular ways. They are also unique in their long-standing interest in gender as constitutive of the self. Gender, in psychoanalytic thinking, has always been one of the principle axes of development, and gender differences and similarities have interested psychoanalytic thinkers from the beginning.

Although many contemporary theorists have criticized Freud, as did his own contemporaries, for some of his sexist and phallocentric views on gender, it is nonetheless the case that many of his insights have stood the test of time and proven useful to other contemporary theorists. Many of his theories retain a flexibility characteristic of few other psychological theories of his time. Freud developed the notion of internal conflict and the concept of an unconscious part of ourselves that motivates us, but of which we are unaware. These concepts have been extremely helpful in understanding the complexity and contradictions of gender. He cautioned against the conflation of gender and sexuality, arguing that one is not predictive of the other. He pointed to the distinction between sex and gender, and contended that they are not the same, that gender is not predetermined, but is shaped by one's experiences in the world.

Second-wave feminist psychoanalytic theorists have developed an important reformulation of psychoanalytic theories of gender. They pointed to the significant role of gender in parenting, and argued that women's mothering and men's lack of involvement in child rearing create and perpetuate particular forms of gender and gender inequality.

They also discussed the ways in which male and female gender are intertwined and co-created, as they are often defined in opposition to one another. They provided compelling accounts of the ways in which gender is constitutive of both individual psyches and the culture at large.

Contemporary feminist psychoanalytic theorists have furthered our understanding of gender by focusing on both personal and cultural roots of gender. In some sense, they have returned to Freud's most compelling early observations of gender—that it is related to but not determinate of sexuality, that it is influenced but not determined by sex, that it is informed by but not caused solely by the body, and that it is always mediated by the personal unconscious. At the same time, they retain a focus on social meanings of gender that both influence and are influenced by personal experiences of gender.

ACKNOWLEDGMENTS

Thanks to Nancy Chodorow, Alex Gronke, Meg Jay, Elena Moser, and the editors of this volume for careful and thoughtful comments on earlier drafts of this chapter.

REFERENCES

Aron, L. (1995). The internalized primal scene. *Psychoanalytic Dialogues*, *5*(2), 195–237.

Bem, S. L., & Lenney, E. (1976). Sex-typing and the avoidance of cross-sex behavior. *Journal of Personality and Social Psychology*, *33*(1), 48–54.

Benjamin, J. (1988). *The bonds of love: Psychoanalysis, feminism, and the problem of domination*. New York: Pantheon.

Benjamin, J. (1995). *Like subjects, love objects: Essays on recognition and sexual difference*. New Haven, CT: Yale University Press.

Benjamin, J. (1998). *Shadow of the other: Intersubjectivity and gender in psychoanalysis*. New York: Routledge.

Bordo, S. (1993). *Unbearable weight: Feminism, western culture, and the body*. Berkeley: University of California Press.

Breuer, J., & Freud, S. (1895). Studies on hysteria. *Standard Edition*, *2* (pp. 1–319). London: Hogarth Press, 1953.

Butler, J. (1990). *Gender trouble: Feminism and the subversion of identity*. London: Routledge.

Chasseguet-Smirgel, J. (1970). Feminine guilt and the Oedipus complex. In J. Chasseguet-Smirgel (Ed.), *Female sexuality: New psychoanalytic views* (pp. 94–134). Ann Arbor: University of Michigan Press.

Chodorow, N. J. (1974). Family structure and feminine personality. In M. Z.

Rosaldo & L. Lamphere (Eds.), *Woman, culture and society* (pp. 43–66). Stanford, CA: Stanford University Press.

Chodorow, N. J. (1978). *The reproduction of mothering: Psychoanalysis and the sociology of gender.* Berkeley: University of California Press.

Chodorow, N. J. (1989). *Feminism and psychoanalytic theory.* New Haven, CT: Yale University Press.

Chodorow, N. J. (1992). Heterosexuality as a compromise formation: Reflections on the psychoanalytic theory of sexual development. *Psychoanalysis and Contemporary Thought, 15*, 267–304.

Chodorow, N. J. (1995). Gender as a personal and cultural construction. *Signs, 20*(3), 516–544.

Chodorow, N. J. (1999a). From subjectivity in general to subjective gender in particular. In D. Bassin (Ed.), *Female sexuality: Contemporary engagements* (pp. 241–250). Northvale, NJ: Jason Aronson.

Chodorow, N. J. (1999b). *The power of feelings: Personal meaning in psychoanalysis, gender, and culture.* New Haven, CT: Yale University Press.

Chodorow, N. J. (2000). Foreword. In S. Freud, *Three essays on the theory of sexuality.* New York: Basic Books.

de Lauretis, T. (1991). Queer theory: Lesbian and gay sexualities. *Differences, 3*, iii–xviii.

Dimen, M. (1991). Deconstructing difference: Gender, splitting, and transitional space. *Psychoanalytic Dialogues, 1*(3), 335–352.

Dimen, M. (1995). The third step: Freud, the feminists, and postmodernism. *American Journal of Psychoanalysis, 55*(4), 303–319.

Dimen, M. (1999). Polyglot bodies: Thinking through the relational. In L. Aron & F. S. Anderson (Eds.), *Relational perspectives on the body* (pp. 65–93). Hillsdale, NJ: Analytic Press.

Dinnerstein, D. (1976). *The mermaid and the minotaur.* New York: Harper & Row.

Elise, D. (1998). Gender repertoire: Body, mind, and bisexuality. *Psychoanalytic Dialogues, 8*(3), 353–371.

Elise, D. (2000). Woman and desire: Why women may *not* want to want. *Studies in Gender and Sexuality, 1*(2), 125–145.

Fast, I. (1984). *Gender identity: A differentiation model.* Hillsdale, NJ: Erlbaum.

Foucault, M. (1978). *The history of sexuality: Vol. 1* (R. Hurley, Trans.). New York: Pantheon.

Freud, S. (1905). *Three essays on the theory of sexuality.* New York: Basic Books, 2000.

Freud, S. (1920). The psychogenesis of a case of homosexuality in a woman. *Standard Edition, 18* (pp. 145–172). London: Hogarth Press, 1955.

Freud, S. (1925). Some psychical consequences of the anatomical distinction between the sexes. *Standard Edition, 19* (pp. 241–258). London: Hogarth Press, 1961.

Freud, S. (1931). Female sexuality. *Standard Edition, 21* (pp. 225–243). London: Hogarth Press, 1961.

Freud, S. (1932). Femininity. In *New introductory lectures on psycho-analysis* (pp. 139–166). New York: Norton, 1964.

Freud, S. (1937). Analysis terminable and interminable. *Standard Edition, 23* (pp. 209–254). London: Hogarth Press, 1964.

Goldner, V. (1991). Toward a critical relational theory of gender. *Psychoanalytic Dialogues, 1*(3), 249–272.

Hall, G. S. (1904). *Adolescence: Its psychology and its relations to physiology, anthropology, sociology, sex, crime, religion and education.* New York: Appleton.

Harris, A. (1991). Gender as contradiction. *Psychoanalytic Dialogues, 1*(2), 197–224.

Harris, A. (1996). Animated conversation: Embodying and gendering. *Gender and Psychoanalysis, 1*, 361–383.

Heilbrun, A. B., Jr. (1984). Sex-based models of androgyny: A further cognitive elaboration of competence differences. *Journal of Personality and Social Psychology, 46*, 216–229.

Heiser, P., & Gannon, L. (1984). The relationship of sex-role stereotypes to anger expression and the report of psychosomatic symptoms. *Sex Roles, 10*, 601–611.

Helson, R., & Picano, J. (1990). Is the traditional role bad for women? *Journal of Personality and Social Psychology, 59*(2), 311–320.

Hochschild, A. R. (1997). *The second shift.* New York: Avon.

Horney, K. (1926). The flight from womanhood. *International Journal of Psycho-Analysis, 7*, 324–339.

Horney, K. (1932). The dread of women. *International Journal of Psycho-Analysis, 13*, 348–360.

Hornstein, G. (1992). The return of the repressed: Psychology's problematic relations with psychoanalysis, 1909–1960. *American Psychologist, 47*(2), 254–263.

Isay, R. (1990). *Being homosexual: Gay men and their development.* New York: Avon.

Jacobson, E. (1968). On the development of the girl's wish for a child. *Psychoanalytic Quarterly, 37*, 523–538.

Jones, E. (1927). The early development of female sexuality. *International Journal of Psycho-Analysis, 8*, 459–472.

Klein, M. (1928). Early stages of the Oedipus conflict. *International Journal of Psycho-Analysis, 9*, 167–180.

McDougall, J. (1985). *Theaters of the mind: Illusion and truth on the psychoanalytic stage.* New York: Basic Books.

McDougall, J. (1995). *The many faces of eros: A psychoanalytic exploration of human sexuality.* New York: Norton.

Mitchell, S. (1981). The psychoanalytic treatment of homosexuality: Some technical considerations. *International Review of Psychoanalysis, 8*, 63–87.

Piaget, J. (1929). *The child's conception of the world.* Totawa, NJ: Littlefield, Adams.

Rivière, J. (1929). Womanliness as a masquerade. *International Journal of Psycho-Analysis*, *9*, 303–313.

Rubin, G. (1975). The traffic in women: Notes towards a "political economy" of sex. In R. Reiter (Ed.), *Toward an anthropology of women* (pp. 157–210). New York: Monthly Review Press.

Sedgewick, E. (1990). *Epistemology of the closet*. Berkeley: University of California Press.

Stoller, R. (1968). *Sex and gender: On the development of masculinity and femininity*. New York: Science House.

Sweetnam, A. (1996). The changing contexts of gender: Between fixed and fluid experience. *Psychoanalytic Dialogues*, *6*(4), 437–459.

Sweetnam, A. (1999). Sexual sensations and gender experience: The psychological positions and the erotic third. *Psychoanalytic Dialogues*, *9*(3), 327–348.

Thompson, C. (1943). "Penis envy" in women. *Psychiatry*, *6*, 123–125.

U.S. Bureau of the Census. (2001). *U.S. Department of commerce news*. Washington, DC: U.S. Government Printing Office.

8

Gender Differences in Relational and Collective Interdependence

Implications for Self-Views, Social Behavior, and Subjective Well-Being

WENDI L. GARDNER
SHIRA GABRIEL

> Man's love is of man's life a thing apart . . . but tis woman's whole existence.
>
> —BYRON (1824), from *Don Juan*, Canto I

Human attachments are a fundamental source of strength and succor for all individuals. However, common beliefs about gender differences often echo Byron's suggestion that men and women differ strongly in the importance of social bonds. For example, one contemporary best-seller targeted to teens includes a chapter titled "Men and Women Are Different," an ostensible attempt to help teens better understand the behavior of the opposite sex, in which one primary gender difference is stated as "women are social, men are individualistic . . . " (Brain, 1997, p. 111). Although obviously a caricature, this portrayal of the sexes does appear to parallel beliefs current college students may hold about gender differences in sociality, as revealed by our recent survey.

We recently asked 50 undergraduates (equal numbers of males and females) which sex was more likely to place more importance on various aspects of life, including some social aspects (e.g., friendships, club memberships, being an individual) and some nonsocial aspects (e.g., succeeding in classes, creative problem solving, being happy with life), on a scale of 1 to 7, with 1 labeled *definitely men*, 7 labeled *definitely women*, and 4 labeled *men and women equally*. For the questions concerning relationships with best friends, family, and romantic partners, the results were in favor of women placing greater importance on these close relationships (*M*'s = 6.2, 5.5, and 6.8, respectively). Similarly, when we asked which sex was more likely to place more importance on their memberships in groups or organizations, such as fraternity–sorority membership, being members of their university, and membership in social clubs, the results were again in favor of women (*M*'s = 4.8, 4.7, and 4.9, respectively). At the opposite end of the social spectrum, when we asked which sex was more likely to place more importance on being an individual, going it alone, and being independent from others, results were in favor of men (*M*'s = 1.9, 2.5, and 2.2, respectively). In contrast to the gender differences seen in the social sphere, the college students we sampled did not expect much of a gender difference in other domains, such as succeeding in classes (*M* = 3.9), being creative problem solvers (*M* = 4.2), or being happy with life (*M* = 3.9).

Such beliefs concerning gender differences in sociality may not be limited to our college student sample. Indeed, when gender stereotypes were sampled in 25 diverse nations, "independent" was identified as a masculine trait in all 25, whereas "affectionate" was identified as a feminine characteristic in 24 of the 25 nations (Williams & Best, 1990). Thus, it appears that one belief about how men and women differ appears to concern the social domain; women may be thought to place greater importance on social interactions and social ties compared to men.

Even in the psychological literature, there is evidence that women are thought to place greater emphasis on relations with others compared to men. For example, one well-explored gender difference concerns itself with gender-linked motivations toward agency or communion that are reflected in and reinforced by the different social roles inhabited by men and women. Men are thought to be oriented toward agency, characterized by traits such as instrumentality, assertiveness, and self-confidence, whereas women are thought to be oriented toward communion characterized by warmth, expressiveness, and concern for others (e.g., Bakan, 1966; Bem, 1974; Wood, Christensen, Hebl, & Rothgerber, 1997). Moreover, these motives have been shown to be internalized into the self-concepts of men and women, with the sex-typed norms of women as warm and expressive, and men as more independent and self-confident, serving as standards for self-evaluation (Wood et al., 1997). And in a recent review of gender differences in the sociality of the self-concepts of men and women, it has been argued that as a result of these norms, men develop and maintain a more independent view of the self (e.g., one grounded in individual abilities, traits, and preferences), whereas women develop and maintain a more interdependent view of the self (e.g., one grounded in social ties with close relationships and groups; Cross & Madson, 1997).

Sex differences in social aspects of the self have rarely been directly examined. However, recent research has begun to focus on this aspect of gender differences, with potentially surprising results. Instead of finding support for the view of men as individualistic and women as more socially attuned, this work exposes the shared importance of social associations to the self; both men and women appear to look to their social ties as a basis for identity. Despite this basic similarity, potentially distinct features of men's and women's interdependent identities have emerged. Specifically, men appear to emphasize collective (group-based) bonds, whereas women appear to emphasize relational (dyadic) attachments. In other words, the most accurate description of gender differences in interdependence might be that men and women appear to be "separate but equal"; men and women differ in the *aspects* of interdependence that are emphasized and elaborated, but do not differ in the overall *extent* of interdependence, nor in the impact of interdependent construals on social cognition and behavior (e.g., Arndt, Greenberg, & Cook, 2002; Baumeister & Sommer, 1997; Gabriel & Gardner, 1999; Gardner, Gabriel, & Hochschild, 2002; Seeley, Gardner, Pennington, & Gabriel, 2003).

This chapter first briefly reviews the cultural literature from which the construct of an interdependent self-construal emerged. We also describe socialization processes that may encourage interdependence to take distinct and gendered forms within North America. Finally, we review the empirical evidence supporting the notion that interdependence is both represented and communicated differently in men and women. The expanded model of gender and interdependence has received support in domains as diverse as spontaneous self-descriptions, values and worldviews, the encoding and recall of social information, self-evaluation and regulation, and the bases of social attachments and well-being.

AN EXPANDED VIEW OF GENDER AND INTERDEPENDENCE

The distinction between an independent versus interdependent construal of the self, characterized as self-definitions grounded within personal traits and attributes (e.g., athletic, tall) versus social roles and close relationships (e.g., mother, husband), came to prominence within social psychology as a framework for understanding the robust differences between members of East Asian and North American cultures in social thought and behavior (e.g., Gardner, Gabriel, & Lee, 1999; Markus & Kitayama, 1991). An independent self-construal is thought to arise from a belief in the inherent separateness of individuals, and to encourage the goal of discovering and expressing what makes one positively distinct from others. In contrast, an interdependent self-construal is thought to arise from a belief in the fundamental embeddedness of every individual in a larger web of close relationships and group memberships, and thus encourages the goal of maintaining harmony with others (e.g., Heine, Lehman, Markus, & Kitayama, 1999; Lee, Aaker, & Gardner, 2000).

As a framework for understanding cultural differences, the distinction between independent and interdependent self-construals has been successful in both predicting and explaining cultural differences in areas as varied as causal attribution (e.g., Menon, Morris, Chiu, & Hong, 1999), social influence (e.g., Ybarra & Trafimow, 1998), self-enhancement and esteem (e.g., Heine et al., 1999), and the bases of subjective well-being (e.g., Suh, 2000). Recently, several researchers have argued that the chronic motives linked to independent and interdependent self-construals may parallel the constructs of agency and communion (Cross & Madson, 1997; Ickes & Barnes, 1978). Others have argued that, to some extent, children grow up in sex-segregated separate cultures, complete with distinct gendered norms and practices (e.g., Hoffman, 1972; Maccoby, 1989, 1990; Maltz & Borker, 1982; Tannen, 1990). Taken in this context, it is understandable that extending the cultural distinction between independent and interdependent self-construals to explore potentially distinct "cultures of gender" would be seen as helpful in understanding sex differences in cognition and behavior.

As previously mentioned, in an interesting and influential article, Cross and Madson (1997) asserted that North American culture encourages the development of a more interdependent focus in women and independent focus in men. Furthermore, they argued that many empirically demonstrated gender differences could be seen as reflecting these differences in self-construal. Certainly much of the developmental literature supports the notion that girls appear to be more strongly attuned to relationships. For example, when asked to describe themselves, young girls spontaneously refer to close relationships and relational characteristics to a greater extent than do their male counterparts (McGuire & McGuire, 1982; Rosenburg, 1989). Moreover, gender differences in sensitivity to close relationships appear to continue into adulthood. Adult women attend to information related to relationships more than do men

(Josephs, Markus, & Tafarodi, 1992; Ross & Holmberg, 1992), and close relationships appear to have a greater impact on women's well-being, in that more women than men describe interpersonal problems as a source of distress (Pratt, Golding, Hunter, & Samson, 1988; Walker, de Vries, & Trevethan, 1987).

However, the broad support for the notion that women appear to maintain relatively more interdependent self-construals and social biases, as reviewed by Cross and Madson (1997), does not necessitate that men must maintain relatively independent self-construals. The indispensability of social ties to well-being is becoming increasingly recognized in medical as well as psychological literature, and the negative consequences of social isolation do not appear to be moderated by gender (e.g., House, Landis, & Umberson, 1986; Mistry, Rosansky, McGuire, McDermott, & Jarvik, 2001). Indeed, the "need to belong"—a need fulfilled only through affiliation with and acceptance from others—is so universally powerful that it has been proposed to be as basic to our psychological makeup as hunger or thirst is to our physical makeup (Baumeister & Leary, 1995; Gardner, Pickett, & Brewer, 2000). Thus, to the extent that the interdependent self rests upon and reflects belonging needs (e.g., Gardner et al., 1999), simply being male should not allow one to escape the importance of regulating and maintaining an interdependent self-view.

In their analysis of belonging as a basic human need, Baumeister and Leary (1995) argued that although the motivation is universal, belonging needs may be satisfied in a number of interchangeable ways, ranging from marital satisfaction to church and community involvement. The "substitution postulate" allows for a reconciliation of a universal need to belong, with the empirical evidence that men appear to be significantly less focused on relationships than are women. In fact, Baumeister and Sommer (1997) persuasively argued that men may value interdependent characteristics that do not fundamentally depend on intimate dyadic relationships.

Given the necessity of social connection, then, men and women should not differ in the overall importance of social bonds to the self. To reconcile this notion with the overwhelming evidence that women are much more strongly attuned to relational information, we recently argued for an expanded model of gender and the interdependent self (Gabriel & Gardner, 1999). We theorized that, given childhood socialization patterns, women and men would be differentially encouraged to emphasize distinct aspects of interdependence as important. Specifically, we drew on the distinction between the relational and collective forms of interdependence (Brewer & Gardner, 1996). Relational interdependence reflects the aspect of the self that is defined in terms of roles in close relationships (e.g., sister, husband) and is analogous to the interdependence described by Cross and Madson (1997). In contrast, collective interdependence reflects the aspect of the self that is defined in terms of membership in important groups (e.g., sorority member, ethnic identity) and is most similar to the construct of social identity (Hogg & Abrams, 1988; Turner, Hogg, Oakes, Reicher, & Wetherell, 1987). We hypothesized that women would maintain a greater relational sense of self compared to men, but that men would maintain a greater collective sense of self compared to women; thus, no differences in overall interdependence would be expected. In other words, we proposed that gender differences in interdependent self-construal represent a distinction of "kinds" rather than of extent.

Extensive support exists for the notion that women maintain a greater relational self-construal than men (see Cross & Madson, 1997, for review); however, the collective aspect of interdependent self-construal has traditionally received far less attention in the gender literature. Even so, a number of sources, ranging from those emphasizing evolutionary selection to those demonstrating gender norms in childhood socialization, are all quite consistent with the notion that relational versus collective interdependence may develop distinct importance for girls versus boys.

Indeed, even the classic distinction between agency and communion may be interpreted as consistent with a more expanded model of interdependence. For example, communal traits, such as "affectionate, supportive, and sympathetic," appear strongly relationally interdependent, without implying increased collective interdependence. Moreover, agentic traits, such as "competitive, aggressive and dominant," are not constrained to an individualist and, therefore, independent interpretation. In fact, Baumeister and Sommer (1997) argued that many agentic characteristics are useful in navigating larger social hierarchies, gaining leadership in groups, and other collectively interdependent rather than independent tasks. Thus, the traditional distinction between masculine and feminine stereotypes may be at least as consistent with an expanded view of gender differences in aspects of interdependence as with Cross and Madson's (1997) interpretation of men as independent and women as interdependent.

THE ORIGINS OF GENDERED FORMS OF INTERDEPENDENCE

As with any observable sex difference, the proposed distinction between relational and collective interdependence may potentially be viewed through multiple perspectives, from the biological to the societal (e.g., Wood & Eagly, 2002). We briefly speculate on the potential origins of these differences by reviewing a number of relevant research areas consistent with the notion of an expanded model of interdependence. Representing multiple perspectives on sex differences, all can be seen as potentially supportive of the notion of gendered forms of interdependence, but, of course, none can be considered definitive.

Viewed through the lens of evolutionary psychology, it is possible that distinct forms of interdependence may at least in part reflect biologically prepared characteristics. Several researchers have speculated on the evolutionary advantages afforded by collective competence in men or relational competence in women (e.g., Baumeister & Sommer, 1997; Taylor et al., 2000; Tiger, 1969). For example, Tiger (1969) argued that survival in early societies might have necessitated men bonding in task-oriented groups to coordinate the complex task of hunting for large prey. That type of large-group bonding may have made it more likely that men would retain genetic tendencies toward group loyalty and collective skills. Additionally, as Baumeister and Sommer (1997) pointed out, skills that increased a male's value to the group would also have increased his attractiveness as a mate.

Taking a similar evolutionary perspective, Taylor et al. (2000) have proposed that women may in part be biologically prepared for relational attachment as a protective mechanism for buffering stress. In a review of the stress and coping literature, they highlight the fact that females respond differently to stress than do males, and that female responses to stress appear to follow a "tend and befriend" pattern, in which nurturant activities reduce psychological and physiological distress. Intriguingly, they link this relational pattern of stress reduction to the release of oxytocin, believed to underlie attachment processes between mothers and offspring, as well as other intimate social bonds. Moreover, "tend and befriend" coping responses put a woman and her offspring at a lower risk than the "fight-or-flight" pattern more typical for males. Finally, because male androgens partially block the soothing effects of oxytocin, these researchers believe that at least some of the benefits of relational support seeking may be specific to women.

Regardless of whether relational and collective interdependence were differentially advantaged in our evolutionary history, gender asymmetries in relational versus collective construals are encouraged by the gender norms of current society. The roles traditionally inhabited by women and men may differ in their emphasis on dyadic relational bonding (e.g., child rearing and other caregiving) versus the emphasis on acceptance and success within larger collectives (e.g., a sports team or corporation). These differing social roles convey gender-linked norms for behavior, and children are ultimately encouraged to internalize and behave in accordance with these norms (Berndt & Heller, 1986; Eagly, 1987; Lytton & Romney, 1991; Maccoby, 1990; Wood et al., 1997).

One robust area of differential treatment is parental encouragement of gender-typed toys, play, and interests (Etaugh & Liss, 1992; Lytton & Romney, 1991). Gender-typed play, in turn, appears to differentially emphasize relational activities for girls, such as playing at mothering dolls, and collective activities for boys, such as team sports (Bradbard, 1985; Miller, 1987). In one particularly compelling demonstration of the power of gender norms in play, gender socialization was communicated through toys at an astonishingly early age (Sidorowicz & Lunney, 1980). In this study, participants were surreptitiously observed while interacting with a 10-month-old baby, who they were told was either a boy or a girl. The baby's crib held a small football, a doll, and a teething ring. Although one might guess a priori that the teething ring was probably the most appropriate toy for a 10-month-old baby, when participants thought the baby was a boy, 65% chose to play with "him," using the football; conversely, when participants thought the baby was a girl, 80% chose to play with "her," using the doll.

Of course, gender socialization is not limited to parents or caregivers; a good deal of research has documented the powerful role of peers as arbiters of gender-typed behavior (Berndt & Heller, 1986; Carter & McClosky, 1984). Starting at the age of 3, children's play becomes sex-segregated (e.g., Lewis & Phillipsen, 1998; Maccoby & Jacklin, 1987; Martin, Fabes, Evans, & Wyman, 1999) and as children age, there is mounting peer pressure to adhere to gender norms (Berndt & Heller, 1986). Moreover, these sex-segregated play groups themselves often differ in both size and purpose; girls are much more likely to interact with peers in close, same-sex dyads (Broderick & Beltz, 1996; Clark & Bittle, 1992; Jones, Bloys, & Wood, 1990), whereas boys spend more time with peers in team and group activities (Belle, 1989; Berndt & Hoyle, 1985; Maccoby, 1989, 1990).

Thus, whether examined from an evolutionary or socialization perspective, gender differences in relational and collective construals are expected to emerge relatively early in childhood and be encouraged and maintained through adulthood. Self-construals are thought to create a powerful interpretive lens through which the social world is viewed (e.g., Gardner et al., 1999; Markus & Kitayama, 1991). Thus, we would expect these accessible constructs to shape both cognition and behavior in ways that may be gender-equivalent in their overall focus on social connection, but relatively distinct in the emphasis placed on close relationships versus social groups. Although the expanded model of gender and interdependence is comparatively new, a growing body of research is beginning to reveal the consequences of these distinctions for self-descriptions, social information processing, and the nature of social motives held by men and women.

GENDER DIFFERENCES IN SELF-CONSTRUAL

The most obvious prediction of the expanded model of gender and interdependence is specific asymmetries in self-descriptions. Importantly, the model predicts that no gender differences will be found in the overall level of interdependent self-descriptors, but significant gender differences in the aspect of interdependence that is central to the self will be obvious. Specifically, women should employ a greater number of relational roles in self-descriptions compared to men, and men should employ a greater number of group memberships compared to women.

In fact, gender differences in the social aspects of self-construals are easily noticeable when people are asked simply to describe themselves to others. For example, in an analysis of children's self-descriptions, the McGuires observed that both boys and girls used social constructs in self-definition, but that the forms expressed were distinct. Consistent with the predictions of the expanded model, girls exceeded boys in self-descriptions centered within close relationships, whereas boys exceeded girls in self-descriptions relying on group memberships (McGuire & McGuire, 1982). In a recent study with young adults, we found parallel gender differences in the spontaneous self-descriptions of college students (Gabriel & Gardner, 1999, Study 1). When we asked men and women to write 20 self-descriptive sentences (Kuhn & McPartland, 1954), we found that whereas women expressed nearly twice as many relational self-descriptors as men (e.g., "I am Pam's sister"; "I am Amanda's best friend"), men expressed approximately twice as many collective self-descriptors as women (e.g., "I am a member of Pi Kappa Alpha"; "I am a Northwestern student"). Importantly, men and women were *not* found to differ significantly in the overall proportion of independent self-descriptors they spontaneously supplied (e.g., "I am ambitious"; "I am good at golf"), providing support for the notion that social self-views are as important to men as to women.

In addition to spontaneous self-descriptions, this same asymmetric pattern has been observed with use of direct measures of relational and collective self-focus (Cross, Bacon, & Morris, 2000; Gabriel & Gardner, 1999). Susan Cross and her colleagues developed and validated a measure of relational construal (Cross, Morris, & Gore, 2002; Cross et al., 2000) that comrpises of endorsements of items such as "When I feel close to someone, it often feels to me like that person is an important part of who I am." We examined gender differences in scores on the RISC, as well as on a scale created to parallel the RISC but measure level of collective construal, with items such as "When I join a group, I usually develop a strong sense of identification with that group." Across several samples of college-age men and women, we found that women consistently endorsed the relational items to a greater degree, whereas men more often endorsed the collective items (Gabriel & Gardner, 1999, Study 2; Gardner, Gabriel, & Hochschild, 2002). Importantly, these studies failed to find gender differences in a measure of general interdependence (Singelis, 1994), demonstrating once again that the notion that women show greater overall interdependence may be mistaken.

A further examination of gendered patterns in the measures of relational and collective interdependence established that these are functionally distinct constructs, linked to masculine and feminine ways of expressing interdependence. Scores on the relational self-construal scale were significantly correlated with levels of psychological femininity (as measured by the Personal Attributes Questionnaire; Spence & Helmreich, 1978) but not with measures of masculinity. Scores on the collective self-construal scale, in contrast, were correlated with measures of psychological masculinity, but not with measures of femininity (Gabriel & Gardner, 1999, Study 2). Given that the measurement of masculinity and femininity relies heavily on participants' endorsements of agentic and communal traits, these findings also lend credence to the view that agentic traits may be associated with activities and motives within a collective (e.g., Baumeister & Sommer, 1997).

Thus, direct measures of the importance of relational and collective connections to identity appear to reliably support the expanded model of interdependence. The self-descriptions of men were found to be as socially centered as those expressed by women. Gender differences were found, however, in aspects of interdependence; men emphasized the collective aspects and women, the relational aspects. This gender-specific pattern held for both the spontaneous self-descriptions of children and young adults, and endorsements on identity scales. Finally, collective interdependence was specifically related to levels of psychological masculinity, and relational interdependence was related to femininity.

GENDER DIFFERENCES IN SOCIAL COGNITION

The expanded model of interdependence is proposed to encompass a broad range of gender differences, in addition to those revealed in self-description. The self has been posited to be the most powerful and elaborated knowledge structure possessed by individuals (Bower & Gilligan,

1979; Linville & Carlston, 1994). As a result, self-schemas and beliefs serve as frequent filters for information; accessible self-constructs shape perceptions of the social world. Indeed, the ability of the self to implicitly guide information processing in the service of chronic concerns and motives is a central tenet in social psychology, backed by decades of empirical evidence (e.g., Markus, 1977; see Baumeister, 1998, for review). To the extent that relational and collective interdependence reflect the differential importance of relationships and groups in satiation of belonging needs, biases in information processing in the service of these needs should be apparent.

Biases in encoding and memory have long been used as indicators of construct accessibility and importance (e.g., Bargh & Tota, 1985; see Higgins, 1996, for review). One paradigm used to assess important concerns capitalizes on biases in the spontaneous recall of information. In one instantiation of this paradigm, individuals are given a diary containing behaviors that differ along dimensions of interest (e.g., gain- vs. loss-focused behaviors; social vs. nonsocial behaviors) and are told to form an impression of the individual described by the diary. After several subsequent filler tasks, a surprise recall task is then used to examine the types of information that individuals remember; biases in recall reflect differential encoding and/or retrieval processes, and have been established as markers of situational motives or chronic concerns (Gardner et al., 2000; Higgins & Tykocinski, 1992).

To investigate whether gender-consistent aspects of self-construal would bias spontaneous cognitive processing, we adapted the diary paradigm to present behaviors that were independent, relational, or collective in nature (Gabriel & Gardner, 1999, Study 4). As expected, results of this study were supportive of the expanded model of interdependence; whereas women to a greater extent than men remembered a greater number of relational behaviors (e.g., a night out with a roommate), men remembered collective behaviors (e.g., a meeting of the church choir) to a greater extent than did women. Gender differences did not emerge for recall of the independent events (e.g., receiving an A on an exam), or for independent versus interdependent events more generally, implying once again that men and women do not appear to differ in the overall accessibility or importance of interdependence per se.

In a recent demonstration of gender differences in accessible interdependence-related constructs, Arndt et al. (2002) have reported gender differences consistent with relational and collective interdependence in studies of terror management theory (Solomon, Greenberg, & Pyszczynski, 1991), which proposes that when death becomes salient, important cultural values become activated and protect the self from fear by reinforcing the notion that the individual is tied to a broader system that is both meaningful and enduring. Research in the domain of terror management theory has found consistent and robust evidence that mortality salience (e.g., becoming aware of one's own mortality by either engaging in thoughts of one's own death or being exposed to situations related to mortality, such as walking past a cemetery) motivates defense of one's values and cultural worldview. These defenses may take varied forms, such as negative judgments of those who do not share one's values, false consensus concerning the number of people who share one's own worldviews, or a general reluctance to violate cultural norms oneself (see Greenberg et al., 1997, for review). Importantly, the activation of central values is thought to provide a self-protective function in the face of recognizing one's own mortality.

In a creative series of studies, Arndt and colleagues (2002) investigated potential gender differences in the types of values that became activated by men and women in response to mortality salience. To the extent that the gender differences in relational and collective aspects of interdependence are internalized, the content activated after a mortality prime would be expected to differ in a manner consistent with the expanded model of interdependence.

In fact, across multiple studies, these researchers found reliable evidence that mortality salience activated more relational constructs for women (e.g., marriage) and more collective constructs in men (e.g., nationalism). What is particularly striking about these findings is the nonconscious nature of the relational or collective responses, indexed, for example, by facilitated recognition of the relational word *romance* in women, or the completion of a word fragment such as f _ _ g with the collective word *flag* rather than *frog* in men. Thus, this research implies that the gender-linked distinction between relational and collective interdependence may lead to similar distinctions in the values and social institutions that, when activated, serve ego-protective functions.

GENDER DIFFERENCES IN SELF-EVALUATION AND REGULATION

Acknowledging the centrality of relational and collective interdependence to the psyche of women and men suggests a powerful role for these constructs in self-evaluations and regulation. Gender norms themselves often serve as internalized standards for behavior (e.g., Wood et al., 1997). Thus, to the extent that gendered aspects of interdependence are internalized as a part of these standards, adherence to relational or collective behavior would clearly be predicted to influence men and women differently.

In one study examining the potential impact of gender differences in interdependence on behavioral regulation, we asked men and women to imagine themselves in various scenarios in which the welfare and interests of others (either a close friend or an important group) were in conflict with their own personal interests (Gabriel & Gardner, 1999, Study 5). For example, one scenario asked participants to imagine themselves in a situation in which they wished to attend a review session for an upcoming exam (personal interest) at the same time that their student organization needed help with an important project (collective interest). In another scenario, participants imagined a situation in which they were on the way to a highly anticipated concert (personal interest) when they spotted a close friend standing on the side of the road next to a car with its hood up (relational interest). Multiple relational and collective scenarios were presented, and after each scenario, participants indicated how they would respond in the situation (e.g., go to the review session vs. helping their organization, or go to the concert vs. helping their friend). We hypothesized, and found, that women were more likely than men to put their own personal desires aside to assist a friend, whereas men were more likely than women to put their personal desires aside to help their groups. In other words, it appeared that gender differences in relational and collective interdependence also influenced standards for appropriate behavior.

Gender differences in aspects of interdependence may also affect the impact of different forms of social comparisons on self-evaluations. The positive performance of relevant others can affect the self-concept in two very different ways. First, one can "bask in the reflected glory" of a relevant other and feel pride in his or her accomplishments (Cialdini et al., 1976). Conversely, one can compare the self to the other(s) and, thus, feel worse about the self (Festinger, 1954). One factor that can affect which reaction occurs is linking of the other to the self. Specifically, assimilating the target to the self makes "basking in reflected glory" more likely and comparison less likely (e.g., Gardner, Gabriel, & Hochschild, 2002; Stapel & Koomen, 2001). Thus, the impact of the performance of a close relation or group on the self should be moderated by whether the comparison target may be assimilated to the self through a relational or collective view of interdependence.

The impact of self-enhancement motives on the process and outcomes of social comparison has been robustly demonstrated in both dyadic and group settings. For example, self-evaluation maintenance theory (SEM) emphasizes these effects at the dyadic level and proposes that whenever a close other (e.g., sibling) performs well in a self-relevant domain, self-esteem suffers (Tesser, 1980; 1988). To avoid these painful consequences, individuals have been shown to willfully bias the process of social comparison by both preferring and predicting poorer performance for close others (Tesser & Campbell, 1982) to protect the self. Similarly, the frog pond effect (FPE) emphasizes the interplay of self-enhancement and social comparison at a group level (Davis, 1966). The FPE proposes that being a "big frog in a small pond," or a success in a relatively unsuccessful group, is preferred over situations in which the performance of an individual's group may outshine the individual's own successes. This, too, can lead to esteem-protecting biases and actions that affect both the individual and the group (Chen, Brockner, & Katz, 1998; Marsh, 1987; McFarland & Beuhler, 1995).

The expanded model of gender and interdependence would predict reliable differences in the impact of various targets for the self-evaluations of men versus women. Specifically, given women's levels of relational interdependence, comparisons with close others should be less threatening (because of the assimilation of the close other to the self) than comparisons with a group. In fact, in an examination of social comparison processes in marriages, Beach et al. (1998) reported that wives exhibited a consistently lower tendency to engage in self-evaluation maintenance behaviors with their spouses than did husbands. This difference between husbands and wives had been interpreted as evidence of a higher general level of interdependence in women; this high general level of interdependence was hypothesized to prevent comparisons with others from being as threatening to women as they are to men (Cross & Madson, 1997; see also Kemmelmeier & Oyserman, 2001). Conversely, the expanded model would predict that although men's focus on collective interdependence may leave them open to the threatening effects of comparisons with relationship partners, the assimilation of the group to the self should buffer the impact of group comparisons.

We recently examined the moderating role of relational and collective interdependence on the impact of social comparisons with friends or ingroups (Gardner, Gabriel, & Hochschild, 2002). We used a self-evaluation maintenance paradigm in which participants brought close friends into the laboratory with them and were then given the opportunity to predict the performance of their friend and a stranger on an important task (analytic problem solving). Results were as hypothesized: Men showed the classic self-evaluation maintenance effect of predicting better performance for the stranger than the friend, whereas women showed the opposite effect, predicting better performance for the friend than for the stranger. Because the SEM refers specifically to close relationships, we hypothesized that gender patterns of social comparison would be reversed within a more group-oriented context. In fact, when we used an FPE paradigm in which participants could compare their performance to an ingroup, we found women engaging in greater comparison. When told that they personally had performed badly, but that their group was performing well, men reported more positive moods than women. Similarly, when told that they personally had performed well but that their group had performed poorly, women reported more positive moods than men.

Perhaps most compelling, the proposed causal role of differential relational and collective self-construals in producing the gender differences received support when we activated relational and collective interdependent self-construal using a priming task. Men primed with relational interdependence in a self-evaluation maintenance paradigm lowered their level of social comparison with a friend to the level of women, and women primed with collective interdependence in an FPE paradigm lowered their levels of social comparison with an ingroup to the level of men. The disappearance of gender differences as a result of activating relational or collective interdependence provides still further evidence that it is the differences in aspects of interdependence, rather than alternative gender-linked constructs, that appear to be responsible for the observed differences in social cognition and behavior.

Taken in combination, results of these reviewed research programs converge on the conclusion that although women and men fail to differ in the general importance of social bonds in self-construal, they appear to differ in the aspects of interdependence emphasized in the social self. Spontaneous self-descriptions, direct measures of relational and collective centrality to the self, biases in memory, indirect measures of relational versus collective construct accessibility, and responses to different types of social comparisons all appeared consistent with the theory that women and men place significantly differential weighting on relationships and groups as a basis for identity, and that these distinctions are internalized as distinct gendered values and standards.

Equally important, the stereotype of women placing greater emphasis on the social sphere in contrast to men's emphasis on individualism was refuted. In every study that provided a measure of general independence and interdependence, gender differences failed to emerge on overall levels of interdependence; men and women displayed equivalent levels of social self-descriptions, socially biased encoding and retrieval, and fundamentally social worldviews.

In the final section of this review, we discuss the implications for daily social life that these gender differences might imply. We investigate the extent to which relational and collective interdependence may reflect different strategies for fulfilling belonging needs. In doing so, we briefly review recent evidence suggesting that men and women differ in the patterns of relational and collective social contact they regularly enjoy, in the factors that lead to loneliness, and in the types of social comfort they seek in times of stress.

GENDER DIFFERENCES IN THE RANGE OF SOCIAL NEEDS

In our initial presentation of the expanded model of interdependence, we focused on evidence that women and men differ in the aspect of the interdependent self that is emphasized, and that, furthermore, these differences result in corresponding cognitive differences in the tendency to focus relatively more on relationships or groups in social information processing (Gabriel & Gardner, 1999). In a recent series of studies, we have begun to explore the consequences of gender differences in interdependence for social attachments and emotional well-being (e.g., Gardner, Seeley, et al., 2002; Seeley et al., 2003). The expanded model of gender and interdependence assumes that gender-linked differences in relational and collective interdependence both result from and reinforce differences in relational versus collective belonging needs. Our more recent research thus examined the hypothesis that gender shapes the way in which belonging needs are both experienced and satisfied.

Obviously, connections with others and an adequate number of positive social relationships are crucial for the well-being of both men and women (e.g., Baumeister & Leary, 1995). The expanded model of interdependence additionally suggests that there may be important differences in the expression and fulfillment of men's and women's social desires. Indeed, the model predicts that women would focus on the relational or dyadic forms of belonging more than men, but that men would focus on the collective or group forms of belonging more than women.

A recent series of studies exploring this possibility have provided persuasive evidence of gender differences in social foci (Gardner, Seeley, et al., 2002). Across four studies of everyday social behavior, coping strategies, precursors of loneliness, and predictors of subjective well-being, we found that men and women differed in their everyday experiences with relationships and groups, as well as in the power that these specific forms of experiences wielded over satisfaction with their social world. For example, in a diary study tracking men's and women's daily events across 2 months, we found the predicted interaction, with women reporting greater relational events than men, and men reporting greater collective events than women. Moreover, women reported experiencing more pleasure in their relational events compared to men, and men enjoyed their collective events more than did women.

Recall that one gender difference in the literature that clearly pointed to the importance of close relationships to women was the finding of Taylor et al. (2000) that women, when faced with stress, exhibit "tend and befriend" coping responses. In other words, they nurture those close to them, and seek comfort and solace in intimate relationships to a greater degree than do men. This "tend and befriend" response emphasizes relational bonds. In a recent study of coping behavior (Gardner, Seeley, et al., 2002), we both replicated Taylor's findings with women (they turned more to close others in times of stress) and found evidence for a collective social solace strategy in men (they turned to spending time in their social groups in times of stress). Furthermore, the extent to which women reported using relational strategies was a predictor of more successful coping. Women who reported turning to friends suffered less depression and anxiety than those who did not. Similarly, collective coping strategies served to buffer men. Men who reported spending more time in groups, while undergoing stress, suffered less depression and anxiety than those who reported spending less time in groups.

Given the differential social comfort found in relational or collective interactions, we thought it likely that when individuals are deprived of one or the other type of interaction, emotional suffering would also fit the expanded model of gender and interdependence. Thus, we examined reports of loneliness in over 1,000 college freshmen to examine whether men and women require different forms of social interaction to ward off loneliness. Results revealed that endorsement of the relational "connectedness" subscale of the UCLA Loneliness Scale (e.g., "There are people who really understand me"; see Russell, Peplau, & Cutrona, 1980) predicted the frequency and intensity of loneliness for women more than for men. In contrast, the more collective "belonging" subscale (e.g., "I feel part of a group of friends") better predicted loneliness for men than for women. Additionally, we found that although women's scores on the connectedness scale were sufficient to predict loneliness (e.g., no additional significant variance was explained by adding the belonging scale), men's loneliness scores were influenced by both the connected and belonging subscales. Interestingly, these findings imply that men may require both a feeling of intimacy with close others and a feeling of belonging to a group to avoid loneliness, which potentially explains the consistent finding in the literature that men experience more loneliness than women (e.g., Koenig, Isaacs, & Schwartz, 1994; Schultz & Moore, 1986; Wiseman, Guttfreund, & Lurie, 1995).

CONCLUSIONS

The desire to be connected and intimate with others is considered primary and essential to the human experience (Baumeister & Leary, 1995). Our goal in this chapter has been to reconcile the universality of social needs with their potentially gendered expressions. The research reviewed in this chapter has established that this important component of existence, interdependence, is different for men and women, with women maintaining greater focus on the close relationships of which they are a part, and men, on the groups to which they belong. We argued that child socialization patterns may encourage the experience and the expression of interdependence to take these gendered forms.

We believe that an expanded view of gender and interdependence has the potential to illuminate mechanisms contributing to a wide array of gender differences in social behavior. Equally important, it refutes the stereotype that men and women differentially value social connection. Importantly, across a multitude of studies, no gender differences were observed in overall levels of independence and interdependence, or autonomy versus sociality. Both men and women defined the self in social ways, were biased toward social information processing, used social networks as part of their protective worldviews, and drew on social values to guide behavior. Both men and women sought social contact, became attached to organizations that fulfilled social needs, and suffered when those needs went unfulfilled. Throughout, gender differences emerged not in the extent of these social needs and processes, but in their expression.

Both men and women are motivated to seek and maintain connection with those around them. The fact that the experience of these connections may be subtly shaped by gender neither alters their shared importance nor limits either sex to a social or autonomous role. Indeed, in recognizing that belonging is an essential component of the human experience, the expanded model of interdependence allows an examination of the way gender differences may be evident on the surface of the social landscape, without losing sight of underlying similarities.

REFERENCES

Arndt, J., Greenberg, J., & Cook, A. (2002). Mortality salience and the spreading activation of worldview-relevant constructs: Exploring the cognitive architecture of terror management. *Journal of Experimental Psychology—General*, *131*, 307–324.

Bakan, D. (1966). *The duality of human existence*. Chicago: Rand McNally.

Bargh, J., & Tota, M. E. (1985). Context-dependent automatic processing in depression: Accessibility of negative constructs with regard to self but not others. *Journal of Personality and Social Psychology, 54*, 925–939.

Baumeister, R. F. (1998). The self. In D. T. Gilbert, S. T. Fiske, & G. Lindzey (Eds.), *The handbook of social psychology* (4th ed., pp. 680–740). New York: Oxford University Press.

Baumeister, R. F., & Leary, M. R. (1995). The need to belong: Desire for interpersonal attachments as a fundamental human motivation. *Psychological Bulletin, 117*, 497–529.

Baumeister, R. F., & Sommer, K. L. (1997). What do men want?: Gender differences and two spheres of belongingness: Comment on Cross and Madson (1997). *Psychological Bulletin, 122*, 38–44.

Beach, S. R. H., Tesser, A., Fincham, F. D., Jones, D. J., Johnson, D., & Whitaker, D. J. (1998). Pleasure and pain in doing well together: An investigation of performance-related affect in close relationships. *Journal of Personality and Social Psychology, 74*, 923–938.

Belle, D. (1989). Gender differences in children's social networks and supports. In D. Belle (Ed.), *Children's social networks and social supports* [Wiley series on personality processes] (pp. 173–188). New York: Wiley.

Bem, S. L. (1974). The measurement of psychological androgyny. *Journal of Consulting and Clinical Psychology, 42*, 155–162.

Berndt, T. J., & Heller, K. A. (1986). Gender stereotypes and social influence: A developmental study. *Journal of Personality and Social Psychology, 50*, 889–898.

Berndt, T. J., & Hoyle, S. G. (1985). Stability and change in childhood and adolescent friendships. *Developmental Psychology, 21*, 1007–1015.

Bower, G. H., & Gilligan, S. G. (1979). Remembering information related to oneself. *Journal of Research in Personality, 13*, 404–419.

Bradbard, M. R. (1985). Sex differences in adults' gifts and childrens' toy requests at Christmas. *Psychological Reports, 56*, 969–970.

Brain, M. (1997). *The teenager's guide to the real world.* Raleigh, NC: BYG.

Brewer, M. B., & Gardner, W. (1996).Who is this "we"? Levels of collective identity and self representations. *Journal of Personality and Social Psychology, 71*, 83–93.

Broderick, P. C., & Beltz, C. M. (1996). The contributions of self-monitoring and gender to preadolescents' friendship expectations. *Social Behavior and Personality, 24*, 35–45.

Byron, G. G. (1988). "Don Juan." In T. G. Steffan, E. Staffan, & W. Pratt (Eds.), *Lord Byron: Don Juan.* New York: Penguin. (Original work published in 1824)

Carter, D. B., & McClosky, L. A. (1984). Peers and the mainteneance of sex-typed behavior: The development of children's conceptions of cross-gender behavior in their peers. *Social Cognition, 2*, 294–314.

Chen, Y., Brockner, J., & Katz, T. (1998). Toward an explanation of cultural differences in in-group favoritism: The role of individual versus collective primacy. *Journal of Personality and Social Psychology, 75*, 1490–1502.

Cialdini, R. B., Borden, R. J., Thorne, A., Walker, M. R., Freeman, S., & Sloan, L. R. (1976). Basking in reflected glory: Three (football) field studies. *Journal of Personality and Social Psychology, 34*, 366–375.

Clark, M. L., & Bittle, M. L. (1992). Friendship expectations and the evaluation of present friendships in middle childhood and early adolescence. *Child Study Journal, 22*, 115–135.

Cross, S. E., Bacon, P. L., & Morris, M. L. (2000). The relational-interdependent self-construal and relationships. *Journal of Personality and Social Psychology, 78*, 191–808.

Cross, S. E., & Madson, L. (1997). Models of the self: Self-construals and gender. *Psychological Bulletin, 122*, 5–37.

Cross, S. E., Morris, M. L., & Gore, J. S. (2002). Thinking about oneself and others: The relational interdependent self-construal and social cognition. *Journal of Personality and Social Psychology, 82*, 399–418.

Davis, J. A. (1966). The campus as a frog-pond: An application of the theory of relative deprivation to career decisions of college men. *American Journal of Sociology, 72*, 17–31.

Eagly, A. H. (1987). *Sex differences in social behavior: A social-role interpretation*. Hillsdale, NJ: Erlbaum.

Etaugh, C., & Liss, M. B. (1992). Home, school, and playroom: Training grounds for adult gender roles. *Sex Roles, 26*, 129–147.

Festinger, L. (1954). A theory of social comparison processes. *Human Relations, 7*, 117–140.

Gabriel, S., & Gardner, W. L. (1999). Are there "his" and "hers" types of interdependence?: The implications of gender differences in collective versus relational interdependence for affect, behavior, and cognition. *Journal of Personality and Social Psychology, 77*, 642–655.

Gardner, W. L., Gabriel, S., & Hochschild, L. (2002). When you and I are we, you are not threatening: The role of self-expansion in social comparison. *Journal of Personality and Social Psychology, 82*, 239–251.

Gardner, W. L., Gabriel, S., & Lee, A. (1999). "I" value freedom, but "we" value relationships: Self-construal priming mimics cultural differences in judgment. *Psychological Science, 10*, 321–326.

Gardner, W. L., Pickett, C. L., & Brewer, M. B. (2000). Social exclusion and selective memory: How the need to belong influences memory for social events. *Personality and Social Psychology Bulletin, 26*, 486–496.

Gardner, W. L., Seeley, E. A., Pennington, G. L., Gabriel, S., Ernst, J., Skowronski, J., & Solomon, J. (2002). *The role of "his" and "her" forms of interdependence in everyday life: Gender, belonging, and social experience*. Manuscript under review.

Greenberg, J., Solomon, S., & Pyszczynski, T. (1997). Terror management theory of self-esteem and social behavior: Empirical assessments and conceptual refinements. In M. P. Zanna (Ed.), *Advances in experimental social psychology* (Vol. 29, pp. 61–139). New York: Academic Press.

Heine, S. J., Lehman, D. R., Markus, H. R., & Kitayama, S. (1999). Is there a universal need for positive self-regard? *Psychological Review, 4*, 766–794.

Higgins, E. T. (1996). Knowledge activation: Accessibility, applicability, and salience. In E. T. Higgins & A. W. Kruglanski (Eds.), *Social psychology: Handbook of basic principles* (pp. 133–168). New York: Guilford Press.

Higgins, E. T., & Tykocinski, O. (1992). Self-discrepancies and biographical memory: Personality and cognition at the level of psychological situation. *Personality and Social Psychology Bulletin, 18*, 527–535.

Hoffman, L. W. (1972). Early childhood experiences and women's achievement motives. *Journal of Social Issues, 28*, 129–155.

Hogg, M. A., & Abrams, D. (1988). *Social identifications: A social psychology of intergroup relations and group processes.* London: Routledge.

House, J. S., Landis, K. R., & Umberson, D. (1988). Social relationships and health. *Science, 241*, 540-545.

Ickes, W., & Barnes, R. D. (1978). Boys and girls together—and alienated: On enacting stereotyped sex-roles in mixed sex dyads. *Journal of Personality and Social Psychology, 78*, 669–683.

Jones, D. C., Bloys, N., & Wood, M. (1990). Sex roles and friendship patterns. *Sex Roles, 23*, 133–145.

Josephs, R. A., Markus, H. R., & Tafarodi, R. W. (1992). Gender and self-esteem. *Journal of Personality and Social Psychology, 63*, 391–402.

Kemmelmeier, M., & Oyserman, D. (2001). The ups and downs of thinking about a successful other: Self-construals and the consequences of social comparisons. *European Journal of Social Psychology, 31*, 311–320.

Koenig, L. J., Isaacs, A. M., & Schwartz, J. A. J. (1994). Sex differences in adolescent depression and loneliness: Why are boys lonelier if girls are more depressed? *Journal of Research in Personality, 28*, 27–43.

Kuhn, M. H., & McPartland, T. (1954). An empirical investigation of self-attitudes. *American Sociological Review, 19*, 58–76.

Lee, A. Y., Aaker, J., & Gardner, W. L. (2000). The pleasures and pains of distinct self-construals: The role of interdependence in regulatory focus. *Journal of Personality and Social Psychology, 78*, 1122–1134.

Lewis, T., & Phillipsen, L. (1998). Interactions on an elementary school playground: Variations by age, gender, race, group size, and playground area. *Child Study Journal, 28*, 309–320.

Linville, P. W., & Carlston, D. E. (1994). Social cognition of the self. In P. G. Devine, D. L. Hamilton, & T. M. Ostrom (Eds.), *Social cognition: Impact on social psychology* (pp. 143–193). San Diego: Academic Press.

Lytton, H., & Romney, D. M. (1991). Parents' differential socialization of boys and girls: A meta-analysis. *Psychological Bulletin, 109*, 267–296.

Maccoby, E. E. (1990). Gender and relationships: A developmental account. *American Psychologist, 45*, 513–520.

Maccoby, E. E. (1989). Gender as a social category. In S. Chess & M. E. Hertzig (Eds.), *Annual progress in child psychiatry and child development* (pp. 127–150). New York: Brunner/Routledge.

Maccoby, E. E., & Jacklin, C. N. (1987). Gender segregation in childhood. *Advances in Child Development and Behavior, 20*, 239–287.

Maltz, D. N., & Borker, R. A. (1982). A cultural approach to male–female miscommunication. In J. J. Gumperz (Ed.), *Language and social identity* (pp. 195–216). New York: Cambridge University Press.

Markus, H. (1977). Self-schemata and processing information about the self. *Journal of Personality and Social Psychology, 35*, 63–78.

Markus, H., & Kitayama, S. (1991). Culture and the self: Implications for cognition, emotion, and motivation. *Psychological Review, 98*, 224–253.

Marsh, H. W. (1987). The big frog little pond effect on academic self-concept. *Journal of Educational Psychology, 79*, 280–295.

Martin, C. L., Fabes, R. A., Evans, S. M., & Wyman, H. (1999). Social cognition on the playground: Children's beliefs about playing with girls versus boys and their relations to sex segregated play. *Journal of Social and Personal Relationships, 16*, 751–771.

McFarland, C., & Beuhler, R. (1995). Collective self-esteem as a moderator of the frog-pond effect in relation to performance feedback. *Journal of Personality and Social Psychology, 68*, 1055–1070.

McGuire, W. J., & McGuire, C. V. (1982). Significant others in self space: Sex differences and developmental trends in social self. In J. Suls (Ed.), *Psychological perspectives on the self* (Vol. 1, pp. 71–96). Hillsdale, NJ: Erlbaum.

Menon, T., Morris, M., Chiu, C., & Hong, Y. (1999). Culture and the construal of agency: Attribution to individual versus group dispositions. *Journal of Personality and Social Psychology, 76*, 701–717.

Miller, C. L. (1987). Qualitative differences among gender-stereotyped toys: Implications for cognitive and social development in girls and boys. *Sex Roles, 16*, 473–487.

Mistry, R., Rosansky, J., McGuire, J., McDermott, C., & Jarvik, L. (2001). Social isolation predicts re-hospitalization in a group of older American veterans enrolled in the UPBEAT Program. *International Journal of Geriatric Psychiatry, 16*, 950–959.

Pratt, M. W., Golding, G., Hunter, W., & Sampson, R. (1988). Sex differences in adult moral orientations. *Journal of Personality, 56*, 373–391.

Rosenberg, M. (1989). The self-concept: Social product and social force. In M. Rosenberg & R. H. Turner (Eds.), *Social psychology: Sociological perspectives* (pp. 593–624). New York: Basic Books.

Ross, M., & Holmberg, D. (1992). Are wives' memories for events in relationships more vivid than their husbands' memories? *Journal of Social and Personal Relationships, 9*, 585–604.

Russell, D., Peplau, L. A., & Cutrona, C. E. (1980). The revised UCLA Loneliness Scale: Concurrent and discriminant validity. *Journal of Personality and Social Psychology, 39*, 472–480.

Schultz, N. R., & Moore, D. (1986). The loneliness experience of college students: Sex differences. *Personality and Social Psychology Bulletin, 12*, 111–119.

Seeley, E. A., Gardner, W. L., Pennington, G., & Gabriel, S. (2003). Circle of friends or members of a group?: Sex-differences in relational and collective attachment to groups. *Group Processes and Intergroup Relations, 6*, 251–264.

Sidorowicz, L. S., & Lunney, G. S. (1980). Baby X revisited. *Sex Roles, 6*, 67–73.

Singelis, T. M. (1994). The measurement of independent and interdependent self-construals. *Personality and Social Psychology Bulletin, 20*, 580–591.

Spence, J. T., & Helmreich, R. L. (1978). *Masculinity and femininity: Their psychological dimensions, correlates, and antecedents.* Austin: University of Texas Press.

Solomon, S., Greenberg, J., & Pyszczynski, T. (1991). A terror management theory of social behavior: The psychological functions of self-esteem and cultural worldviews. In M. P. Zanna (Ed.), *Advances in experimental social psychology* (Vol. 24, pp. 93–159). New York: Academic Press.

Stapel, D. A., & Koomen, W. (2001). I, we, and the effects of others on me: How self-construal level moderates social comparison effects. *Journal of Personality and Social Psychology, 80*, 766–781.

Suh, E. M. (2000). Self, the hyphen between culture and subjective well-being. In E. Diener & E. M. Suh (Eds.), *Culture and subjective well-being* (pp. 63–86). Cambridge, MA: MIT Press.

Tannen, D. (1990). *You just don't understand: Women and men in conversation.* New York: Morrow.

Taylor, S. E., Klein, L. C., Lewis, B. P., Gruenewald, T. L., Gurung, R. A., & Updegraff, J. A. (2000). Biobehavioral responses to stress in females: Tend-and-befriend, not fight-or-flight. *Psychological Review, 107*, 411–429.

Tesser, A. (1980). Self-esteem maintenance in family dynamics. *Journal of Personality and Social Psychology, 39*, 77–91.

Tesser, A. (1988). Toward a self-evaluation maintenance model of social behavior. *Advances in Experimental Social Psychology, 21*, 181–222.

Tesser, A., & Campbell, J. (1982). Self-evaluation and the perception of friends and strangers. *Journal of Personality, 59*, 261–279.

Tiger, L. (1969). *Men in groups.* London: Nelson.

Turner, J. C., Hogg, M., Oakes, P., Reicher, S., & Wetherell, M. (1987). *Rediscovering the social group: A self-categorization theory.* Oxford, UK: Blackwell.

Walker, L. J., de Vries, B., & Trevethan, S. D. (1987). Moral stages and moral orientations in real-life and hypothetical dilemmas. *Child Development, 58*, 842–858.

Williams, J. E., & Best, D. L. (1990). *Measuring sex-stereotypes: A thirty nation study.* Beverly Hills, CA: Sage.

Wiseman, H., Guttfreund, D. G., & Lurie, I. (1995). Gender differences in loneliness and depression of university students seeking counselling. *British Journal of Guidance and Counselling, 23*, 231–243.

Wood, W., Christensen, P. N., Hebl, M., & Rothgerber, H. (1997). Conformity to sex-typed norms, affect, and the self-concept. *Journal of Personality and Social Psychology, 73*, 523–536.

Wood, W., & Eagly, A. H. (2002). A cross-cultural analysis of the behavior of women and men: Implications for the origins of sex differences. *Psychological Bulletin, 128*, 699–727.

Ybarra, O., & Trafimow, D. (1998). How priming the private self or collective self affects the relative weights of attitudes and subjective norms. *Personality and Social Psychology Bulletin, 24*, 362–370.

9

On the Construction of Gender, Sex, and Sexualities

Jeanne Marecek
Mary Crawford
Danielle Popp

"Sexy Babes! Live 1-on-1!" Perhaps you've seen the ads in newspapers and magazines, with their promise of "Hot Live Talk!" followed by a toll phone 900-number, "$2.99 per minute," and easily dismissed restrictions, such as "18+" or "Adults Only." What ideas do these ads bring forward about sex, gender, and sexualities? One way to account for phone sex services is that they exist because men have powerful sex drives that must be satisfied even when a partner is not readily available. The 900-numbers provide an outlet for men's innate needs. Another explanation might center on the idea that there are two kinds of women: good women who would never dream of earning money from "hot talk" with strangers, and bad women—sluts or whores—who do. Still another explanation might emphasize that sexual services for hire constitute exploitation of women. Perhaps the women who deliver such services are mentally disturbed, destitute, or drug abusers, and they take these degrading jobs out of desperation. Yet another account is that sex work is a job like any other job, and what people choose to do sexually is no one's business but their own so long as no one is harmed. Women are free agents, and those who do phone sex must like it or they would not do it. Perhaps readers can think of still other ways of understanding why some men pay for "hot talk" with "sexy babes," and why some women provide this service.

Phone sex is only one of innumerable social phenomena that involve sex, gender, and sexuality. Phone sex raises many questions about gender and sexuality, and there are many ways a psychologist might study phone sex. Here, we use phone sex as a ready example to begin describing how social constructionists approach an object of study. Social constructionists would not seek the correct interpretation of phone sex, or the true motives of the male callers and the "sexy babes" who answer the phones. Nor would they hope to discover what men really get from a phone encounter. They might instead examine the range of interpretations of phone sex that have credence in the culture. Which representations of phone sex workers (e.g., "deluded victims" or "nymphomaniacs") make sense to a community of listeners, and which (e.g., "wanton sinners") do not? Social constructionists might also observe the social processes by which different explanations are put forward and warranted. How does it come about that certain accounts of phone sex come to be regarded as obvious or common sense? Social constructionists might also seek to understand how participating in phone sex (as a caller, as a "sexy babe," or perhaps only as a reader of ads) shapes one's ideas about sexual desire, male–female relations, and masculinity and femininity.

Social constructionism raises novel and intriguing questions about social phenomena related to sex, gender, and sexualities. The family of ideas and research tools associated with social constructionism provides a robust approach to understanding the social world and processes by which meanings are devised, validated, and contested. We begin with an overview of some important themes of social constructionism, then describe social constructionists' work on gender, sex, and sexualities.

SOCIAL CONSTRUCTIONISM: AN OVERVIEW

Social Constructionism Is a Theory of Knowledge

Social constructionists hold that what we take to be knowledge is an account of reality produced collaboratively by a community of knowers. Such accounts of reality arise through a process of social interchange and negotiation. Social constructionists are interested in the terms and forms in use among the members of a social group. How do people make use of those terms and forms to compose accounts that make sense to others in their social group? When, as social constructionists, we say that gender or sexuality is "socially constructed," we do not mean that it is social rather than biological, learned rather than innate, or the result of environment rather than heredity. Rather, we mean that the assumptions and linguistic constructs that enable people to talk and think about the phenomena are products of social negotiation and are therefore not universal or fixed. Thus, for example, in some social groups, it is common sense that people are straight, gay, or bisexual. However, this particular way of accounting for sexual practices—which entails a large set of implicit propositions about sexuality and identity—is only one of many possible accounts. It contrasts, for example, with accounts offered by queer and transgender activists (Parlee, 1998).

For social constructionists, concepts and categories are not direct, unequivocal, and unproblematic reflections of reality. Rather, what people consider to be reality takes its form and meaning from the concepts and categories available to them. Whether we construe the sale of phone sex as a necessary outlet for men, a job like any other, or a degrading and immoral practice, we draw on an array of constructs that precedes and shapes the story we tell: "male sex drive," "slut," "free choice," "women as victims," "false consciousness," and perhaps even "decline of civilization."

Knowledge Is a Social Product

For social constructionists, who emphasize the collective character of knowledge, knowledge is not the product of individual mental processes. Accounts of reality, as well as the concepts and categories that organize them, are specific to a particular time and place. Some researchers study the social and cultural codes that frame such accounts of reality. For example, double standards for the sexual behavior of women and men may be expressed in religious teachings, moral discourses, and media representations. They are also brought forward in everyday language, such as slang ("studs" vs. "sluts") and proverbs (Crawford & Popp, 2003). In the recent past, teenage boys were encouraged to "sow their wild oats," whereas girls were warned that a prospective husband "won't buy the cow if he can get the milk for free." Other researchers study the ways that conversation partners jointly construct an account of specific events. For example, Orenstein's (1994) study of middle school students provided an anecdote in which male students construct and communicate sexual double standards under the eyes of a teacher in a sex education class. The teacher, Ms. Webster, was trying to illustrate the risk of sexually transmitted diseases:

> "We'll use a woman," she says, drawing the Greek symbol for woman on the blackboard. "Let's say she is infected, but she hasn't really noticed yet, so she has sex with three men."

> As she draws symbols for men on the board, a heavyset boy in a Chicago Bulls cap stage whispers, "What a slut," and the class titters.
>
> "Okay," says Ms. Webster, who doesn't hear the comment. "Now the first guy has three sexual encounters in six months." She turns to draw three more women's signs, her back to the class, and several of the boys point at themselves proudly, striking exaggerated macho poses.
>
> "The second guy was very active, he had intercourse with five women." As she turns to the diagram again, two boys stand and take bows.
>
> During the entire diagramming process, the girls in the class remain silent. (p. 61)

Accounts of reality, as well as concepts and categories, have histories. They arise in particular times and places, and change as circumstances and social realities change. This is true of both scientific and everyday concepts. Parlee (1994) has traced the struggles among doctors, social scientists, drug manufacturers, and feminist health activists over the meanings of the term *premenstrual syndrome* (PMS). At issue were its name and, more important, whether it was to be defined as a psychiatric condition, a gynecological disorder, or a normal variant of female functioning. As one might surmise, both money and power were at stake. Assembling the histories of concepts and constructs—genealogies of knowledge, as Foucault (1972) called them—is an important part of social constructionist scholarship. Such scholarship documents the invention of constructs, overt controversy over their meaning, and slippages and shifts in meaning over time.

Social Constructionists Attend to Power and Hierarchy

For social constructionists, power, along with its associated differences in status, entitlement, efficacy, and self-respect, is a central dimension of social life. Viewed from afar, power may appear entrenched. Yet power is not a fixed and invariant property of individuals; rather, it is a network of noncentralized forces. It is continually produced, contested, resisted, and subverted. By examining social interchanges in close detail, social constructionists document the micropolitics of subordination, dominance, and resistance. Furthermore, power is not limited to external forces that restrict, prohibit, and constrain people. Modern systems of power operate by heightening self-surveillance and self-control. Foucault, who referred to these systems of power as "technologies of the self," pointed out how individuals come to take pride and pleasure in the ways that they exert discipline and restraint over themselves. For example, because current North American norms of masculinity prescribe restricted emotionality for men, boys monitor their own and other boys' emotional displays in order to suppress them. In a study of white, suburban teenage boys, Oransky and Marecek (2002) noted that the boys valued the ability to distance themselves from negative feelings, to be able to "take it like a man." They also valued teasing and bullying, because such hostile interactions helped them to toughen up, to learn to "suck it up."

Social constructionists' insistence on the social character of knowledge opens the way to consider the politics of knowledge. Some accounts of reality become dominant discourses, assuming the status of truth or common sense; others remain muted or unavailable. What are the interactional processes by which some accounts get shunted off to the side, whereas others prevail? Whose accounts are authorized and supported? Whose accounts are marginalized and subjugated? By connecting the circulation of power in immediate interpersonal encounters to the larger culture, social constructionists hope to offer an account of how particular language practices and discourses gain their meaning and potency.

Language Makes a Difference

To use language is to participate in culture. To speak intelligibly is to make use of the linguistic genres available within the culture. It is to participate in a system that is already constituted (Gergen, 1985). In this way, language precedes and outlives an individual. The classifications and categories provided by language establish distinctions that "make a difference." Such classifications guide our actions and carry implications for how we should evaluate and react to individuals or events (Hare-Mustin & Marecek, 1990). They also, of course, regulate our own actions. Such classification systems are power-laden in the sense that they often create hierarchies of value, prestige, morality, and authority (good vs. evil, beautiful vs. ugly, smart vs. dumb).

Language is a representation of reality, not a direct replica of it. Concepts and categories embed shared, culture-specific meanings. For example, categories such as "gay," "straight," and "bisexual" embed a particular account of sexual desire. They are more or less discrete classifications that are relatively enduring. Moreover, they render sexual desire as a key aspect of personal identity. As we discuss, other accounts bring forward more fluid and expansive forms of desire. Moreover, in this category system, the sex of one's partner is the key dimension of desire; other dimensions are rendered unimportant. This category system helps to establish homosexual and bisexual desire as different and "other," thus shoring up the superiority and "normalcy" of heterosexuality.

Concepts and categories associated with gender, sex, and sexuality work to regulate social behavior and identity. The concept of a male sex drive and its role in construing sexual encounters is one example. The construct of an implacable male urge for sex figures in accounts used by some men to pressure women to have sex with them (Hollway, 1989). It also figures in accounts that some women give to explain why they agreed to sex they did not want (Gavey, 1992). It has also figured in post hoc accounts that serve to excuse men and boys who have engaged in violent or coercive sex.

Social constructionists do not hold a determinist view of language. As practitioners of language, individuals can shift or undermine its meanings. For example, speakers may use irony, humor, and other linguistic and paralinguistic devices to subvert the dominant meanings of language (Crawford, 1995). In recent decades, homosexual activists have undermined the homophobic epithets "gay" and "queer" by reappropriating and investing them with positive meaning. Social constructionist research on language brings forward the paradox that people are enmeshed in a web of linguistic meanings, yet are able to use language in ways that resist or undermine established meanings.

In summary, to speak is to take part in culture, but individuals can put linguistic forms to novel and subversive uses. Moreover, communications among people not only convey messages but also make claims about who the speakers are relative to one another, and about the nature of their relationships. Relations of power are negotiated through the medium of language (Crawford, 1995; Potter & Wetherell, 1987). Thus, language is an activity with practical, material consequences.

Social Constructionism Focuses on Processes

From a social constructionist perspective, meanings are not fixed, but are instead always emergent in human interactions. (This is what constructionists mean when they say that meanings are "co-constructed.") Moreover, people do not passively imbibe cultural messages without awareness, nor do they simply parrot cultural discourses unreflectively. Social constructionists examine the social activities, language practices, and other social processes through which people account for themselves as gendered and sexed actors. They expect that people will not sustain coherent and unchanging accounts of themselves. Social constructionists often are specifically interested in how people shift among different accounts as they move through differing situations and relationships. The ongoing production of meanings is part of the flow of social life. People produce meanings of gender, sex, and sexualities that are provisional, contingent, and specific to particular settings. Therefore, social constructionists do not attempt to assert universally applicable or enduring claims about gender, sex, or sexual orientation. This sets social constructionist accounts of gender and sexuality apart from those of theoretical approaches such as evolutionary psychology. Moreover, social constructionists are skeptical of technologies, such as scales or inventories, that attempt to measure masculinity and femininity as enduring personal qualities.

Individual and Society Are Indissoluble

The Western philosophical tradition of liberal humanism views the self as bounded and separate from society (cf. Henriques, 1998). In this view, social life is the context that surrounds individuals and influences their thoughts and actions. Social constructionists, in contrast, construe the individual and society as mutually constitutive. Berger and Luckmann (1966) express this as a paradoxical trilogy of statements:

> Society is a human product.
> Society is an objective reality.
> Man is a social product. (p. 61)

Social constructionists favor terms such as *culture-in-mind* or *social mind* to describe the indissolubility of psyche and culture. Many prefer not to use the term *self*, because it signifies an independent and unitary entity. Instead, some speak about subjectivity. Others view people as taking up different subject positions as they move through various settings. Cole's (1996) definition of context is akin to the social constructionist view:

> In seeking uses of the term *context* which avoid the pitfalls of context as that which surrounds, I have found it useful to return to the Latin root of the term, contextere, which means "to weave together." A similar sense is given in the *Oxford English Dictionary*, which refers to context as the connected whole that gives coherence to its parts. (p. 135)

Social Constructionists Look at Phone Sex

Let us return to the phenomenon of phone sex to illuminate some of the ideas introduced in our overview. We draw on the interviews with phone sex workers conducted by Hall (1995). Interviewees said that they consciously strove to create themselves as the fantasy women their clients desired by manipulating their language. As sellers of a commodity, the workers were aware of the kind of women's language that is marketable as "sexy talk." They created sexy talk by using feminine or flowery words, inviting comments, and a dynamic intonation pattern (breathy, excited, varied in pitch, lilting). In North American culture, listeners often interpret these features of language as submissive or powerless (Lakoff, 1975). However, the workers on the fantasy lines did not feel powerless; they generally felt quite superior to their male callers, whom they characterized as unintelligent and socially inept.

Hall's study of phone sex illustrates a number of social constructionist themes. First, meaning is co-constructed through linguistic practice. The callers and the workers shared particular ideas of what constituted "sexiness." Workers drew on this shared cultural knowledge to present themselves as "sexy babes." Second, the phone conversations not only reproduced gendered power relations but also complicated and resisted such relations. On the fantasy lines, sex workers made deliberate use of feminine talk. Such talk is usually heard as submissive and powerless, but phone workers used it as a resource to exert some power. They enticed callers to part with their money. Perhaps they also exercised some control over callers' sexual arousal and, in that way, were able to prolong the time spent on the phone, thus earning more money. Third, the phone sex workers constructed accounts of social reality that enabled them to feel superior to their clients and effective in their jobs. They viewed their customers as inept. By their own accounts, phone workers' jobs had a number of advantages. The workers exercised some creativity as they generated characters and scripts. They earned a lot of money and had low overhead (e.g., they did not need expensive clothing, and they could work from home). And they could play at sex anonymously and at a distance, with no risk of violence, sexually transmitted diseases, or social sanctions. However, although individual workers gain some power, phone sex does not enhance the status or power of women collectively.

Hall's study invites still further constructionist questions. To the male callers, the fantasy woman constructed entirely through language was presumably satisfying. Callers paid well for the service, and many requested the same worker on repeat calls. But what accounts might callers offer of their own motives and behavior? How do they classify the women on the other end of the line? Whose accounts of phone sex and of phone sex workers are more likely to be heard, those of the callers or the workers? Furthermore, phone sex illustrates the constructionist contention that gender arrangements and categories are historically and culturally situated. Phone sex did not exist in the United States until recently, and it is absent in many other societies. Indeed, even the term *phone sex* is a recent coinage, and not every English speaker is privy to its meaning. Does the visibility of phone sex—even to those who do not participate in it—shift ideas about and evaluations of sex (perhaps especially masturbation)? Do phone sex, Internet sex, and other forms of anonymous, distanced sexual encounters undermine the link between emotional intimacy and sexuality (a linkage that, at least in our time and place, has been especially important to women)?

Finally, the phone sex study challenged several categories and constructs often used in producing accounts of sexual relationships. For example, one of the most successful phone sex workers was a man who impersonated a woman. Clearly, this man was adept in performing linguistic femininity. How can we account for his performance and the satisfaction he provided to male callers? Is he a stud? Is he a slut? Are the sexual encounters in which he engages homosexual ones? Heterosexual ones? Such categories cannot easily stretch to encompass a sexual encounter between two men, in which one poses as a woman and the other falsely believes his partner is a woman.

SOCIAL CONSTRUCTIONISM AND THE PSYCHOLOGY OF GENDER

Feminists adopted the term *gender* in the late 1970s to distinguish between biological mechanisms and the social aspects of maleness and femaleness. Unger, who introduced this formulation to mainstream psychology in 1979, defined gender as "those characteristics and traits socio-culturally considered appropriate to males and females," which she termed *masculinity* and *femininity* (p. 1085). In this formulation, sex is to gender as nature is to nurture; that is, sex pertains to what is biological or natural, whereas gender pertains to what is learned or cultural. The sex–gender dichotomy enabled psychologists to examine constructs such as sex roles, sex role socialization, and cultural norms of masculinity and femininity. The dichotomy is now commonplace in mainstream psychology. Indeed, it has been the basis for much psychological research intended to determine what is learned and what is inherent; what is malleable and what is not. An example is research on the femininity, masculinity, and sexual orientation of people with variations in hormonal or chromosomal components of biological sex. It has also fueled political and moral debates about what is natural and proper for each sex.

Social constructionists proceed from different formulations of both sex and gender. They reject the definition of gender as individual-level characteristics and traits set in place by social imperatives and cultural conditioning. They also question the idea that sex is the biological bedrock and gender is a mere cultural overlay. More specifically, social constructionists question the following aspects of the conventional sex–gender model: (1) the idea of gender as a property of individuals; (2) the idea of gender as static and enduring aspects of individuals; (3) the formulation of sex and gender as a dichotomy; and (4) the claim that biological sex is a bedrock that stands apart from and untouched by language and culture. Social constructionists take a dynamic approach to gender. Rather than regarding gender as individual personality or trait differences, they construe gender as a social process—the shared labor through which we are continually producing one another as male or female people. The phrase "doing gender" reflects the social constructionist view. As West and Zimmerman (1987) say,

> The "doing" of gender is undertaken by women and men whose competence as members of society is hostage to its production. Doing gender involves a complex of socially guided perceptual, interactional, and micropolitical activities that cast particular pursuits as expressions of masculine and feminine "natures." . . . Rather than as a property of individuals, we conceive of gender as an emergent feature of social situations: both as an outcome of and a rationale for various social arrangements and as a means of legitimating one of the most fundamental divisions of society. (p. 380)

Social constructionists also have a distinctive conception of biological sex. They do not take sex to be the immutable bedrock that precedes gender and remains after gender is stripped away. They do not regard sex, biology, and bodies as ahistorical and prediscursive "givens." What any cultural group takes to be natural does not reside outside the realm of interpretation and language. What are taken as biological facts are actually situated understandings lodged within webs of assumptions that shift from one cultural setting to another, from one epoch to another, and from perhaps from one subgroup to another within the same culture (e.g., Fausto-Sterling, 2000; Laqueur, 1990). Social constructionists set themselves the task of investigating the cultural meanings of bodies, biological processes, and embodied practices. In the next section, we show how a social constructionist approach offers new and generative ways to think about gender, sex, and sexuality.

THE PRODUCTION OF GENDER IN SOCIAL LIFE

Performing Gender

We begin by focusing on the individual and how he or she might enact gender in accord with the codes of his or her cultural surround. Let us return to phone sex to consider the gender performances that take place there. The phone lines are sites where shared ideas about women's language are overtly manipulated. The sex worker never meets the caller and knows nothing about him, yet she (or he) must convince him that she (or he) is a "hot babe," ready and willing to enjoy fantasy sex with him. Because the telephone as a medium does not allow for visual stimulation, the fantasy must be created in words alone. To create the illusion, Hall's (1995) phone workers drew on the idioms of pornography. Training manuals for the job told them to create stereotypical characters—bimbo, nymphomaniac, mistress, slave, lesbian, virgin. They were also instructed to be "bubbly, sexy, interesting, and interested" (pp. 190–191).

Another example of gender enactment comes from an early social constructionist project that examined how male-to-female transsexual individuals "pass" as a gender inconsistent with their biological sex.[1] Drawing on interviews, Kessler and McKenna (1978) showed the importance of speech style—vocabulary, intonation, and other pragmatic aspects. In addition, transsexual individuals self-consciously mimicked and practiced feminine modes of walking, standing, sitting, and gesturing. Cameron (1996) has nicely summarized the constructionist view of gender as a social performance:

> If I talk like a woman this is not just the inevitable outcome of the fact that I am a woman; it is one way I have of becoming a woman, producing myself *as* one. There is no such thing as "being a woman" outside the various practices that define womanhood for my culture—practices ranging from the sort of work I do to my sexual preferences to the clothes I wear to the way I use language. (p. 46)

Of course, gender performances are not limited to femininity. Indeed, femaleness and femininity can be enacted only in contrast to maleness and masculinity. For gender to remain a social classification system of some import, there must be people who enact masculinity. In a study of male U.S. college students' conversation while watching a televised basketball game, Cameron (1997) noted that, in addition to sports talk, the young men talked about daily events—going to classes, shopping for food—and their sexual exploits with women. (The male student who collected the data summarized their talk as "wine, women, and sports.") Another important topic was gossip about other (despised) men, whom they called "gay." Cameron interpreted such gossip as a way for the students to display their own heterosexual masculinity. These men distin-

[1] In 1978, when Kessler and McKenna wrote *Gender*, the term *transsexual* was standard usage to refer to people whose psychological gender identity was incongruent with their biological sex assignment, and who attempted to change the latter through hormonal treatment, surgery, or behavioral "passing."

guished themselves from "unmasculine" men by denigrating those men as "artsy-fartsy fags" and "homos." Cameron noted that this kind of discursive strategy "is not only *about* masculinity, it is a sustained performance *of* masculinity" (p. 590).

People have strong investments in particular ways of doing gender and in accounting for themselves as particular kinds of women or men. The basketball game viewers, for example, were invested in accounting for themselves not just as men but as *heterosexual* men. People may hold firm to certain accounts of themselves even when their behavior offers disconfirming evidence. In such cases, they may fabricate ingenious narratives that reconcile a preferred self-account with disconfirming behavior. For example, in a study of dating violence in young heterosexual couples, Parker (2002) found that some young women were adamant that they would not tolerate being hit by a boyfriend ("He hits me once and I'm out of there"). They were invested in constructing themselves as strong, autonomous, feminist women. When they were hit, they brought forward mitigating narratives that excused the violent incident as an exception ("He was drunk"; "He had a rough week"; "His family was giving him a lot of grief"). These narratives enabled a woman to remain in a relationship with a violent partner and still retain an image of herself as a strong woman who would not permit herself to be hit. Social constructionists take special interest in the discursive processes at hand to resolve such apparent contradictions. Focusing on these processes may shed light on the complex relationships among gender norms, gendered identities, and gender performances.

Cultural Repertoires of Gender

Members of a culture understand themselves and others through shared repertoires of meaning. Many social constructionists have studied aspects of everyday interactions that create and reaffirm gender difference, separateness, and hierarchy. To observe how gender is produced through joint social labor in everyday interactions, consider the talk of adolescent girls. Girls do many different things in talk. One of their most important accomplishments is to create and sustain friendships by sharing experiences and feelings in supportive ways. Girls also jointly construct their femininity: They enact what it is to be a girl in their particular community and culture. Coates (1996) recorded a conversation among four 16-year-old British girls about one girl as she tried on another girl's makeup. In complimenting her ("Doesn't she look really nice?"; "She does look nice"; "You should wear makeup more often"), they were being supportive friends. At the same time, however, they were drawing on, and jointly reaffirming, a cultural repertoire in which looking good is very important, and working on one's appearance is expected and rewarded.

Another example is girls' use of the cultural repertoires concerned with body size and shape. In a study of high school girls in Arizona, Nichter (2000) examined adolescent girls' talk about their bodies. Regardless of their weight and body size, the white girls complained regularly about being too fat ("I'm so fat"; "Look at these thighs"; "I look terrible in this"). Nichter analyzed the social uses of this incessant "fat talk." Girls' complaints about their weight served many social purposes. For example, "fat talk" called for support and reassurance from friends ("No, you look great"). It expressed solidarity and rapport with others. For example, a thin girl might complain about being fat as a means of establishing her sameness with other girls and showing that she does not think she is better than they are. A declaration of being fat might also constitute an apology for indulging in "fattening" food and a means to ward off others' condemnation ("I know I shouldn't be eating this; I'm so fat"). Yet even as such "fat talk" lubricates the gears of girls' social life, the litany of complaints and rebuttals about fat, and the continual references to fat, reaffirm body size as a key dimension on which women and girls are judged.

Contemporary repertoires of gender serve both to maintain the boundaries and distinctions between men and women and to keep women subordinated to men. They often naturalize or conceal unequal power relations, injustice, and even violent coercion. For example, women's suppression of their own needs and interests to meet those of their spouses and children may be attributed to maternal instinct, an ethic of care, female relationality, or a biological predisposition to "tend and befriend." Such formulations locate the origins of such behaviors within the individual, not in the matrix of social relations. Moreover, they imply that the behaviors are natural (and perhaps inevitable) expressions of female nature.

Even at the level of grammatical structures, forms of talk may maintain gender difference and domination. For example, speakers and writers across a variety of settings tend to use passive-voice constructions and euphemisms that excuse or minimize men's culpability for violence against women. Rather than saying that a man raped a woman, one says, "She was raped," "A rape was committed," or even more euphemistically, "The incident occurred." Indeed, one study quoted a physician's report that stated, "Patient was hit in the face by a fist" (Phillips & Henderson, 1999). Such grammatical practices have been noted in medical and behavioral science writing, newspaper reports, accounts by convicted rapists, courtroom transcripts, and in the talk of experts on rape prevention (Crawford, 1995; Lamb, 1991).

The Production of Sexual Bodies

Social constructionists do not deny that genes, hormones, and brain physiology may have effects on behavior and morphology. However their interest lies in the accounts that people give about sexual bodies, the cultural meanings inscribed on the body, and the social implications of those meanings. Kessler (1998) studied intersexed children (i.e., children born with ambiguous genitalia), pediatricians, and parents. In the United States, it is standard medical practice to alter surgically an infant's genitals when they are deemed ambiguous. The procedures are difficult, painful, sometimes protracted, and may produce infertility or permanent loss of the capacity for sexual pleasure. The assignment of an intersexed infant to the category male or female, and the surgical interventions that follow, are based primarily on the size of the infant's phallic structure. The size difference between a medically acceptable penis and a medically acceptable clitoris is a mere 1½ centimeters—a difference that might not even be noticeable to laypeople. The purpose of "corrective" surgery is to create male and female genitals as unmistakably different structures. Surely, this is a radical example of social construction: The physical body is reconstructed to match what is considered to be the proper appearance of male or female anatomy.

The episode of the "Hottentot Venus" affords another example of how bodies are inscribed with social significance. The Hottentot Venus, a southern African woman given the name Saartjie Baartman, had genitals and buttocks that became the focus of overwhelming interest and curiosity in late 19th-century Europe. Baartman was described in the scientific literature of the day as having labia that reached her knees and abnormally large buttocks. European doctors, public health officials, and anthropologists regarded these physical characteristics as "primitive" and indicative of the uncontrolled sexual appetites of African women (Gilman, 1985). Baartman was crudely exhibited in the nude at scientific meetings, then as a public spectacle. She (and black African women in general) thus served as an example of moral degeneracy, a model of what a white woman was not and should not be (Hammonds, 1997). Claims about Baartman's primitive sexuality also bolstered Europeans' claims of the civilizing influence and moral "upliftment" brought to Africa by European imperialism. In the United States, claims of black women's hypersexuality entered into Reconstruction era debates about whether blacks in America were entitled to citizenship (Giddings, 1984).

Sex Categories

Thus far, we have reviewed constructionist explorations of the cultural meanings ascribed to anatomy. Now, we turn to a more fundamental cultural construction, the sex categorization system itself. In contemporary Western societies, biological sex and sex category are conflated; that is, the agreed-upon criterion for classification as a member of one or the other sex is male or female external genitalia. Moreover, the idea of two, and only two, sex categories has achieved the status of biological, psychological, and moral certainty. Nonetheless, genitalia are usually not available for public inspection. In fact, the demonstrable existence of one or another kind of genitalia is actually irrelevant to the ascertainment of sex category in everyday life. People rely instead on insignias of sex (apparel, names, hair length) as proxies for the genitals that cannot be seen.

Social constructionists have challenged the commonsense idea that there can be only two sexes, as determined by genital dimorphism. They have pointed to social settings in which this does not hold. First, there are individuals who deliberately display a sexual insignia that is discordant with their genitals. These individuals range from some whose displays are relatively transitory—such as the male phone-sex worker who convinced callers that they were interacting with a woman—to others who "pass" for most of their lives. The Internet is a site where some people experiment with sex categories. Some chat room denizens manipulate sexual insignias (names, biographies, verbal style) to assume a sexual identity other than their off-line one. The motive may be playful experimentation, encouraged by the anonymity and distance that the Internet provides (Herrup, 2001). But the deception may also have less innocent goals. For example, a male psychiatrist posing as a woman named Joan initiated numerous on-line intimate relationships with women. His motive was a voyeuristic interest in "lesbian cybersex" (Van Gelder, 1985).

The conventional Western view that there can be only two sexes is not universally shared. For example, in India, *hijras* constitute a third sex category. It is not genitalia that determine whether one is a *hijra*. Some *hijras* are physical hermaphrodites, others have male genitalia, and still others were born with male genitalia but elected to undergo castration. *Hijras* adopt female names and wear women's clothing. However, they do not attempt to pass as women. Their manner of displaying female insignias—heavy makeup; long, unbound hair; sexualized gestures—sets them apart from women in general and marks them as *hijras* (Nanda, 1990).

In Thailand, *kathoeys* represent a third sex. A *kathoey* has male genitalia but dresses in women's clothing. But a *kathoey* is not a man who wishes to be (or become) a woman. Nor do *kathoeys* believe that they have "a woman's mind" trapped inside the "wrong body" (an account that some American and European transsexuals give of themselves). According to Herdt, a *kathoey* "takes some pride in his male genitals" (1997, p. 149). Moreover, most *kathoeys,* like most *hijras*, do not wish to pass unobtrusively as women. They behave and dress in dramatic, loud, brash ways that violate the norms of femininity in Thai culture, thus distinguishing them from women. Transgender and transsexual activists in the United States also maintain that it is possible to have more than two sex categories and that a sex category need not be defined by biological sex. The increasingly visible and vocal "trans" movement has put forward an abundance of sex categories: "FTM [Female-to-Male], MTF [Male-to-Female], eonist, invert, androgyne, butch, femme, Nellie, queen, third sex, hermaphrodite, tomboy, sissy, drag king, female impersonator, she-male, he-she, boy-dyke, girlfag, transsexual, transvestite, transgender, cross-dresser" (Stryker, 1998, p. 148).

"Trans" activism has produced not only a bumper crop of new gender–sex categories but also competing accounts of what they mean. The term *transsexual* once referred to someone in transition from one sex to the other. However, some who identify as transsexual or transgendered do not regard themselves as either "in between" one sex and another or "in transition" from one to another. Rather, they regard "trans" as another sex category (Bornstein, 1994; Elliot & Roen, 1998). Like *hijras* and *kathoeys*, they do not wish to pass as men or women. Rather, they wish to make their crossing visible, to pose it as a counter to the dominant account that there are only two sexes. The alternate designation, *genderqueer*, which some prefer, makes this aspect of identity more salient. As Jeffrey Weeks (1995, p. 104) says, the intent is "to upset the dominant cultural codes and reveal their irrationality, partiality, and illegitimacy." Indeed, the transgender movement can be seen as guerilla warfare against dominant constructions of sex, gender, and sexuality—dramatized enactments of social constructionism.

Sex, like gender, draws meaning from shifting cultural understandings and ever-changing social practices. Sex categorization is a matter of insignias and performances (as in on-line manipulations). These categorizations are culture-bound: Westerners, for example, often do not recognize *hijras* when they interact with them; to locals, however, *hijra*s are unmistakable. In the United States, the rising visibility of trans individuals in popular culture, along with an increase in "trans" activism and political organizations, suggests that our system of sex categorization is destabilizing, shifting, and expanding.

The Construction of Sexuality

Humans engage in a variety of sexual and erotic practices whose meanings and morality vary across historical era and cultural context

(D'Emilio & Freedman, 1988). What is erotic and arousing in some cultures may be offensive and repellent in others. Romantic attraction to members of one's own sex category has different meanings worldwide. Sexual activity between people of the same sex (which may or may not involve romantic attraction or emotional intimacy) also has different meanings. For example, in many societies, sexual activity between young unmarried men is considered developmentally normal and appropriate. In some societies, adult–child sexual stimulation is considered appropriate. For the Sambia of New Guinea, for example, boy-insemination was a common practice until a few decades ago. Semen transfer from older male relatives to prepubescent boys was regarded as necessary to bring boys to mature manhood (Herdt, 1997). Although bodily pleasure may have been involved, the primary motive was familial obligation on the part of the adult partner. In summary, the meanings of same-sex activity and the values attached to it vary widely across cultures.

The meanings and values attached to same-sex activity within European and American societies have also varied widely across time. For example, in the 19th century, many women in North America had intense friendships, in which they spent weeks at each others' homes, slept in the same beds, and exchanged passionate and tender letters describing the joys of perfect love and the agonies of parting. Heterosexual marriage ended many of these relationships, but others endured over a lifetime. At the time, no one—including the individuals involved—labeled these women homosexuals or lesbians (Faderman, 1981; Smith-Rosenberg, 1975). Their relationships clearly involved romance, attachment, and physical intimacy, though we have no way of knowing how many involved genital contact. Were these women "really" lesbians? From a constructionist point of view, the answer is emphatically "no." Imputing the definitions, meanings, terms, and concerns of our day to the past is an error.

If our contemporary categories of sexual desire (heterosexual, homosexual, bisexual) do not carve nature at its joints, then what are their meanings? Let us look briefly at some recent definitions of the term *lesbian* by lesbian women:

> . . . a woman who loves women, who chooses women to nurture and support and to create a living environment in which to work creatively and independently, whether or not her relations with these women are sexual. (Cook, quoted in Golden, 1987, p. 20)

> . . . a woman who has sexual and erotic–emotional ties primarily with women or who sees herself as centrally involved with a community of self-identified lesbians. (Ferguson, quoted in Golden, 1987, p. 21)

> It is not having genital intercourse with a woman that is the criterion. There are lesbian women who have never had genital or any other form of sexual contact with a woman, while there are also women who have had sex with other women but who are not lesbian. (Lorde, quoted in Wekker, 1997, p. 18)

A further example is *political lesbians*, a term for women who choose to have relationships with women because heterosexual relationships constitute "sleeping with the enemy" (Kitzinger, 1987).

These varying definitions of the term *lesbian* have been a matter of lively dispute. Some lesbians regard political lesbians as inauthentic and set them apart from "true" lesbians. Others object to characterizations such as Lorde's, because they downplay eroticism and sexuality in lesbians' lives—in their view, a concession to the "nice girl" standards of traditional femininity. The category "lesbian" is a contested one, with multiple meanings related to erotic practices, choice of a sexual partner, emotional attachments, political commitments, and resistance to male dominance. Different individuals endorse different meanings, and the same individual might endorse different meanings at different times.

Researchers and clinicians often rely on the typology of heterosexual, homosexual, and bisexual orientations to categorize and describe sexualities. But everyday understandings and practices concerned with sexual identity and sexualities are considerably more variegated, complex, and ambiguous. The term *sexual orientation* implies a deep-seated and enduring inclination. This way of accounting for sexuality is not universal; rather, it is specific to our time and place. The idea that one's erotic attractions, sexual activities, or emotional attachments necessarily confer a social identity is similarly an account limited to particular cultural contexts. (In Sri Lanka, sexual activity between young men is common and unremarkable, but "homosexuality" is regarded as a vile and decadent product of the West.) Moreover, even in our own society, there is reason to question the notion of such enduring "orientations." Diamond (2000), for example, found that among young women she interviewed, fully 50% of those who described themselves as lesbian or bisexual at the time of the first interview had changed their sexual identity (i.e., their self-described sexual predisposition) more than once by the time of a follow-up interview 2 years later. Golden (1987) found that a substantial portion of the college-age women she interviewed regarded their choice of sexuality as elective and, thus, open to change. Moreover, people's accounts of their sexual identities (e.g., straight, gay, lesbian, bisexual) can be discordant with their sexual practices. For example, Bart (1993) found that many women who identified themselves as lesbians continued to do so even when they were involved in a sexual relationship with a man. Similarly, some men identify themselves as heterosexual even though they have sex with both men and women. In other words, in everyday practice, the social category "lesbian" is not the same as "women who have sex with women," and the social category "male homosexual" is not the same as "men who have sex with men." Self-categorization (e.g., as straight, gay, lesbian, or bisexual) and selection of a sexual partner are separable.

In some cultural groups in the United States, members hold alternative meanings of categories of sexual identity or use different categories altogether. In some Latino subcultures, the Spanish term equivalent to *homosexual* refers only to men who assume the passive, receiver role (coded as feminine) in sexual relations with men (Almaguer, 1991; Carrier, 1976). Also, some people identify themselves as bisexual to announce that they are attracted to people and not to gender categories. Others label themselves as *ambisexual*; they reject the term *bisexual* as inherently conservative, because it encodes the idea of two and only two sexes. Others adopt the term *spectrum person* to indicate that they see sexuality on a continuum and refuse to be pigeonholed into any category. Still others identify as *queer*, a term that does not refer to any particular sexual/erotic practice, but rather signifies a commitment to "dismantl[ing] the standardizing apparatus that organizes all manner of sexual practices into 'facts' of sexual identity" (Berlant & Freeman, 1993, p. 196).

These on-the-ground accounts of sexual identity and sexual practice are of great interest to social constructionists. It is in terms of these accounts that people live their lives, form identities, forge close relationships, and make judgments about others. Understanding the narratives of sexual lives and identities that flow from these accounts is a project with considerable practical import (e.g., for HIV/AIDS prevention programs). It is also a project for which constructionist research tools are ideally suited. Social constructionists are also concerned with the political implications of different typologies and category systems. For example, some people substitute the term *sexual preference* for *sexual orientation*; others reject that term on the grounds that it implies that one's sexuality is chosen, thus supporting conservatives' efforts to "reform" gay and lesbian people. Some use the term *affectional preference* to indicate that their relationships are not limited to sexual activity; others reject that term as glossing over physical desire and sexual acts, thus contributing to the continued invisibility of sexual diversity.

The proliferation of categories and meanings of sexual identities reflects contemporary grassroots resistance to authoritative pronouncements about sexuality. But, as is often the case, such resistance is double-edged. On the positive side, it signifies emancipation from received categories and a refusal to live with stigmatized and pathologized identities. On the negative side, however, the destabilization of categorization schemes may inhibit social change. Without a collective identity, a marginalized group cannot easily mobilize for social change. If sexuality is socially constructed as unstable, fluctuating, and unmoored from identity, the movement for equal rights for sexual minorities could lose its core membership and its political purpose.

THE VALUE OF SOCIAL CONSTRUCTIONISM

We have introduced social constructionism as a theory of knowledge and have discussed a variety of constructionist inquiries into gender, sex, and sexuality. We have suggested that it has opened important areas of investigation. Furthermore, it has served as the epistemological grounding for some new social movements related to sex and gender. We now consider in general terms the value of social constructionism for advancing the psychology of gender. We identify four areas of contributions that social constructionists have made thus far.

Pragmatic Empiricism

Constructionists' projects are often designed to yield knowledge that is of immediate practical use. Several projects we have described were born out of a commitment to social transformation; some incorporated an action component. External validity, often a scarce commodity in laboratory research, is a forte of constructionist inquiry. By investigating mundane activities and forms of talk in real-life locales, researchers come to grips with social reality in an intimate and firsthand way. The interventions that flow from these projects may be tailored to the specific situations and social groups that the researcher has investigated. Moreover, because researchers draw their constructs and categories directly from the lexicon of their research participants, their findings are more readily communicated to the communities from which the participants were drawn.

Social constructionists do not seek to make generalized claims about human behavior that transcend a particular time, place, and social group. Nonetheless, their projects may contribute to general knowledge. The constructs and themes emerging from a particular investigation may serve as sensitizing devices for subsequent investigations, action projects, or therapeutic interventions. More generally, by calling attention to what is taken for granted, social constructionists can bring into view what was heretofore unseen. By "denaturalizing" what might have seemed natural and inevitable, social constructionists' knowledge can make a space for political debate, and perhaps for social and political change.

Building Bridges to Other Disciplines and to Global Psychologies

In our view, social constructionism can be a bridge to other disciplines, psychologies, and intellectual movements. It has aspects in common with the influential intellectual movements grouped under the rubric postmodernism; thus, it can link psychology to disciplines such as cultural studies, feminist/gender studies, and critical theory. Social constructionism is also kin to rich and fruitful sociological and anthropological traditions such as symbolic interactionism, practice theories, and ethnomethodology (cf. Holstein & Gubrium, 2003). Social construction theory and practice may also serve to connect psychology in the United States to intellectual developments in the psychologies of the United Kingdom, Europe, Australia, and New Zealand. Indeed, much of the research that we have cited was carried out in these countries.

Conceptual Innovation and Critique

Social constructionists study the meanings, category systems, and narrative logic of the conceptual worlds that people inhabit. Understanding these conceptual worlds is crucial to understanding how people explain themselves and others, and how they justify and interpret various forms of conduct. In many cases, these everyday construals do not map closely onto formal scientific categories (e.g., recall the plethora of emerging categories designating alternative genders and categories of sexuality).

Social constructionists have also turned attention to the scientific categories and constructs used by psychologists. They have investigated how cultural ideologies, social forces, and historical events shape these categories and constructs, as well as the production of knowledge in psychology more generally. They have also examined how psychological knowledge reaffirms certain cultural ideologies and justifies certain social practices by imbuing them with scientific legitimacy. Feminist social constructionists have been critical of a variety of constructs and categories pertaining to gender and sexuality. For instance, they have challenged the ontological status of categories such as female masochism, male sex drive, PMS, and the human sexual response cycle.

For social constructionists, knowledge is always situated and partial; inevitably, it reflects the perspectives, position, and investments of the knower. For this reason, many constructionist researchers make themselves visible in their research reports by describing who they are and what political commitments they have. In this way, they engage readers in an inquiry into how researchers' subjectivity may have shaped the research process and its outcomes. Some researchers have experimented with innovative procedures designed to accommodate and make use of the partial and perspectival nature of knowledge. For example, to analyze open-ended narratives collected from gay men and lesbians, Russell (2000) assembled a team of five gay and straight people from diverse educational, religious, and socioeconomic backgrounds. The team's prolonged discussion of divergent coding schemes was central to the interpretive work and to Russell's analytical stance. For a social constructionist, a researcher's standpoint influences not only the interpretation of the findings but also the choice of research questions, the way the questions are framed, and preferred methodological strategies for collecting data.

Critical Reflection on Psychology

Social constructionism invites critical reflection on knowledge-making practices. Such critical reflection goes beyond an evaluation of methodological adequacy to encompass value-based, ethical, and political concerns as well. These reflections start with the recognition that psychologists, like other members of the culture, cannot divorce themselves from the cultural surround or from its system of meanings. Categories of psychological knowledge are not a priori givens but are historically specific acts of meaning. Some investigations have excavated the history of psychological concepts (e.g., intelligence, development, self, and stress). These investigations also trace the social structures and practices that such scientific constructs served to justify. Other investigations concern the historical and sociological processes that have formed the discipline. For example, Morawski (1988) and others have investigated the rise of experimentation in North American psychology. Porter (1955) has probed the historical circumstances that led to the reliance on quantification and trust in statistics. Danziger (1977) has examined psychology's predilections for naming and measuring the mind. Such critical reflections can make the generation of knowledge more sophisticated conceptually, empirically, and politically, no matter which methods of inquiry researchers use.

REFERENCES

Almaguer, T. (1991). Chicano men: A cartography of homosexual identity and behavior. *Differences: A Journal of Feminist Cultural Studies*, *3*, 76–100.

Bart, P. (1993). Protean women: The liquidity of female sexuality and the tenacity of lesbian identity. In S. Wilkinson & C. Kitzinger (Eds.), *Heterosexuality: A "Feminism and Psychology" reader* (pp. 246–252). London: Sage.

Berger, P. L., & Luckmann, T. (1966). *The social construction of reality.* New York: Anchor.

Berlant, L., & Freeman, E. (1993). Queer nationality. In M. Warner (Ed.), *Fear of a queer planet* (pp. 193–229). Minneapolis: University of Minnesota Press.

Bornstein, K. (1994). *Gender outlaw: On men, women and the rest of us.* New York: Routledge.

Cameron, D. (1996). The language–gender interface: Challenging co-optation. In V. L. Bergvall, J. M. Bing, & A. F. Freed (Eds.), *Rethinking language and gender research: Theory and practice* (pp. 31–53). New York: Addison-Wesley/Longman.

Cameron, D. (1997). Performing gender identity: Young men's talk and the construction of heterosexual masculinity. In S. Johnson & U. H. Meinhof (Eds.), *Language and masculinity* (pp. 47–64). Oxford, UK: Blackwell.

Carrier, J. M. (1976). Cultural factors affecting urban Mexican male homosexual behavior. *Archives of Sexual Behavior*, *5*, 103–124.

Coates, J. (1996). *Women talk.* Oxford, UK: Blackwell.

Cole, M. (1996). *Cultural psychology.* Cambridge, MA: Harvard University Press.

Crawford, M. (1995). *Talking difference.* London: Sage.

Crawford, M., & Popp, D. (2003). Sexual double standards: A review and methodological critique of two decades of research. *Journal of Sex Research*, *40*, 13–26.

Danziger, K. (1997). *Naming the mind: How psychology found its language.* Thousand Oaks, CA: Sage.

D'Emilio, J., & Freedman, E. B. (1988). *Intimate matters: A history of sexuality in America.* New York: Harper & Row.

Diamond, L. M. (2000). Sexual identity, attractions, and behavior among young sexual-minority women over a two-year period. *Developmental Psychology*, *36*, 241–250.

Elliot, P., & Roen, K. (1998). Transgenderism and the question of embodiment. *GLQ—A Journal of Lesbian and Gay Studies*, *4*, 231–261.

Faderman, L. (1981). *Surpassing the love of men: Romantic friendship and love between women from the Renaissance to the present.* New York: Morrow.

Fausto-Sterling, A. (2000). *Sexing the body.* New York: Basic Books.

Foucault, M. (1972). *The archaeology of knowledge.* New York: Pantheon.

Gavey, N. (1992). Technologies and effects of heterosexual coercion. *Feminism and Psychology, 2,* 325–351.

Gergen, K. G. (1985). The social constructionist movement in modern psychology. *American Psychologist, 40,* 266–275.

Giddings, P. (1984). *When and where I enter.* New York: Bantam.

Gilman, S. L. (1985). Black bodies, white bodies: Toward an iconography of female sexuality in late 19th century art, medicine, and literature. *Critical Inquiry, 12,* 204–242.

Golden, C. (1987). Diversity and variability in women's sexual identities. In Boston Lesbian Psychologies Collective (Eds.), *Lesbian psychologies* (pp. 18–34). Urbana: University of Illinois Press.

Hall, K. (1995). Lip service on the fantasy lines. In K. Hall & M. Bucholtz (Eds.), *Gender articulated: Language and the socially constructed self* (pp. 183–216). New York: Routledge.

Hammonds, E. M. (1997). Toward a genealogy of black female sexuality: The problematic of silence. In M. J. Alexander & C. T. Mohanty (Eds.), *Feminist genealogies, colonial legacies, democratic futures* (pp. 152–170). New York: Routledge.

Hare-Mustin, R., & Marecek, J. (1990). *Making a difference: Psychology and the construction of gender.* New Haven, CT: Yale University Press.

Henriques, J. (1998). Social psychology and the politics of racism. In J. Henriques, W. Hollway, C. Urwin, C. Venn, & V. Walkerdine (Eds.), *Psychology and the social regulation of subjectivity* (pp. 60–89). London: Methuen.

Herdt, G. (1997). *Same sex, different cultures.* Boulder, CO: Westview Press.

Herrup, M. J. (2001). Virtual identity. In M. Crawford & R. Unger (Eds.), *In our own words: Writings from women's lives* (2nd ed., pp. 210–216). Boston: McGraw-Hill.

Hollway, W. (1989). *Subjectivity and method in psychology.* London: Sage.

Holstein, J. A., & Gubrium, J. F. (2003). *Inner lives and social worlds.* New York: Oxford University Press.

Kessler, S. J. (1998). *Lessons from the intersexed.* New Brunswick, NJ: Rutgers University Press.

Kessler, S. J., & McKenna, W. (1978). *Gender: An ethnomethodological approach.* Chicago: University of Chicago Press.

Kitzinger, C. (1987). *The social construction of lesbianism.* London: Sage.

Lakoff, R. (1975). *Language and woman's place.* New York: Harper & Row.

Lamb, S. (1991). Acts without agents. *American Journal of Orthopsychiatry, 61,* 250–257.

Laqueur, T. (1990). *Making sex: Body and gender from the Greeks to Freud.* Cambridge, MA: Harvard University Press.

Morawski, J. G. (1988). *The rise of experimentation in American psychology.* New Haven, CT: Yale University Press.

Nanda, S. (1990). *Neither man nor woman: The* hijras *of India.* Belmont, CA: Wadsworth.

Nichter, M. (2000). *Fat talk*. Cambridge, MA: Harvard University Press.

Oransky, M., & Marecek, J. (2002). *Doing boy*. Unpublished manuscript, Swarthmore College, PA.

Orenstein, P. (1994). *Schoolgirls: Young women, self-esteem, and the confidence gap*. New York: Doubleday.

Parker, L. M. (2002). *Love me long time*. Unpublished doctoral dissertation, University of Waikato, New Zealand.

Parlee, M. B. (1994). The social construction of premenstrual syndrome: A case study in scientific discourse as cultural contestation. In M. G. Winkler & L. B. Cole (Eds.), *The good body: Asceticism in contemporary culture* (pp. 91–107). New Haven, CT: Yale University Press.

Parlee, M. B. (1998). Situated knowledges of personal embodiment: Transgender activists' and psychological theorists' perspectives on "sex" and "gender." In H. J. Stam (Ed.), *The body and psychology* (pp. 120–140). London: Sage.

Phillips, D., & Henderson, D. (1999). "Patient was hit in the face by a fist . . . ": A discourse analysis of violence against women. *American Journal of Orthopsychiatry*, *69*, 116–121.

Porter, T. M. (1995). *Trust in numbers: The pursuit of objectivity in science and public life*. Princeton, NJ: Princeton University Press.

Potter, J., & Wetherell, M. (1987). *Discourse and social psychology*. London: Sage.

Russell, G. M. (2000). *Voted out: The psychological consequences of anti-gay politics*. New York: New York University Press.

Smith-Rosenberg, C. (1975). The female world of love and ritual: Relations between women in nineteenth-century America. *Signs*, *1*, 1–30.

Stryker, S. (1998). The transgender issue. *GLQ—A Journal of Lesbian and Gay Studies*, *4*, 145–158.

Unger, R. K. (1979). Toward a redefinition of sex and gender. *American Psychologist*, *34*, 1085–1094.

Van Gelder, L. (1985). The strange case of the electronic lover. In C. Dunlop & R. Kling (Eds.), *Computerization and controversy: Value conflicts and social choices* (2nd ed., pp. 364–375). Boston: Academic Press.

Weeks, J. (1995). *Invented moralities: Sexual values in an age of uncertainty*. New York: Columbia University Press.

Wekker, G. (1997). Mati-ism and black lesbianism: Two idealtypical expressions of female homosexuality in black communities of the Diaspora. *Journal of Lesbian Studies*, *1*, 11–24.

West, C., & Zimmerman, D. H. (1987). Doing gender. *Gender and Society*, *1*, 125–151.

10

Gender As Status

An Expectation States Theory Approach

CECILIA L. RIDGEWAY
CHRIS BOURG

In human societies, gender always expands beyond biological traits and behaviors that are related to sexuality and reproduction. It becomes a social *system* of difference and similarity that acts as one of a society's major principles for organizing social relations among individuals and groups across the full range of human activity. A society's widely held gender stereotypes are the "genetic code" of this gender system, because such stereotypes contain the cultural rules or schemas for defining what is socially expected of men and women, and for organizing social relations on the basis of enactments of these definitions. Expectation states theory points out that gender stereotypes contain at their core *status beliefs* that socially evaluate men as generally more superior and diffusely more competent than women, while granting each sex its specialized skills (Ridgeway, 2001a; Wagner & Berger, 1997). The theory argues that because gender is associated with status in cultural beliefs, it becomes a principle for organizing social relations in terms of not only difference but also of hierarchy and inequality.

Expectation states theory is a sociological theory of status and influence hierarchies rather than of gender per se (Berger, Fisek, Norman, & Zelditch, 1977; Berger & Zeldtich, 1998). As such, however, the theory is distinctively positioned to explain how gender becomes a pervasive, if often subtle, basis for inequality in everyday social encounters. It offers a well-documented account of how gender, through the status beliefs associated with it, affects who is listened to in social encounters, who is judged to have the best ideas or the most ability, who rises to leadership, and who is directed toward or away from positions of power and influence in society.

The theory's predictions about the impact of gender status beliefs on men's and women's behaviors and evaluations have points in common with some of those recently proposed by social role theory (Eagly & Karau, 2002; Eagly, Wood, & Johannesen-Schmidt, Chapter 12, this volume). The status approach, however, allows us to examine systematically the extent to which observed gender differences in social behavior are unique to gender or are due to common status processes that also produce behavioral differences along other status distinctions such as occupation, race, or education. As we see, some common gender differences actually covary more strongly with status position than with sex category of the actor. By directing our attention to the way gender status beliefs embed a hierarchical element into our very understanding of "who" men and women are or should be, expectation states theory provides special insight into the processes through which the enactment of gender also becomes the enactment of inequality.

The status approach also has some elements in common with social dominance theory's analysis of gender and power (Sidanius & Pratto, 1999; Pratto & Walker, Chapter 11, this volume). Like social dominance theory, the status approach views the association between gender and power as a dynamic process that is affected by processes at both the interpersonal and social structural levels. Gender status beliefs, according to expectation states theory, function much like the consensual ideologies emphasized by social dominance theory, in that they prescribe and legitimate status and power differences between men and women. Expectation states theory, however, develops a detailed account of the circumstances and processes through which gender status beliefs create power and influence differences between men and women. Unlike social dominance theory, the status approach makes no assumptions about individual or gender differences in personal propensities to dominance, although it is not incompatible with such assumptions. Rather, the status approach emphasizes the way people's cultural beliefs about status shape their behaviors and evaluations, independent of their own personal traits.

In this chapter, we review expectation states theory's account of how the status culturally linked to gender organizes social relations between men and women, and constructs gender as a system of inequality in social outcomes, as well as difference in social behavior. As we see, expectation states theory is primarily about *how* gender inequality is enacted and sustained in contemporary society, rather than an effort to trace the origins of gender inequality. We begin with an examination of the nature of status beliefs and their relationship to the content of gender stereotypes. Next, we turn to the core arguments of expectation states theory and its predictions about the impact of gender status on social behaviors and evaluations. To examine the validity of these predictions, we review the research literature on gender differences in task-related behaviors and influence, evaluations of competence and inferences of ability, the emergence and exercise of leadership, and the legitimacy of authority. Then, we take up the question of the emergence of status beliefs. Finally, we consider expectation states theory's arguments about policies for counteracting the effects of gender status and reducing gender inequality.

STATUS BELIEFS

Status beliefs are widely shared cultural beliefs that inform people of the status relationship between one social group and another in their society. Status beliefs are most often associated with social groups created by distinctions, such as occupation, gender, race, education, or ethnicity, that are important for organizing social relations in a given society. Status beliefs attach greater social significance and competence, as well as differing specific skills, to persons in one category of a social distinction (professionals, men, whites) compared to those in another (laborers, women, people of color) (Berger et al., 1977). By linking competence to evaluative significance, status beliefs legitimate inequality between people from different social categories.

Expectation states theory refers to social distinctions associated with status beliefs in a society as *status characteristics*. There is clear evidence that gender is a status characteristic in the United States and most societies. Gender stereotypes include largely shared beliefs that associate greater overall status and competence with men than with women, particularly in socially valued arenas of instrumental competence, while granting each sex specialized skills, such as mechanical ability for men and nurturing skills for women (e.g., Broverman, Vogel, Broverman, Clarkson, & Rosenkrantz, 1972; Fiske, Cuddy, Glick, & Xu, 2002; Spence & Buckner, 2000; Williams & Best, 1990). Although women are currently evaluated at least as favorably as men in the United States and Canada, the growing positive associations with women are largely based on women's presumed communal qualities which, in turn, are seen as less socially valued than men's instrumental qualities (Eagly & Mladinic, 1994).

People acquire status beliefs about important social distinctions in their society, including gender, in the same way that they learn other taken-for-granted cultural beliefs and rules: primarily through socialization processes, such as those involving peers, parents, and the media. Although gender status beliefs are widely held by adolescents and adults in the United States (e.g., Fiske et al., 2002; Spence & Buckner, 2000), it is not clear at what age children fully take on gender status beliefs. There is evidence that, as early as 2 or 3 years of age, boys show greater preference for same-sex activities and companions than girls, and children of this age appear to recognize the differential social evaluation attached to male and female roles (see Bussey & Bandura, Chapter 5, this volume). Yet evidence is mixed about whether boys and girls in elementary school have fully developed gender status beliefs that differentially shape their assumptions about competence and their willingness to speak up in class or accept influence from others (Leal-Idrogo, 1997; Lockheed, Harris, & Nemceff, 1983). By secondary school, however, children generally act as though they have fully taken on gender status beliefs (see Persell, James, Kang, & Snyder, 1999, for a review).

As beliefs about the evaluative relation between social groups, status beliefs are distinctive in that they are *consensual* rather than competitive beliefs about ingroup superiority (Tajfel & Turner, 1986). Both those who are advantaged and those who are disadvantaged by a status belief accept, as a matter of social reality, that "most people" believe that persons in the advantaged group are more respected and competent than those in the disadvantaged group (Jackman, 1994; Jost & Burgess, 2001; Ridgeway, Boyle, Kuipers, & Robinson, 1998). Members of the dominant rather than subordinate group may be more likely to endorse status beliefs personally rather than merely accept them as descriptive beliefs (Ridgeway et al., 1998). Whether or not individuals personally endorse culturally predominant status beliefs, however, the assumption that most people share these beliefs leads individuals to assume that others will judge them by those beliefs. As a result, these individuals must take culturally predominant status beliefs into account in their own behavior (Seachrist & Stangor, 2001). The cultural presumption that status beliefs are widely shared gives them force in organizing social relations.

Consensual status beliefs, rather than beliefs favoring each competing ingroup, are most likely to develop among groups whose members must regularly cooperate to achieve what they want or need (Glick & Fiske, 1999; Jackman, 1994; Ridgeway et al., 1998). Compared to other group distinctions, gender has a number of unusual characteristics that cause men and women to interact frequently under conditions of cooperative interdependence (Ridgeway & Smith-Lovin, 1999). Sexuality and reproduction uniquely increase interaction and interdependence between the sexes. Also, gender divides people into two, roughly equal-size groups, which increases the chance of interaction, and gender crosscuts kin relations, which further encourages interaction and cooperation. Although cooperative interdependence alone does not produce status beliefs, when it exists as a structural feature of interaction between two or more groups, it dramatically increases the likelihood that status beliefs about the groups will develop. In this way, the unusual cooperative interdependence between men and women has played an important role in the development of status beliefs about gender in most societies (Williams & Best, 1990).

STATUS AND STEREOTYPE CONTENT

When status beliefs develop about a social distinction such as gender or race, the beliefs form an element in the cultural stereotypes of the groups delineated by the distinction, although these stereotypes contain nonstatus elements as well. Expectation states theory argues that the specific skills associated in status beliefs with one group compared to another reflect the particular history and social structural circumstances of the groups' relationship with one another and may change over time. Gender, racial, and occupational stereotypes differ in many ways, for instance. Yet each of these stereotypes retains a characteristic, core status content that advantages one category of the social distinction over others in status worthiness and competence at the things that count most in society at the time. Because of the similar core status content in their stereotypes, expectation states theory argues, different social distinctions such as gender, race, and occupation can have comparable effects on the hierarchical organization of social relations among people who differ on these social distinctions (Webster & Foschi, 1988).

Growing evidence indicates that the core status content that becomes embedded in some group stereotypes derives partly from people's shared conceptions of the nature of status relations between individuals (Conway, Pizzamiglio, & Mount, 1996; Geis, Brown, Jennings, & Corrado-Taylor, 1984; Gerber, 1996; Wagner & Berger, 1997). Status relations are unusual in that they exist both between social groups in a society, as expressed in cultural status beliefs, and between individuals in interpersonal hierarchies based on respect, influence, and social esteem. When people interact in regard to collective goals, inequalities quickly develop in how much each person participates, the attention and evaluations their efforts receive, and how influential they become (see

Ridgeway, 2001b, for a review). The emergence of these status and influence hierarchies casts the participants into characteristic behavior profiles that affect how they are perceived (Wagner & Berger, 1997). On the one hand, the more influential participants appear proactive and agentic. The less influential people, on the other hand, are cast into the role of reactors whose attention is directed toward others, and who respond to and support the suggestions of others, making them appear more expressive and communal.

In support of this argument, Gerber (1996) studied same- and mixed-sex police teams, and found that partners agreed that the higher status partner was more instrumental and the lower status partner was more expressive, regardless of the partners' sex. Conway et al. (1996) reported evidence that the advantaged and disadvantaged in status distinctions as different as gender, occupation, and hypothetical tribal status were similarly perceived in terms of agency and instrumental competence versus expressive communality. They speculated that people may have a general cultural schema for interpersonal status relations that shapes perceptions of status differences between groups as well. In a related argument, Fiske et al. (2002) reported that the stereotypes of cooperatively interdependent groups in society tend to have a characteristic, "ambivalent" content, in which one group is perceived as higher status and more competent, whereas the other is perceived as lower status but warm.

The stereotypes of men and women in Western societies correspond unusually closely to the pattern of agency and instrumental competence versus reactive communality fostered by interpersonal status relations. Perhaps, on the one hand, this is not surprising given that men and women most commonly encounter one another under the conditions of cooperative interdependence in which interpersonal status hierarchies develop. On the other hand, women, compared to other low-status groups in our society, are viewed not only as expressive and communal but also as nurturing and kind. Social role theory likely is correct in assuming that the nearly exclusive assignment of nuturing roles to women in our society is responsible for the usually high degree of warmth attributed to women (Eagly et al., Chapter 12, this volume).

Although gender may begin as a group distinction rooted in biology, once widely shared status beliefs become embedded in gender stereotypes, these status beliefs root social superiority–inferiority in the sex category itself rather than in specific physical differences associated with biological sex, such as size, strength, or lactation. Thus, gender status beliefs create a social disadvantage even for women who are just as large and strong as the men with whom they are interacting, and who are not lactating mothers. In this way, gender status beliefs generalize the significance of being a man or woman beyond biological differences. Gender status beliefs transform gender into a general purpose, taken-for-granted cultural tool that can be used to organize social hierarchies across a wide range of social activities.

EXPECTATION STATES THEORY

Scope of the Theory

Expectation states theory and its variant, status characteristics theory, ask how status beliefs affect people's behavior and evaluations of one another in situations in which people are working together on a collective goal or task (Berger et al., 1977; Webster & Foschi, 1988). When people cooperate to achieve a goal, their need for some way to evaluate whose contributions are likely to be more or less useful causes status considerations to come into play. Consequently, the theory's traditional scope covers collective goal-oriented settings rather than settings in which people have no focused task or shared goal.

Given the unusual degree of cooperative interdependence between the genders, men and women frequently encounter one another in just these conditions in which expectation states theory is assumed to apply. Cross-gender interactions in work and school settings are readily seen as collectively goal-oriented, but cross-gender interactions in other settings frequently also meet these conditions even though they entail less formal goals. When men and women interact within family or social settings, activities, such as cooking a meal or planning a social outing, contain shared goals toward which the actors are usually collectively oriented. Expectation states theory argues that status beliefs are a major determinant of gender inequality precisely because men and women interact so frequently under the conditions in which status beliefs shape people's behavior and evaluations.

Recent research suggests that the conditions in which status beliefs affect behavior and evaluations may be even broader than interpersonal goal-oriented settings. Erickson (1998) and Correll (2001b) have shown that expectation states theory's scope conditions can be expanded also to include situations in which individuals work alone on socially significant tasks designed to rank people, such as college entrance exams or math ability tests, whose results will be accepted as valid by others. When gender status beliefs become salient in these situations, they can have significant effects not only on task performance but also on the ability that men and women attribute to themselves in important social arenas (Correll, 2001a).

Core Arguments

Expectation states theory argues that when people come together to work toward a shared goal, they look for cues to help define the situation and to anticipate how to behave. To decide whether to speak up or hold back, people form implicit assumptions or guesses about the likely value of what they themselves have to offer compared to what they guess others can offer to the task. These implicit *self–other performance* expectations, as the theory terms them, are not necessarily conscious, are always relative to salient others in the setting, and are specific to the task or goal at hand.

As expectations often do (Miller & Turnbull, 1986), according to the theory, performance expectations, once formed, have self-fulfilling effects on people's task-oriented behaviors and evaluations in the situation. The theory argues, specifically, that the differences between actors' task-related behaviors and evaluations in a situation are a direct function of the degree to which performance expectations formed for them advantage or disadvantage one actor compared to the other (Berger et al., 1977). For instance, the lower one's expectation for oneself compared to another, (1) the less likely that one offers one's own task suggestions, (2) the more likely that one asks for the other's ideas, (3) the more likely that one evaluates positively the ideas the other suggests, and (4) the more likely that one accepts influence from the other by changing to agree with him or her. In this way, the implicit performance expectations that people form for themselves compared to others create and sustain a behavioral status hierarchy. Those for whom higher performance expectations are held tend to participate more, receive more attention, be more positively evaluated, and be more influential than others.

We know from research in social cognition that the search for cues that creates performance expectations involves the often automatic process of categorizing self and other according to relevant and/or socially significant social dimensions. Gender is both visibly accessible and culturally meaningful, making it one of the primary categorization systems used in Western societies (Fiske, 1998). Research shows that actors unconsciously sex-categorize any specific other with whom they interact (Brewer & Liu, 1989; Stangor, Lynch, Duan, & Glass, 1992). Thus, the process of categorizing and defining self and other to create performance expectations involves sex categorization, which in turn primes gender stereotypes and the gender status beliefs they contain, as research shows (Banaji & Hardin, 1996).

A distinctive claim of the theory, however, is that although sex categorization primes status beliefs in virtually all settings, gender status beliefs only affect performance expectations (and, thus, behavior and evaluations) when gender is effectively *salient* in the situation, because it is diagnostic for behavior (Wagner & Berger, 1997). Status characteristics, the theory argues, are salient in a situation in which the actors either differ on the characteristic (e.g., a mixed-sex group) or the characteristic is relevant in that it is culturally linked to the shared task (e.g., a gender-typed task, setting, or activity).

When gender or another status characteristic is salient in a situation, the theory predicts that a *status generalization* process will occur. The assumptions about general competence and specific skills evoked by salient status beliefs shape actors' self–other performance expectations in the situation and, therefore, their task-related behavior and evaluations. Any status characteristic that differentiates actors, no matter how seemingly irrelevant, affects actors' performance expectations, unless something in the situation specifically disassociates the characteristic from the task. This is one of the ways that gender status beliefs affect a wide range of mixed-sex settings in which gender is logically irrelevant to the shared goal or task. The strength of a status characteristic's impact on performance expectations, however, is proportional to its relevance to the situation. The theory argues, then, that gender status beliefs usually have a stronger effect on expectations and behavior in gender-typed settings or tasks than in mixed-sex but gender-neutral situations.

Although people sex-categorize each other in nearly all situations, they almost always categorize one another in other ways as well (Fiske, 1998). These categorizations often make other status characteristics, such as race, occupation, or institutional role, salient in the situation, along with gender. The theory claims that actors use all available status information in forming expectations for self and other (Berger et al., 1977). As additional status characteristics become salient, actors combine the new information, both consistent and inconsistent, with existing information to form aggregated performance expectations that shape behavior and evaluations. Actors do behave as though they form aggregate expectations in this way, as research shows (Balkwell, 1991; Berger, Norman, Balkwell, & Smith, 1992).

This combining argument is consistent with social cognition research, which indicates that as additional categorizations are made beyond sex category, they are cognitively nested within the prior understanding of the person as male or female (Brewer & Liu 1989; Stangor et al., 1992). The new categorizations take on a slightly different meaning as a result (e.g., a female judge). In many settings, identities other than gender—institutional roles such as student, boss, or employee—are more relevant to the situation and task, and have a stronger impact on expectations and behavior. Yet if the situation is mixed-sex or gender-relevant, gender will remain diffusely salient in the background, shaping expectations and moderating the performance of institutional roles in degrees ranging from subtle to substantial. In fact, gender is such a broadly defined social distinction that it most often shapes behavior in goal-oriented situations as a *background identity* that is not explicitly part of actors' definition of "what is happening here." The implicit, background nature of gender status effects in such situations can make it difficult for women to pin down what is happening to them, even when they sense that something prejudicial is occurring.

Predictions

Taken together, these core arguments of expectation states theory yield a specific set of predictions about the effects of gender status on men's and women's performance expectations for one another and, therefore, their task-related behaviors and evaluations. In mixed-sex settings with a gender-neutral task, gender status modestly advantages men in performance expectations over women who are otherwise similar to them. When the task is masculine in association (car repair), men's advantage over women is greater. When the task is stereotypically feminine (cooking), women have a slight advantage over otherwise similar men, because the disadvantaging general competence implications of gender status beliefs combine with the positive implications of more task-relevant specific skills to give women a small net advantage over men in performance expectations (Wagner & Berger, 1997). In same-sex contexts, however, gender status is not salient unless the task is gender-typed. Therefore, men's and women's task-related behaviors and evaluations should be similar in same-sex groups with gender neutral tasks.

GENDER STATUS, BEHAVIOR, AND EVALUATIONS: RESEARCH EVIDENCE

If expectation states theory's arguments are valid, then we should see the theory's predicted pattern of gender status effects across a wide range of task-related behaviors and evaluations. Task-related behaviors include the verbal and nonverbal behaviors through which people enact interpersonal status hierarchies, such as participation, task suggestions, visual dominance, assertive gestures, assertive versus tentative speech, and influence. Task-related evaluations include agreeing with or positively evaluating others' ideas, evaluating task performances, and inferring ability from performance of a given quality. Because leadership in task-oriented situations is enacted through task behaviors, influence, and evaluations, we also should see the theory's predicted pattern of gender status effects in regard to leadership emergence and effectiveness (Ridgeway, 2001a).

In an achievement-oriented society, such task-focused behaviors and judgments are a major basis on which people are encouraged to advance or are held back; are directed toward or away from social rewards; are hired, promoted, and granted power and influence. They are fundamental to the enactment of inequality. The task-directed behaviors and evaluations addressed by the theory do not include all aspects of interpersonal or gendered behavior, however. They entail agentic behaviors and some communal behaviors, such as agreeing, being responsive to others, and supporting others' positions, but they do not include purely social behaviors such as joking, laughing, and smiling.

Studies of the behaviors by which people enact interpersonal status hierarchies in goal-oriented encounters at work, school, or home conform rather closely to the predictions of expectation states theory. Other things being equal, men in mixed-sex groups talk more (Dovidio, Brown, Heltman, Ellyson, & Keating, 1988; James & Drakich, 1993), make more task suggestions (Wood & Karten, 1986), display more visual dominance (Ellyson, Dovidio, & Brown, 1992) and assertive gestures (Dovidio et al., 1988), use less tentative speech (Carli, 1990), and are more influential than women (Carli, 2001; Pugh & Wahrman, 1983; Wagner, Ford, & Ford, 1986). Yet in same-sex groups with a gender-neutral task, as predicted, no differences exist between men and women in participation and task suggestions (Carli, 1991; Johnson, Clay-Warner, & Funk, 1996; Shelly & Munroe, 1999) or in willingness to accept influence from others (Pugh & Wahrman, 1983).[1] Finally, Dovidio et al. (1988) demonstrated that, as the theory predicts, when mixed-sex dyads shifted from a neutral- to a masculine-typed task, men's advantage over women in participation, visual dominance, and assertive gestures increased. Yet when the same dyads shifted to a feminine-typed task, women's participation, visual dominance, and assertive gestures increased, whereas men deferred, so that women gained a modest advantage over men in these task behaviors.

In support of the theory's argument that these are status effects is evidence that men's higher rates of assertive and task-related behaviors in mixed-sex groups are mediated by status-based assumptions that men are more competent. Wood and Karten (1986) demonstrated that when

[1] In contrast to this pattern of findings, studies that code behavior according to Bales's (1970) interaction process analysis (IPA) find marginally larger differences between men and women in the percentage of their behavior that is task related in same-sex rather than mixed-sex groups. This apparent contradiction, however, has been shown to be an artifact of the IPA coding scheme (for reviews, see Carli, 1991; Ridgeway & Smith-Lovin, 1999).

performance expectations for men and women in mixed-sex groups are equalized, gender differences in task-related behaviors disappear. Further supporting the status argument, similar differences in task-related behaviors have been documented for other status characteristics as well, including race and education (see Webster & Foschi, 1988, for a review). Evidence shows that these, too, are mediated by status-based performance expectations (Driskell & Mullen, 1990).

Expectation states theory predicts that gender status will create similar patterns of inequality in evaluations of men's and women's task performances, both by themselves and by others. The meta-analysis of evaluation studies by Swim, Borgida, Maruyama, and Meyers (1989) does indeed reveal this pattern. They reported a modest tendency for the same task performance to be evaluated less positively when produced by a woman; this tendency strengthened significantly when the task was male-typed, and it disappeared when the task was associated with women. Also, as the theory predicts, Carli (1989, reported in Carli, 1991) found that when men and women rated the quality of the ideas they had contributed after either a mixed-sex or same-sex discussion, women evaluated their ideas as lower quality than those of men in the mixed-sex context but equally positively in the same-sex setting.

Gender status beliefs shape task behaviors and evaluations by biasing the performance expectations that men and women form for themselves and others. Foschi (1989, 2000) argues that status characteristics such as gender have another effect as well. When salient in a situation, status characteristics evoke double standards for inferring ability from a performance of a given, recognized quality. Studies confirm Foschi's argument that lower status groups such as women and African Americans are held to higher standards to prove high ability than are higher status groups such as men and whites (Biernat & Kobrynowicz, 1997; Foschi, 2000). That such effects occur for both race and gender supports expectation states theory's argument that these are status effects rather than unique gender effects.

In further support of the theory's claim that these are status effects, gender biases in the attribution of ability from performance are affected by gender's relevance to the task more or less as the theory predicts. A meta-analysis has shown that biases in the attribution of success to ability rather than effort clearly favor men for masculine tasks and disappear for feminine tasks (Swim & Sanna, 1996). These studies show that to prove high ability in a gender-neutral or masculine-typed domain, often a condition for advancement to positions of power and authority in our society, women must actually perform better than similar men. Although women do not suffer this disadvantage, and may even be slightly advantaged, in proving ability in feminine domains, these domains themselves are less valued by society and less likely to lead to positions of authority and high social rewards (Padovic & Reskin, 2002).

Recently, Correll (2001a, 2001b) combined Foschi's double standards concept with Erickson's (1998) extension of expectation states theory to individual performance on socially important tasks designed to rank people. Correll used these combined arguments to posit that gender status filters women out of scientific and technical careers by evoking double standards for judging math ability, despite the social rewards attached to such careers. This occurs, argued Correll, because math is widely seen as a masculine task (cf. Nosek, Benaji, & Greenwald, 2002), which makes gender status salient in math-testing contexts in a manner that disadvantages women (Spencer, Steele, & Quinn, 1999).

Following the status argument, Correll (2001b) demonstrated experimentally that when a task was labeled *masculine,* women rated their ability lower than did men for the same performance. Yet, as the theory predicts, when the same task was explicitly disassociated from gender, no differences existed between men's and women's ability inferences from performance. Correll (2001a) then used longitudinal data from a representative sample of junior and senior high school students to show that girls attributed less math ability to themselves than did boys, based on the same math test scores and grades. The math ability that students attributed to themselves further affected the likelihood that they went on to advanced study in math and science.

If gender status beliefs bias task behaviors, evaluations, and inferences of ability in mixed-sex and gender-relevant settings, then they are likely to bias the emergence of leadership and its perceived effectiveness in these settings, too. Leaders are high-ranking members of interpersonal status hierarchies who take on additional duties and rights to direct, rather than merely influence, their group's activities. Gender biases in the emergence of leadership should follow the same pattern as that predicted for other gender status effects. Eagly and Karau's (1991) meta-analysis of emergent leadership in mixed-sex contexts did indeed find that men were moderately more likely than women to be selected as leaders. The effect was stronger for masculine tasks but was still present even for feminine tasks. When leadership was defined in more masculine terms as strictly task-oriented, the tendency for men to emerge as leaders was stronger. When leadership was defined in social rather than task terms, men's advantage disappeared, and there was a slight tendency for women to emerge as leaders. Similarly, Eagly, Karau, and Makhijani (1995), in a meta-analysis of leadership effectiveness, reported only a slight overall tendency for men to be rated as more effective leaders. In male-dominated and military contexts, however, men were substantially more likely than women to be seen as effective. Women were moderately more likely than men to be viewed as effective leaders in contexts linked more closely with women, such as educational, government, and social service domains.

Overall, then, the research evidence about gender's impact on a wide range of task-related behaviors and evaluations corresponds fairly well with the predictions of expectation states theory. The theory is especially successful in accounting for the way these effects vary across situations in both direction and strength, depending on the sex composition and gender relevance of the context. Evidence that gender differences in task behaviors and evaluations do not develop under certain circumstances (same-sex groups with gender-neutral tasks), and can be eliminated when they do occur by equalizing performance expectations between men and women, and change from favoring men to disappearing or slightly favoring women under other circumstances (a feminine task) lends particular credence to the fact that these differences are status effects. Evidence exists that some similar effects occur for race, education, and other status characteristics as well. In their agentic instrumentality or reactive agreement and deference, task behaviors are closely connected to our cultural conceptions of the differences between men and women. Yet the status account draws our attention to the fact that these behaviors vary more strongly in accordance with an actor's specific position in the particular interpersonal status hierarchy that characterizes a given context than with the sex category of the actor.

GENDER STATUS AND AUTHORITY: THE QUESTION OF LEGITIMACY

The repeated activation of gender status processes across a wide variety of goal-oriented contexts, usually under circumstances in which gender status disadvantages women, creates a web of subtle barriers for women who seek influence, recognition, power, and social rewards commensurate with that of their male peers. Yet more and more women are determined to resist the pressure of gender-evoked negative performance expectations by developing skills of which they can be confident and acting assertively to achieve positions of respect and influence. When they do so, however, expectation states theory predicts that women may sometimes encounter a resistive "backlash" reaction from others (Berger, Ridgeway, Fisek, & Norman, 1998; Ridgeway & Berger, 1986). Such reactions, the theory argues, should be most likely in contexts in which gender status is salient and disadvantages women, that is, mixed-sex situations, with a gender-neutral or masculine-typed task.

Why should assertive behavior evoke a negative reaction? The theory views it as a problem of legitimacy. When widely shared status beliefs cause others implicitly to presume that a person is less competent and less appropriate for high status than others in the situation, it "does not seem right" when that person acts assertively to gain influence or to wield authority. The behavior violates the essential hierarchical nature of the status belief, and the competence assumptions that legitimate it. As a result, others react negatively and often dislike the assertive low-status person. The legitimacy effects of gender status beliefs, according to expectation states theory, give gender stereotypes what some have called a "prescriptive" quality (Eagly & Karau, 2002; Glick & Fiske, 1999).

According to the theory, women's assertive behavior may evoke legitimacy problems in two sorts of situations. In the first, a woman in a mixed-sex group attempts to attain influence over others by assertively putting her ideas forward. Carli (1990) studied this situation and found that, as the theory predicts, whereas assertive language increased influence for men in both mixed- and same-sex dyads, and for women in same-sex dyads, it actually reduced influence for women in mixed-sex dyads and caused them to be viewed as less trustworthy and likable. Other studies have revealed similar reactions to women who engage in assertive, self-promoting behavior (Ridgeway, 1982; Rudman & Glick, 2001).

Legitimacy problems put women in such double-bind situations, because women cannot gain influence without asserting themselves, yet if they do assert themselves, they risk evoking resistance. There is a way around this bind, but it is not without costs. If a woman who performs the group task competently speaks up assertively to gain influence but combines her assertions with socioemotional "softeners" that present her as cooperative rather than self-interested, research shows she can assuage others' resistance and persuade them to grant her influence (Carli, 2001; Ridgeway, 1982). The downside of this otherwise useful technique is that it requires women, but not men, to be both competent *and* nice, in order to be influential in mixed-sex groups. In the process, it encourages behavior that inadvertently confirms gender stereotypes that expect communality from women.

A second situation in which assertive behavior may provoke resistance involves women placed in a position of leadership over others. If it is a mixed-sex context with other than a feminine task, expectation states theory predicts that when such a woman moves beyond persuasion to exercise directive authority, she will encounter more resistance than would a man in a similar situation. Even if she has demonstrated task skills to overcome presumptions that she is less competent, the theory argues, her low gender status will still provide less cultural support for her leadership than a man would have. A variety of studies demonstrate that women leaders in mixed-sex contexts do face greater resistance to their directive use of power (see Eagly & Karau, 2002, for a review). In a meta-analysis of the evaluation of leaders that held constant leadership behaviors, Eagly, Makhijani, and Klonsky (1992) found a slight overall tendency to evaluate women leaders less positively. As we would expect, however, this tendency was stronger in male-dominated contexts. As the legitimacy argument also predicts, women leaders were devalued more strongly than similar men when they wielded their authority in a directive, autocratic style.

What is the evidence that such resistive reactions to assertive women are status effects rather than unique gender effects produced by specific cultural expectations for women? To examine this question, Ridgeway, Johnson, and Diekema (1994) studied reactions to directive assertions by actors who were advantaged or disadvantaged by status characteristics other than gender. They found that when high-ranking members of a group hierarchy were disadvantaged in age and education, despite being more skilled at the task than their partners, they were resisted when they engaged in highly directive behavior. They gained less influence from such behavior than equally high-ranking members of groups that had age and education advantages over their partners. Because status characteristics other than gender provoke similar reactions, it is likely that such reactions are indeed a result of status-based legitimacy problems.

HOW DO GENDER STATUS BELIEFS ARISE?

If gender status beliefs are such a pervasive source of inequality between men and women, then it becomes important to ask how such beliefs arise. Status beliefs about social distinctions probably develop in many ways, but status construction theory uses ideas from expectation states theory to suggest one set of processes by which this could occur (Ridgeway, 1991; Ridgeway & Erickson, 2000).

Status construction theory argues that when people must regularly cooperate across a group boundary to achieve mutual goals (as men and women must), there is a chance that they will associate the influence hierarchies that develop in their interactions with their group distinction, and form fledgling status beliefs about that distinction. They are likely to carry these fledgling status beliefs to subsequent encounters with people from the other group and, by treating others according to those beliefs, "teach" the belief to at least some others. In this way, beliefs that develop in local encounters have the potential to spread widely and become consensual.

Which group will be favored in these beliefs, and whether the beliefs become widely shared or dissipate in a cultural confusion of conflicting beliefs, depend on the structural conditions in which people from each group encounter one another. The theory argues that if some factor (e.g., material resources, technology, or physical advantage) gives people from one group a systematic advantage in gaining influence over persons from the other group in intergroup encounters, then widely shared status beliefs favoring the advantaged group are likely develop.

Growing evidence indicates that this argument is plausible. Experiments have shown that when participants who were told they differed on a stable personal trait had repeated experiences of working on a cooperative task in which persons from one trait group consistently became influential, the participants formed status beliefs favoring the more influential trait group (Ridgeway & Erickson, 2000); that is, the participants formed beliefs that "most people" would rate the typical person from the influential trait group as higher status, more respected, more competent, but not as considerate as the typical person from the other group. These status beliefs were consensual in that both participants who belonged to the influential trait group and those who did not agreed that "most people" would see the influential group as higher status and more competent, if not as considerate, as the other group. Ridgeway and Erickson also demonstrated that participants could spread these status beliefs about the trait difference to others by treating them according to the beliefs. Finally, simulations indicate that if people do form and spread status beliefs, as these experiments show, then the development of widely shared status beliefs favoring the structurally advantaged group is a logical outcome (Ridgeway & Balkwell, 1997).

Many theories have been proposed to explain the origins of male dominance (e.g., Wood & Eagly, 2002). Several, however, posit some physical factor, such as superior strength or mobility constraints faced by lactating mothers, that at particular points in history would have affected the role assignment and division of labor between men and women (Eagly et al., Chapter 12, this volume). Status construction theory adds the suggestion that such factors might also have given men a systematic advantage over women in gaining influence in everyday interdependent dealings. If this were the case, then status construction theory would predict that any one of these factors would give rise to shared cultural status beliefs favoring men. By grounding hierarchy and inequality in the sex category itself, rather than in individual strength or lactation status, gender status beliefs transform male dominance from a situationally specific physical advantage to a general cultural system for organizing social relations between men and women on hierarchical terms.

Once established, gender status beliefs may help preserve the hierarchical structure of the gender system in the face of changing economic and technological conditions that could potentially undermine the factors that fostered gender inequality at an earlier time (Ridgeway, 1997). People interacting at the edge of economic and technological change develop new ways of doing things and new forms of social organization. Material conditions tend to change more rapidly than widely shared cultural beliefs, however. Consequently, as people interact to create new social practices, they draw on their existing cultural beliefs, including gender status beliefs. Because gender status beliefs implicitly shape what they do, people may inadvertently reinscribe gender inequality into the new social structures they develop.

COUNTERING THE EFFECTS OF GENDER STATUS

Expectation states theory provides a detailed account of the many processes through which gender status beliefs organize everyday encounters between men and women on unequal terms and create an array of subtle barriers for women who seek positions of status, authority, and reward commensurate with those of their male peers. Status construction theory suggests some means by which gender status beliefs that disadvantage women might develop. Can these theories tell us anything about how the effects of gender status beliefs might be undermined? To some degree, yes, they can. These theories point to social processes and policies through which gender inequality might be reduced, both for individuals in specific situations and, over time, for society more generally (Ridgeway & Correll, 2000).

Recall that actors use all available status information when forming aggregate performance expectations for self and other. Recall also that when performance expectations for men and women in a situation are equalized, gender differences in task-related behaviors and evaluations disappear (e.g., Wood & Karten, 1986). One way to reduce the negative impact of gendered expectations on women in interaction, then, is to create situations such that status characteristics on which women have higher or equal status with men are effectively salient. For example, in a setting in which education is relevant to the task at hand, a woman who is more highly educated than her male task partner will suffer less gender disadvantage in the interaction if her educational advantage becomes known. Comparable worth is a social policy whose goal is reduction of the gender gap in wages by the requirement of equal pay for jobs of comparable worth to the employer. As such, comparable worth policies seek to make salient the skills and experience required for female-dominated occupations as a justification for raising pay levels for these occupations compared to men's jobs. By making women's unacknowledged skills levels salient, this policy would also help to reduce performance expectation differences between men and women in many workplace interactions, increasing women's influence and their access to valued positions in these contexts.

Another social intervention that should reduce gender inequality in the workplace, according to expectation states theory, is a policy of open pay information for employees (Ridgeway & Correll, 2000). The theory argues that self–other performance expectations create anticipation of a corresponding distribution of social rewards in a situation (Berger, Fisek, Norman, & Wagner, 1985). Consequently, if gender status is salient in a situation and pay information is not open, women may implicitly expect and, without realizing it, accept lower reward levels than do their male peers. Research on the "depressed entitlement effect" among women documents this (Bylsma & Major, 1992; Jost, 1997).

According to expectations states theory, however, if performance expectations create reward expectations, by the same token, the distribution of rewards can create corresponding performance expectations (Berger et al., 1985). Research indicates that actors do infer competence differences based on how valued rewards are distributed among people in goal-oriented contexts (Harrod, 1980; Stewart & Moore, 1992). Therefore, any policy that equalizes reward levels between men and women will help to lessen differences in performance expectations as well, reducing inequalities in task behaviors and evaluations.

Open-pay policies make gender differences in pay less sustainable by giving people a better idea of what they can ask for, and creating general pressure for equity. Comparable worth policies, of course, also reduce gender differences in pay. When men and women with equal resources interact, their performance expectations for self and other are jointly determined by their gender status and reward levels. In this way, policies that equalize resources can substantially reduce, although not eliminate, the gender disadvantage in expectations and influence that women usually suffer in interactions with similar men (Ridgeway & Correll, 2000).

The principles of expectation states theory also suggest ways in which the effects of reducing gender inequality in multiple individual contexts might accumulate over time to reduce gender inequality more broadly. The theory argues that individuals carry status and expectation information gained in one interaction into subsequent ones (Markovsky, Smith, & Berger, 1984). This means that, as research indicates, a man who interacts with a woman whom he perceives to perform the task better than he does will carry that expectation into subsequent encounters with other women (Pugh & Wahrman, 1983). On the one hand, this positive effect on the performance expectations he forms for other women tends to wear off over time without a "booster" experience

(Markovsky et al., 1984). On the other hand, social change that increases the number of women with high skills levels, equal resources, and positions of power in the workforce will increase the number of such "booster" experiences that men and women have. Status construction theory suggests that, over time, such iterative pressures on people's performance expectations for individual men and women will put growing pressure on the competence assumptions embedded in gender status beliefs and reduce the size of the implied gender difference.

Finally, some researchers have argued that the best way to reduce the gender inequality that results from gender categorization is through the disruption of sex categories and sex categorization (e.g., Bem, 1995; Butler, 1990; Connell, 1995; Risman, 1999). One way that sex categorization is disrupted is when an actor is unable to sex-categorize another accurately. This type of "gender mistake" can occur in a variety of situations, such as when reading an e-mail or résumé from someone with a gender-neutral name, when interacting with an "effeminate"-looking man or a "masculine"-looking woman, or when interacting over the Internet rather than face-to-face. When mistakes occur, research shows that the incorrect status information continues to affect the perceiver's performance expectations for the other, even after the mistake is corrected. In particular, if an actor mistakes a high-status person for a low-status person, he or she grants that person less power and prestige than if he or she had known the person's true status all along, even after the mistake is corrected (Bourg, 2002). If gender mistakes have similar lingering effects on interaction, then a man who is originally mistaken for woman will have less power and prestige in that interaction than he would have if the mistake had not occurred. The cumulative impact of many men being sex-categorized incorrectly, therefore, has the potential eventually to lead to some reduction in gender inequality in multiple social exchanges. As non-face-to-face interactions, through the Internet and other media, become more common, the likelihood of such gender mistakes increases.

CONCLUSIONS

Status beliefs about gender differences in social significance and general competence lie at the heart of our shared cultural understandings of who men and women are, because they are embedded in widely accepted gender stereotypes. Men and women interact with one another continually, often under cooperative, goal-oriented conditions that make these gender status beliefs salient. As a result, as expectation states theory shows us, much of men's and women's knowledge of and experiences with one another is shaped through self-fulfilling expectations that have been biased by gender status beliefs. The theory's greatest accomplishment is to give us a detailed, well-documented account of how such self-fulfilling, status-biased expectations continually construct and reconstruct gender inequality across the diverse range of social activities in which men and women cooperate in goal-oriented ways. The effects of gender status beliefs on any given encounter are often modest and so taken for granted as to be unrecognized by the participants. Yet these effects accumulate as they are repeated over multiple contexts and encounters to create significant inequalities in men's and women's social outcomes in society. By showing us that a good portion of men's and women's interpersonal behaviors are actually produced by the status culturally ascribed to gender, the theory offers us insight into how much of our very understanding of men's and women's natures is status-based rather than unique to gender.

REFERENCES

Bales, R. F. (1970). *Personality and interpersonal behavior.* New York: Holt, Rinehart, & Winston.

Balkwell, J. W. (1991). From expectations to behavior: An improved postulate for expectation states theory. *American Sociological Review, 56,* 355–369.

Banaji, M. R., & Hardin, C. (1996). Automatic stereotyping. *Psychological Science, 7,* 136–141.

Bem, S. L. (1995). Dismantling gender polarization and compulsory heterosexuality: Should we turn the volume up or down? *Journal of Sex Research, 32,* 329–334.

Berger, J., Fisek, M. H., Norman, R. Z., & Wagner, D. G. (1985). The formation of reward expectations in status situations. In J. Berger & M. Zelditch (Eds.), *Status, rewards, and influence* (pp. 215–261). San Francisco: Jossey-Bass.

Berger, J., Fisek, H., Norman, R., & Zelditch, M. (1977). *Status characteristics and social interaction.* New York: Elsevier.

Berger, J., Norman, R. Z., Balkwell, J. W., & Smith, L. (1992). Status inconsistency in task situations: A test of four status processing principles. *American Sociological Review, 57,* 843–855.

Berger, J., Ridgeway, C. L., Fisek, M. H., & Norman, R. Z. (1998). The legitimation and delegitimation of power and prestige orders. *American Sociological Review, 63,* 379–405.

Berger, J., & Zelditch, M. (1998). *Status, power, and legitimacy: Strategies and theories.* New Brunswick, NJ: Transaction.

Biernat, M., & Kobrynowicz, D. (1997). Gender and race-based standards of competence: Lower minimum standards but higher ability standards for devalued groups. *Journal of Personality and Social Psychology, 72,* 544–557.

Bourg, C. (2002). *Gender mistakes and inequality.* Paper presented at the 98th annual meeting of the American Sociological Association, Chicago, IL.

Brewer, M., & Lui, L. (1989). The primacy of age and sex in the structure of person categories. *Social Cognition, 7,* 262–274.

Broverman, I., Vogel, S., Broverman, D., Clarkson, F., & Rosenkrantz, P. (1972). Sex-role stereotypes: A reappraisal. *Journal of Social Issues, 28,* 59–78.

Butler, J. (1990). *Gender trouble: Feminism and the subversion of identity.* New York: Routledge.

Bylsma, W., & Major, B. (1992). Two routes to eliminating gender differences in personal entitlement. *Psychology of Women Quarterly, 16,* 193–200.

Carli, L. (1990). Gender, language and influence. *Journal of Personality and Social Psychology, 59,* 941–951.

Carli, L. L. (1991). Gender, status, and influence. In E. J. Lawler, B. Markovsky, C. L. Ridgeway, & H. Walker (Eds.), *Advances in group processes* (Vol. 8, pp. 89–113). Greenwich, CT: JAI Press.

Carli, L. L. (2001). Gender and social influence. *Journal of Social Issues, 57,* 725–742.

Connell, R. W. (1995). *Masculinities.* Berkeley: University of California Press.

Conway, M., Pizzamiglio, M. T., & Mount, L. (1996). Status, communality, and agency: Implications for stereotypes of gender and other groups. *Journal of Personality and Social Psychology, 71,* 25–38.

Correll, S. J. (2001a). Gender and the career-choice process: The role of biased self-assessments. *American Journal of Sociology, 106,* 1691–1730.

Correll, S. J. (2001b). *The gendered selection of activities and the reproduction of gender segregation in the labor force.* Doctoral dissertation, Stanford University, CA.

Dovidio, J. F., Brown, C. E., Heltman, K., Ellyson, S. L., & Keating, C. F. (1988). Power displays between women and men in discussions of gender linked tasks: A multichannel study. *Journal of Personality and Social Psychology, 55,* 580–587.

Driskell, J. E., & Mullen, B. (1990). Status, expectations, and behavior: A meta-analytic review and test of the theory. *Personality and Social Psychology Bulletin, 16,* 541–553.

Eagly, A. H., & Karau, S. J. (1991). Gender and the emergence of leaders: A meta-analysis. *Journal of Personality and Social Psychology, 60,* 685–710.

Eagly, A. H., & Karau, S. J. (2002). Role congruity theory of prejudice towards female leaders. *Psychological Review, 109,* 573–579.

Eagly, A. H., Karau, S. J., & Makhijani, M. G. (1995). Gender and the effectiveness of leaders: A meta-analysis. *Psychological Bulletin, 117,* 125–145.

Eagly, A. H., Makhijani, M. G., & Klonsky, B. G. (1992). Gender and the evaluation of leaders: A meta-analysis. *Psychological Bulletin, 111,* 543–588.

Eagly, A. H., & Mladinic, A. (1994). Are people prejudiced against women?: Some answers from research on attitudes, gender stereotypes, and judgments of competence. In W. Stroebe & M. Hewstone (Eds.), *European review of social psychology* (Vol. 5, pp. 1–35). New York: Wiley.

Ellyson, S. L., Dovidio, J. F., & Brown, C. E. (1992). The look of power: Gender differences and similarities. In C. L. Ridgeway (Ed.), *Gender, interaction, and inequality* (pp. 50–80). New York: Springer-Verlag.

Erickson, K. G. (1998). *The impact of cultural status beliefs on individual task performance in evaluative settings: A new direction in expectation states research.* Doctoral dissertation. Stanford University, CA.

Fiske, S. T. (1998). Stereotyping, prejudice, and discrimination. In D. T. Gilbert, S. T. Fiske, & G. Lindzey (Eds.), *The handbook of social psychology* (4th ed., Vol. 2, pp. 357–411). Boston: McGraw-Hill.

Fiske, S. T., Cuddy, A. J. C., Glick, P., & Xu, J. (2002). A model of (often mixed) stereotype content: Competence and warmth respectively follow from perceived status and competence. *Journal of Personality and Social Psychology, 82,* 878–902.

Foschi, M. (1989). Status characteristics, standards, and attributions. In J. Berger, M. Zelditch, Jr., & B. Anderson (Eds.), *Sociological theories in progress: New formulations* (pp. 58–72). Newbury Park, CA: Sage.

Foschi, M. (2000). Double standards for competence: Theory and research. *Annual Review of Sociology, 26,* 21–42.

Geis, F. L., Brown, V., Jennings, J., & Corrado-Taylor, D. (1984). Sex vs. status in sex-associated stereotypes. *Sex Roles, 11,* 771–185.

Gerber, G. L. (1996). Status in same gender and mixed gender police dyads: Effects on personality attributions. *Social Psychology Quarterly, 59,* 350–363.

Glick, P., & Fiske, S. T. (1999). Sexism and other "isms": Interdependence, status, and the ambivalent content of stereotypes. In W. B. Swan, J. H. Langlois, & L. A. Gilbert (Eds.), *Sexism and stereotypes in modern society* (pp. 193–221). Washington, DC: American Psychological Association.

Harrod, W. J. (1980). Expectations from unequal rewards. *Social Psychology Quarterly, 43,* 126–130.

Jackman, M. R. (1994). *The velvet glove: Paternalism and conflict in gender, class, and race relations.* Berkeley: University of California Press.

James, D., & Drakich, J. (1993). Understanding gender differences in amount of talk: A critical review of research. In D. Tannen (Ed.), *Gender and conversational interaction* (pp. 281–312). New York: Oxford University Press.

Johnson, C., Clay-Warner, J., & Funk, S. J. (1996). Effects of authority structures and gender on interaction in same-sex task groups. *Social Psychology Quarterly, 59,* 221–236.

Jost, J. T. (1997). An experimental replication of the depressed–entitlement effect among women. *Psychology of Women Quarterly, 21,* 387–393.

Jost, J. T., & Burgess, D. (2000). Attitudinal ambivalence and the conflict between group and system justification in low status groups. *Personality and Social Psychology Bulletin, 26,* 293–305.

Leal-Idrogo, A. (1997). The effect of gender on interaction, friendship, and leadership in elementary school classrooms. In E. G. Cohen & R. A. Lotan (Eds.), *Working for equity in heterogeneous classrooms* (pp. 77–91). New York: Teachers College Press.

Lockheed, M. E., Harris, A. M., & Nemceff, W. P. (1983). Sex and social influence: Does sex function as a status characteristic in mixed sex groups of children? *Journal of Educational Psychology, 75,* 877–888.

Markovsky, B., Smith, L. F., & Berger, J. (1984). Do status interventions persist? *American Sociological Review, 49,* 373–382.

Miller, D. T., & Turnbull, W. (1986). Expectancies and interpersonal processes. *Annual Review of Psychology, 37,* 233–256.

Nosek, B. A., Banaji, M. R., & Greenwald, A. G. (2002). Math = male, me = female, therefore math ≠ me. *Journal of Personality and Social Psychology, 83,* 44–59.

Padovic, I., & B. Reskin. (2002). *Women and men at work* (2nd ed.). Thousand Oaks, CA: Sage.

Persell, C. H., James, C., Kang, T., & Snyder, K. (1999). Gender and education in global perspective. In J. H. Chafetz (Ed.), *Handbook of the sociology of gender* (pp. 81–104). New York: Kluwer/Plenum.

Pugh, M., & Wahrman, R. (1983). Neutralizing sexism in mixed-sex groups: Do women have to be better than men? *American Journal of Sociology, 88,* 746–762.

Ridgeway, C. L. (1982). Status in groups: The importance of motivation. *American Sociological Review, 47,* 76–88.

Ridgeway, C. L. (1991). The social construction of status value: Gender and other nominal characteristics. *Social Forces, 70,* 367–386.

Ridgeway, C. L. (1997). Interaction and the conservation of gender inequality: Considering employment. *American Sociological Review, 62,* 218–235.

Ridgeway, C. L. (2001a). Gender, status, and leadership. *Journal of Social Issues, 57,* 627–655.

Ridgeway, C. L. (2001b). Social status and group structure. In M. A. Hogg & S. Tindale (Eds.), *Blackwell handbook of social psychology: Group processes* (pp. 352–375). Maulden, MA: Blackwell.

Ridgeway, C. L., & Balkwell, J. (1997). Group processes and the diffusion of status beliefs. *Social Psychology Quarterly, 60,* 14–31.

Ridgeway, C. L., & Berger, J. (1986). Expectations, legitimation, and dominance behavior in groups. *American Sociological Review, 51,* 603–617.

Ridgeway, C. L., Boyle, E. H., Kuipers, K., & Robinson, D. (1998). How do status beliefs develop?: The role of resources and interaction. *American Sociological Review, 63,* 331–350.

Ridgeway, C. L., & Correll, S.J. (2000). Limiting gender inequality through interaction: The end(s) of gender. *Contemporary Sociology, 29,* 110–120.

Ridgeway, C. L., & Erickson, K. G. (2000). Creating and spreading status beliefs. *American Journal of Sociology, 106, 579–615.*

Ridgeway, C. L., Johnson, C., & Diekema, D. (1994). External status, legitimacy, and compliance in male and female groups. *Social Forces, 72,* 1051–1077.

Ridgeway, C. L., & Smith-Lovin, L. (1999). The gender system and interaction. *Annual Review of Sociology, 25,* 191–216.

Risman, B. (1999). *Gender vertigo: American families in transition.* New Haven, CT: Yale University Press.

Rudman, L. A., & Glick, P. (2001). Prescriptive gender stereotypes and backlash toward agentic women. *Journal of Social Issues, 57,* 743–762.

Seachrist, G. B., & Stangor, C. (2001). Perceived consensus influences intergroup behavior and stereotype accessibility. *Journal of Personality and Social Psychology, 80,* 645–654.

Shelly, R. K., & Munroe, P. T. (1999). Do women engage in less task behavior than men? *Sociological Perspectives, 42,* 49–67.

Sidanius, J., & Pratto, F. (1999). *Social dominance.* New York: Cambridge University Press.

Spence, J. T., & Buckner, C. E. (2000). Instrumental and expressive traits, trait stereotypes, and sexist attitudes: What do they signify? *Psychology of Women Quarterly, 24,* 44–62.

Spencer, S. J., Steele, C. M., & Quinn, D. M. (1999). Under suspicion of inability: Stereotype threat and women's math performance. *Journal of Experimental Social Psychology, 35,* 4–28.

Stangor, C., Lynch, L., Duan, C., & Glass, B. (1992). Categorization of individuals on the basis of multiple social features. *Journal of Personality and Social Psychology, 62,* 207–218.

Stewart, P. A., & Moore, J. C. (1992). Wage disparities and performance expectations. *Social Psychology Quarterly, 55,* 78–85.

Swim, J., Borgida, E., Maruyama, G., & Meyers, D. G. (1989). Joan McKay versus John McKay: Do gender stereotypes bias evaluations? *Psychological Bulletin, 105,* 409–429.

Swim, J., & Sanna, L. J. (1996). He's skilled, she's lucky: A meta-analysis of observer's attributions for women's and men's successes and failures. *Personality and Social Psychology Bulletin, 22,* 507–519.

Tajfel, H. H., & Turner, J. C. (1986). The social identity theory of intergroup behavior. In S. Worchel & W. G. Austin (Eds.), *The psychology of intergroup behavior* (pp. 7–24). Chicago: Nelson-Hall.

Wagner, D. G., & Berger, J. (1997). Gender and interpersonal task behaviors: Status expectation accounts. *Sociological Perspectives, 40,* 1–32.

Wagner, D. G., Ford, R. S., & Ford, T. W. (1986). Can gender inequalities be reduced? *American Sociological Review, 51,* 47–61.

Webster, M., & Foschi, M. (1988). *Status generalization: New theory and research.* Stanford, CA: Stanford University Press.

Williams, J. E., & Best, D. L. (1990). *Measuring sex stereotypes: A multination study.* Newbury Park, CA: Sage.

Wood W., & Eagly, A. H. (2000). A cross-cultural analysis of the behavior of women and men: Implications for the origins of sex differences. *Psychological Bulletin, 128,* 699–727.

Wood, W., & Karten, S. J. (1986). Sex differences in interaction style as a product of perceived sex differences in competence. *Journal of Personality and Social Psychology, 50,* 341–347.

11

The Bases of Gendered Power

FELICIA PRATTO
ANGELA WALKER

With the possible exception of childbearing, no aspect of social life is more strongly associated with gender than power. In no known societies do women dominate men. In all societies that accumulate wealth, men, on average, enjoy more power than women, on average, and this appears to have been true throughout human history (Brown, 1991; Lenski, 1984). As we show, understanding how power is gendered is important for understanding not only gender inequality but also inequalities based on race, ethnicity, class, and sexual orientation.

Ironically, most theories of group-based power have neglected gender, focusing instead on interracial, international, colonial, or interethnic relations (Jackman, 1994, p. 47). Power between such groups is generally viewed as intergroup conflict, in which segregated groups are in zero-sum competition for resources and legitimacy. Many apply this approach to sexism, conceiving of sexism as a form of racism or classism directed against women (e.g., Reskin, 1988). But the intergroup conflict approach is inadequate to explain the association between gender and power for several reasons. First, though the genders are segregated in many "public" arenas (e.g., government, paid occupations), gender is integral to many intimate or "private" relationships, notably, families (cf. Rosaldo, 1974). Second, segregation and other aspects of gender roles reduce conflict and coordinate men's and women's behaviors (e.g., Sanday, 1981). Third, many shared cultural beliefs reduce overt conflict by coordinating behavior and disguising power inequalities (Jackman, 1994; Pratto & Walker, 2000). Fourth, the conflict model implies more instability than is typical of gender relations. Fifth, gender inequality is not independent of other forms of group-based inequality; rather, these forms have a dynamic relation with one another.

Social dominance theory views gender inequality differently than do other intergroup theories (see Pratto, 1996; Sidanius & Pratto, 1999, Ch. 10). Along with inequality based on race, class, or other socially defined groups, social dominance theory views gender inequality as a characteristic feature of group-dominance societies. (For short, group distinctions such as ethnicity, nationality, religion, class, or race are called "arbitrary set" groups.) The relatively stable inequality of these societies is a function of coordinated discrimination in the allocation of resources, especially through institutional practice. Systematic coordination and discrimination are prescribed by widely known cultural ideologies, such as moral edicts about resource allocation and stereotypes, which also help to assign people to social roles. Notably, men and women generally play different roles in the maintenance of arbitrary set hierarchies. Moreover, because of the intersections of gender with race, class, and sexual orientation, gender and arbitrary set inequality are dynamically related and mutually sustaining. In particular, men in dominant groups often use coercive and ideological power to expropriate resources from men in subordinate groups, and from women. Such men can sometimes use this power to establish relationships in which they and their children receive care from women. In this way, the power dynamics of heterosexual relationships hinge in part on arbitrary group inequality (see Pratto, 1996). In this chapter, we detail how power is gendered, and how gendered forms of power help maintain arbitrary set inequality.

WHAT IS POWER?

Often power is confused with other constructs (e.g., prestige, wealth) and seen as a fixed property of persons or groups. Power, however, pertains to a dynamic relationship. This implies that saying "men have power" is only sensible as shorthand for what men have power to do and to whom. What, then, are the fundamental bases of power?

Classical political theories of intergroup relations have identified three bases for power, whereas a theory of interpersonal relationships identified a fourth basis. Most obviously, the threat of violence can induce others to obey one's demands. Thus, the potential to harm—

force—is a source of coercive power. More subtly, Marx and Engels (1846) identified control over the means of production of value as the basis of two different kinds of power: First, "real" (material), or economic, power pertains to control of the production of exchangeable material (e.g., food, manufactured goods, energy). Limiting another's access to valued resources, or to a role in their production, provides a second basis for coercion.

Marx and Engels (1846) also argued that the elites who control the means of production control the *desire* for manufactured goods, which partly determine their value. Elites influence the "market value" of goods and of people (!) by promoting ideologies that suggest who or what is desired or disdained. For example, magazine advertisements depicting beautiful women may both create a desire for particular beauty products and imply which women are valuable and for what reasons. As long as no one dissents from these ideologies, the "market value" for a good or person is the same in every stall. Consensus on ideologies makes those influenced by ideologies seem to consent rather than to be coerced, which often obscures the fact that ideology is a basis of power.

Interdependence theory describes power as an asymmetry in how much each party in a relationship needs the other (Thibaut & Kelley, 1959). Controlling more resources than the other party, as men typically do (Engels, 1884/1902; Sacks, 1974), creates this power asymmetry, making it easier for the controller to exit or to set the terms of the relationship. Some feel that women's sexuality is a scarce and desired resource, giving women a source of power in their bodies that can change the balance of power in heterosexual relationships. This, however, forces women to trade in sexuality, in violation of some moral–cultural prescriptions. The other major way to constrain power is through codified social obligations, which can be found in family law, norms of politeness, and family and gender roles. Being advantaged in asymmetrical obligations—being owed more than one owes—is a mark of high power. This source of power has a limiting condition, namely, that having no obligations often implies having no relationships, without which one can neither use power nor receive certain benefits. As we see, many legal systems and gender role prescriptions provide more advantage through obligations to men than to women.

The next four sections of this chapter provide an overview of how and why the previously outlined bases of power—force, resource control, consensual ideologies, and asymmetric social obligations—are gendered, and how each basis pertains to racism and heterosexism. The dynamics of power are demonstrated when one basis of power influences another; examples are provided within each section. Then, we provide evidence that roles associated with each form of power are gendered. Finally, we review how each basis of power can or cannot be exchanged with other bases, so that we can describe the kinds of social changes that are necessary to produce greater equality.

GENDER AND FORCE

Violence is a significant aspect of the power struggles and relationships both between men and women, and between dominant and subordinate arbitrary set groups. Women commit slightly more violent acts against men than the reverse, but men more often than women inflict debilitating injuries and death (Archer, 2000). The threat of men's physical and psychological violence against women has been analyzed as a major source of gender inequality (Schwendinger & Schwendinger, 1983). Assault, rape, sexual harassment, and emotional abuse not only are damaging to women but also limit women's power by reducing their ability to exit from harmful domestic or employer relationships (Fitzgerald, Gelfand, & Drasgow, 1995; Sagrestano, Heavey, & Christensen, 1999). Although many heterosexual relationships are free of this kind of coercion, a woman may feel compelled to remain with a man who does not abuse her, because she fears another mate might. As a result, her current mate has more power over her than he would if other men were not violent.

Analyzing the power of violence cannot end, then, with the actions of the abuser in question. When societies establish few alternatives to women other than marriage, whether because economic provisions are unavailable for women outside of marriage, because women are ostracized or lose their children and family support outside of marriage, or simply because alternatives are not conceivable, laws and social customs conspire to keep women in abusive or exploitative marriages. Likewise, when sexual harassment and gender bias in the workplace are not recognized as wrongs and receive no negative sanctions, social and legal customs combine with economic necessity to trap women in untenable work situations (O'Connell & Korabik, 2000; Riger, 1991; Terpestra & Baker, 1986). In this regard, male violence against women depends on sexist laws and customs. For example, in rural Mexico at present, the town elders who arbitrate law rarely understand that rape is a crime, punish a man much more seriously for stealing a cow than for raping a girl, and perhaps worse, feel that forcing a girl to marry her rapist is an appropriate remedy (Jordan, 2002). A French businesswoman who reported being gang-raped to police in Dubai was charged with adultery under Shari'a and had her passport confiscated for six months, during which time she was required to pay her own personal and legal expenses. After a number of legal maneuvers, she was convicted in absentia and without legal representation (Association de Soutien à Touria, 2003).

Feminist activists in some countries have succeeded in establishing rape as a crime and have decreased the stigmatization of women who pursue prosecution. However, women remain vulnerable to sexual violence worldwide. The World Health Organization estimates that 20% of women experience sexual violence during their lifetimes but notes that certain girls and women (as well as some boys and men) are repeatedly sexually assaulted, especially if they are poor or abused at home (World Health Organization, 2002a). Rates of sexual assault over the lifetime range from 5% of women (Philippines) to 58% of women (Turkey), with most countries reporting percentages in the 20s, 30s, and 40s (United Nations Statistics Division, 2002a). Consistent with social dominance theory's view that gender inequality is functionally related to other forms of inequality, Schwendinger and Schwendinger (1983) found that rape and other forms of male violence against women are more frequent in male-dominated societies than in nonstratified societies. Moreover, rape and other sexual violence against women is horrifically common during arbitrary group war (e.g., Human Rights Watch, 2001a).

More detailed research about the proximal causes of interpersonal violence suggests two seemingly contradictory things about power and violence: Abused wives report that their husbands have more power than they do (e.g., Babcock, Waltz, Jacobson, & Gottman, 1993; Frieze & McHugh, 1992), but husbands who abuse report feeling less powerful than their wives (Johnson, 1995; Sagrestano et al., 1999). In fact, men with lower economic, educational, or occupational status than their wives (Hornung, McCullough, & Sugimoto, 1981), and men who perceive themselves to have lower decision-making power than their wives (Babcock et al., 1993), are more likely to use violence (see also World Health Organization, 2002b). This ironic situation suggests that men use violence to "correct" perceived power inequities.

Another form of violence directed at 2 million girls each year, female genital mutilation, is common in several African countries and among African immigrants (World Health Organization, 2002b). Genital mutilation can cause serious health problems and death, and remove the possibility of most sexual pleasure for women, but it may also confer tribal and feminine identity. Women not only perform but often advocate these practices, and recipients may not feel that they are coerced; in fact, "the change" is perceived as the gateway to marriage (e.g., Sanderson, 1981). Numerous other cultures have harmful feminine body modification practices (e.g., footbinding, starvation dieting, skin bleaching, tatooing) that are promoted by women in intimate relationships (grandmothers, aunts, mothers, friends). Such practices are meant to prepare women's bodies for heterosexual relationships and also mark women's arbitrary group memberships (e.g., social class).

Not all men profit from male violence, because men are most often the victims of severe male violence, whether legal or extralegal. For example, during 2000, 76% of U.S. murder victims and 90% of identified murderers were men (Federal Bureau of Investigation, 2001), following a worldwide pattern (Daly & Wilson, 1988; Sidanius & Pratto, 1999, pp. 256–257). Much male-on-male violence is clearly part of arbitrary set dominance contests, in that men, rather than women, are disproportionately targeted by racist, heterosexist, and other intergroup violence. For example, of the 4,951 Americans lynched between 1882 and 1927, 3,437 were black men (White, 1969). In 2000, there were 1,089 male victims and 230 female victims of hate crimes based on sexual orientation in the United States (Federal Bureau of Investigation, 2001, p. 60). All of the recent cases of racially motivated police brutality have victimized men. The practice of using men as military combatants also illustrates that male-on-male violence is a significant aspect of intergroup relations. Even the horrific practice of raping women of conquered groups is often seen as a symbolic method of demeaning men (e.g., Rodrigue, 1993).

In summary, men commit severe violence at much higher rates than do women. When men are violent to women with whom they live, they may be trying to regain power that sexist beliefs prescribe. Men are often and dangerously violent toward men, especially as part of intergroup and status-striving conflicts. Male violence against women in intergroup conflicts is often sexualized. Much of the violence women commit against themselves and other women is to transform the feminine body to become "suitable" for men. Thus, gendered violence both within and between the sexes reflects the intersection of gender, arbitrary set distinctions, and sexual orientation.

GENDER AND RESOURCE CONTROL

As with force, domestic arrangements and legal customs not only bias resource control in favor of men rather than women in hierarchical societies but also lead to particular dangers for some men. In different economic systems, primary resources differ. In agrarian economies, land is the primary resource, but local customs and laws often bar women from land ownership, even when they are the stewards and primary farmers (e.g., Qvist, 1998). In industrialized nations, wages are the primary resource, and more men have paid and full-time jobs, and earn more than women (e.g., Wirth, 2001). Men are paid more than women doing manufacturing work in all but two nations (United Nations Statistics Division, 2002b).

Gender segregation by occupation is a primary cause of the gender wage gap. Numerous studies have shown that occupations in which men predominate, on the whole, are better paid and associated with more prestige than occupations in which women predominate. There are several indications that this is not coincidental; rather, it is an aspect of power relations between men and women. First, this holds even for occupations requiring the same level of skills (Acker, 1989). Second, when occupations change from being male-dominated to being female-dominated (e.g., secretary), salaries and prestige associated with them decline (Reskin, 1988; Sanday, 1974). Third, even women in high-status, well-paid occupations are paid less than men in those occupations. For example, among U.S. physicians, 21% are women, and their median annual salary is $120,000, whereas that of male physicians is $175,000; sizable gaps are found within each range of years in practice (American Medical Association, 2002). Fourth, within an occupation, men are concentrated into the higher paying sectors. For example, in the United States, 85% or more of federal judges, law firm partners, law school deans, general counsels, and managers of large law firms are men, who have a median annual income $19,000 higher than women lawyers (American Bar Association Commission on Women in the Profession, 2001).

Employment data are most often collected by occupation rather than by job. But the few existing studies of job segregation show even more direct evidence of sexism and of racism in employment than do occupation studies. Women who work at jobs with few or no men make substantially less money than women who work at jobs where men are also employed (Tomaskevic-Devey, 1993; see also Bielby & Baron, 1984, 1986). This is not due to women's choice, or because they have small children, less education, or lower qualifications (Tomaskevic-Devey, 1993). Men who work in jobs with many women are also paid less than men who work in male-dominated jobs, illustrating that men have a salaried stake in working in gender-segregated environments.

Though men generally benefit from gender segregation on the job, their outcomes vary substantially with their social status. At the high end, 97% of top executive jobs around the world are held by men (Wirth, 2001). These jobs are associated with very high salaries, prestige, and political power. Next down, professional jobs in which men predominate also have relatively high compensation and personal safety. On the low end, blue-collar jobs, in which men also predominate, are associated with high levels of job injuries and fatalities. For example, U.S. occupational injuries and fatalities are highest among miners, timber cutters, airplane pilots, construction workers, agricultural workers, and operators, fabricators, and laborers in manufacturing, and these jobs are held almost exclusively by men (U.S. Bureau of Labor Statistics, 2001a, 2001b, 2001c).

In summary, systems of economic remuneration, which are associated with prestige, safety, health, and freedom, favor men over women in a variety of economic systems and sectors. Yet resource outcomes for men are highly variable. As we see in the next section, the resources women enjoy depend substantially on their family relationships with men.

GENDER AND SOCIAL OBLIGATIONS

Most of humans' basic physical needs for sustenance, sanitary living conditions, and basic social needs of belonging and attention are met through a social system of obligation for meeting those needs, namely, the family. Marriage and child rearing organize a division of labor by gender such that men generally acquire resources and women provide care (Brown, 1991). This division is one solution to the necessity of both chronic caregiving and resource acquisition to accomplish child rearing. It may also be a solution to gender inequality outside the family. Given that the costs of paid work, including sexual harassment, gender harassment, and wage discrimination, are higher for women than for men, it may seem to benefit heterosexual families for the wife to work in the home and the husband to earn wages (Becker, 1981). One problem with this system is that seemingly complementary divisions of labor are rarely complementary in terms of power, because both the asymmetrical costs and benefits of family obligations are a source of power inequality themselves and asymmetrical consequences of obligations are aided by and contribute to other forms of gendered power. Another problem is that complementary divisions of labor by gender make heterosexuality "compulsory" and exclude those not desiring such families.

Consider the relation between force and obligation. Some marriage laws provide for an asymmetry in men's and women's obligation to continue marriage by granting men more freedom to exit marriage than women. In Israel, many Jewish women continued to be *gunot,* or "chained," by husbands who refuse to divorce them, and in Uzbekistan, women must obtain permission from local authorities for a divorce (Human Rights Watch, 2001b). Such customs endanger women in abusive marriages whether they flee or stay.

Another asymmetry concerning family obligations is that wherever women's ability to control resources is more limited than men's, as is the case when women cannot own land, have paid jobs, or are underpaid compared to men, marriage offers women access to more resources than they would otherwise have. Generally, then, men and women do not have equal freedom to enter marriage. Furthermore, performing domestic labor and/or bearing children is sometimes a condition for women to stay in marriages (e.g., Solomon, 2003). Thus, receiving the advantages of marriage may be contingent on women's caregiving obligations. The chronic and intimate nature of these obligations not only demands that women contribute their own time and effort without remuneration, but obligatory caregiving also limits their ability to gain control over other resources. For example, 39% of American women and 3% of American men list caretaking responsibilities as their reason for not participating in paid work (Weismantle, 2001). In turn, employers fail to hire or promote women, because they assume that women's family obligations and values are incompatible with career advancement (Wirth, 2001).

The tenuousness of caregiving positions is shown at the margins of social well-being. For example, the reason most American women become homeless is that they have been evicted or can no longer depend on a relationship; the reason most men become homeless is loss of a job, residence in an institution, or substance abuse (Tessler, Rosenheck, & Gamache, 2001). Caregiving duties during marriage, in lieu of paid employment, often make divorce either untenable or a financial disaster for women. American women experience substantial decreases in their standards of living following divorce, whereas men experience increases (e.g., Peterson, 1996; Weitzman, 1985). Twenty-nine percent of custodial mothers live below the poverty line compared to 11% of custodial fathers (Grall, 2002). The no-fault divorce laws now in effect are partly responsible for disadvantaging women and children, because alimony is rarely paid, and division of marital property typically leads to forced sale of the family home (Hanson, McLanahan, & Thomsen, 1998). Such laws declare a legal equality for men and women to exit their marriages, but their power is not the same with regard to resources and obligations. As difficult as divorce is for custodial mothers, never-married mothers have the highest rates of poverty (e.g., U.S. Bureau of the Census, 2002), and their obligations for child care compete directly with their ability to get adequate-paying jobs (e.g., Bassuk, 1993). Women in China and Taiwan usually lose custody of children if they divorce, which implies that no one will care for these women when they are old (Ebrey, 1990). In many ways, then, gender family roles provide asymmetrical costs and benefits of obligations to men and women.

The obligation to provide care may well constitute the center of the feminine gender role. Indeed, American women do substantially more caregiving outside their families than do men (e.g., Gerstel, 2000). Caregiving may provide some benefits to women: affection, intimacy, a sense of belonging, self-affirmation, and access to resources. Men with no social obligations are often bereft of relationships and can suffer greatly without them, as is the case with widowers and homeless men (e.g., Gove & Shin, 1989; Tessler et al., 2001). However, the benefits that accrue to caregivers are rarely, if ever, *exchangeable,* and for that reason, those benefits do not confer *power.* In summary, then, social obligations have a complex but important relation to power. People with no obligations usually cannot experience the benefits of relationships (unless they are extremely high in power, and others are obliged to them), but within relationships, the party with less obligation has higher power.

CONSENSUAL IDEOLOGIES INFLUENCING GENDER INEQUALITY

Shared cultural ideologies prescribe how people should behave, how violators should be sanctioned, and how resources should be allocated (e.g., Pratto, 1999). The most obvious form of ideologies relevant to gender is gender stereotypes. A consistent body of international research has found that women are stereotyped as warm or communal (e.g., as understanding, helpful, affectionate; Spence, Helmreich, & Stapp, 1975; Williams & Best, 1990). Such presumptions make women appear suited to caretaking roles, such as housewife, mother, nurse, or secretary (Glick, Zion, & Nelson, 1988). Stereotypes, in turn, derive from knowledge that women typify such roles (Conway, Pizzimiglio, & Mount, 1996). In contrast, men are usually stereotyped as competent or agentic (e.g., as rational, intelligent, efficacious), making them appear suited to professional and leadership roles (e.g., Cejka & Eagly, 1999; Eagly & Steffen, 1984).

Gender stereotypes legitimize and cause gender differences in power, then, in several ways. First, they saddle women especially with caregiving obligations that, as we have seen, limit their power by monopolizing their lives, and limiting both their freedom to exit relationships and their resource control. Second, coupled with meritocratic beliefs, the stereotype that men are competent implies that they are entitled to resources and to control over resources, such as prestigious and high-paying jobs and land ownership, whereas men's presumptive agency implies that they are entitled to power. A subset of men's stereotypical traits, including aggressive, cold, rational, and nonemotional, makes them appear suited to leadership and especially to war-making roles. In the light of ideologies that legitimize violence against outgroup threats, such as nationalism, militarism, anti-communism, and antiterrorism, men become heroes, and their authoritative power is legitimized.

Another notable set of ideologies relevant to gendered power concerns women's sexuality and their bodies. Many societies' ideologies explicitly prescribe that although women should not control their own sexuality, they may be judged by their appearance. These prescriptions may not only be part of gender stereotypes but may also be aspects of ethnic or national identity, racial prejudice, religious orthodoxy, rape myths, fashion, or decorum. For example, covering women's heads and other body parts has been prescribed as part of Christian, Jewish, and Muslim orthodoxy, and Victorian manners. Ideologies about white women's "chastity" and the "exoticism" of women of color were used to legitimize lynching of black men and to debase women of color (e.g., Davis, 1981; White, 1985). Revealing and emphasizing body and face parts is prescribed so much in modern fashion that sexual objectification of women may be considered the norm (Frederickson & Roberts, 1997). The existence of the seemingly oppositional "orthodox" and "modern" flavors of these objectifying ideologies should not disguise the fact that such ideologies legitimize violence against women (e.g., Burt, 1980; Pratto et al., 2000; White, 1985) and cause them physical and psychological harm (Fredrickson & Roberts, 1997; see also Eagly, Wood, & Johannesen-Schmidt, Chapter 12, this volume). For example, being preoccupied with physical appearance decreases women's academic performance (Fredrickson, Roberts, Noll, Quinn, & Twenge, 1998). When men consider women to be sex objects, they behave in more dominating and sexist ways toward women they interview for jobs (Rudman & Borgida, 1995).

Cultural ideologies relevant to gender are exemplified not only in the law, in social roles, in occupational segregation, in religion, and in interpersonal behavior, but also in public discourse. Examination of the influential mass media informs us about gendered power. Mass media depict many more men than women (e.g., Davis, 1990, Sommers-Flanagan, Sommers-Flanagan, & Davis, 1993). Men on television are usually middle-aged, intelligent, experienced, and attracted to women, and often hold critical, high-status jobs (e.g., as doctors; Davis, 1990). This bias not only reinforces the conception that men are important and merit authoritative positions but also conflates masculinity with being powerful, white, upper class, and straight.

In contrast, women frequently appear on television as sex objects. Female television characters are disproportionately blonde, young, single, and provocatively dressed (Davis, 1990). In magazine photographs, men's faces are more prominent compared to their bodies than are women's faces (e.g., Archer, Iritani, Kimes, & Barrios, 1983). When women are not portrayed as "eye candy," they are cast in caretaking roles as wives, housewives, and mothers. In contrast, one cannot tell whether most male television characters have a family (Davis, 1990). The dearth of nonwhite and nonstraight television characters is well-known.

Finally, experiments show that men who watch sexual violence, as depicted in popular movies, become less bothered by sexual and nonsexual violence against women (Linz, Donnerstein, & Adams, 1989; Linz, Donnerstein, & Penrod, 1989; Malamuth & Check, 1981; Mullin & Linz, 1995) and behave more aggressively toward women (Donnerstein, 1980). We have seen, then, that the mass media reinforce all four of the gendered bases of power: Men's use of forceful power and sexual violence in authoritative positions, men's greater resource control through high-paying jobs, women's greater obligations to caretaking in housewife roles, and men's advantage via cultural ideologies, in that men and their points of view are typically represented.

GENDER AND ROLES RELEVANT TO POWER

As many theories emphasize, gendered roles are a proximate cause of differential outcomes for men and women, especially status differences (see Eagly et al., Chapter 12, this volume; Ridgeway & Bourg, Chapter 10, this volume). One of social dominance theory's particular insights is that roles that tend to maintain or enhance inequality within societies tend to be held disproportionately by men, whereas roles that tend to attenuate inequality within societies tend to be held disproportionately by women (Pratto, Stallworth, Sidanius, & Siers, 1997). By definition, hierarchy-enhancers maintain or enhance status distinctions and group boundaries in part by channeling desirable things (e.g., resources, prestige, legal privileges) to those who are better off and undesirable things (e.g., refuse, low-quality education) to those who are worse off. Hierarchy-attenuators try to reduce status boundaries and power differences, usually by trying to gain desirable things (e.g., legal rights or representation, health care) for those worse off. We examined the representation of men and women in hierarchy-enhancing and -attenuating roles relevant

TABLE 11.1. Percentage of Women and Mean Annual Wages Associated with Various Hierarchy-Enhancing and Hierarchy-Attenuating Occupations, United States

Relation to power	Occupation	% women	Median weekly earnings ($)
	Hierarchy-enhancing occupations		
Wields forceful power	Judges and lawyers	29	1,380
	Police	14	782
	Correctional officers	22	573
Wields economic power	Securities sales	30	980
	Executive, managerial	46	867
Wields ideological power	Marketing managers	39	1,095
	Editors, reporters	51	762
	Hierarchy-attenuating occupations		
Undoing harm	Social workers	72	644
	Counselors	68	766
	Volunteers	62	0
Empowering with information	Teachers	74	730
	Librarians	85	726
Cares for others	Childcare providers	97	246
	Nurses	93	829
Provides personal services	Secretaries	98	475
	Wait staff	76	331
	Cleaners, servants	96	254

Note. Percentage for volunteers is from Independent Sector (1999). All other percentages are from U.S. Bureau of Labor Statistics (2001c). Wages are from U.S. Bureau of Labor Statistics (2001d).

to the four forms of power discussed in this chapter, and the pay associated with them, by using the most accessible data available to us, based mainly on the U.S. Bureau of the Census (see Table 11.1).

Roles That Wield Forceful Power

Physical and emotional violence have received the most attention as the means by which men hold destructive power over women. Another way that men hold the reins of destructive power is in possession and command over social roles that threaten or actually carry out physical force under the legitimacy of law or religious decree, for example, government and military, leadership, the war-making arms of government, and legal prosecution and judicial functions (whether state-based or religious). With the exception of small changes in recent years, such roles are almost universally held by men (Keegan, 1993; Vianello & Siemienska, 1990).

For example, in 2000, nine heads of state (less than 5% of the total), 8% of the world's cabinet members, and 11% of parliamentarians were women. Women are still tokens in virtually all national legislatures, holding 15% of seats. Two African nations with recent progressive revolutions, South Africa and Mozambique, have 30% women in their national legislatures, as do Germany and New Zealand; elsewhere, only Nordic countries have more than token representation by women, with 37% of parliamentary seats in Finland and Denmark, 35% in Iceland, 36% in the Netherlands and Norway, and 43% in Sweden held by women. Of 196 nations, forty-five have no women at all in ministerial decision-making positions, and in only 15 nations do women hold more than 20% women of cabinet positions (see United Nations Statistics Division, 2002c).

In the United States as elsewhere, men predominate in the judicial system. Women comprise 16% of U.S. Circuit Court judges, 2% of U.S. District Court judges, and 22% (2) of the U.S. Supreme Court justices (American Bar Association Commission on Women in the Profession, 2001). The top three lines of Table 11.1 show the percentages of women in occupations that wield forceful power, with associated salaries. Comparison with the rest of the occupations indicates that the percentage of women in these roles is low, whereas the associated wages are high. The higher paid, higher grade positions within the U.S. military are also held disproportionately by men, as are command positions (U.S. Department of Defense, 1998).

Masculine control of "legitimate" force is a significant proximal cause of sexism, in that legal systems institutionalize many forms of sexism and often do little to protect women (e.g., from economic exploitation, rape, sexual harassment), and governments and militaries are supported by public funds but provide jobs and political power disproportionately to men. At the same time, legal and military institutions foment arbitrary set dominance by targeting or exploiting subordinate-group men within their society and in other, subordinate societies, especially male combatants and criminals (see Sidanius & Pratto, 1999, pp. 202–204, 223).

Roles That Wield Resource Control

Women comprise 16% of corporate officers in the 500 largest American companies (Catalyst, 2002) and hold 1–3% of top executive jobs around the world (Wirth, 2001). In the United States, those who control and manage resources within corporations are disproportionately men, and they earn much higher salaries than persons in hierarchy-attenuating jobs (see Table 11.1). Women are also a small minority on the governing boards of the International Monetary Fund, the World Bank, and related financial organizations that have been widely criticized for lending policies that require developing nations to neglect basic care, such as health and education, in favor of debt service (e.g., Women's Environment and Development Organization, 2001). An elite group of men holds tremendous power over the rest of us through control of corporations and financial agencies that have global reach.

Roles That Wield Ideological Power

Roles that control the content and dissemination of ideologies are held predominantly by men. This appears as true for the traditional purveyors of norms of morality, namely, religious and political leaders, as for modern marketing and mass-media hucksters. Marketing managers tend to be highly paid men (see Table 11.1). Although the number of female editors and reporters is proportional to the number of women in the workforce (see Table 11.1), men are much more predominant as media decision makers. Only 13% of executives in U.S. telecommunications, broadcast media, and e-companies are women; women constitute only 9% of board members and hold 3% of titles with "clout" (e.g., CEO or Chairman; Jamieson, 2001). The salaries commanded by these positions are matched by the ideological reach of such companies; a representative of *Fortune* says that the magazine is redefining "how we shop, communicate, advertise, entertain ourselves, plan our lives, and manage our finances" (Jamieson, 2001). Women comprised 17% of all executive producers, directors, writers, cinematographers, and editors working on the 250 top-grossing films of 2001 (Lauzen, 2002), and 26% of news directors and 17% of general managers at U.S. television stations (Jamieson, 2001). Their increasing representation on camera hides the fact that women are not in control of broadcast media.

Roles That Undo Harm

Some people labor to undo the harm caused to people who are needy, undereducated, sick, victimized by violence, and prone to other ills associated with low power. One category of hierarchy-attenuators, then, includes social workers, counselors, and charity volunteers, who, as shown in Table 11.1, are disproportionately women who are paid significantly less than any of the male-dominated hierarchy-enhancing roles shown in Table 11.1.

Roles That Empower Others with Information

In the United States, a founding principle of public education and public libraries is to make knowledge widely available. Helping to disseminate knowledge and provide people with the tools to find, evaluate, and create knowledge might be seen as a populist and hierarchy-attenuating counter to control over mass discourse. For this reason, we consider teachers and librarians to be hierarchy-attenuators. As shown in Table 11.1, these positions are mainly held by women, but the pay is far less than that for those in control of media content.

Roles That Provide Care and Personal Services to Others

Our theoretical analysis shows why providing care to others is a mark of low power. In addition to unpaid homemaking, provision of direct care or personal services is overwhelmingly supplied by women, and among such occupations, only nursing cannot be considered to have a low salary (see Table 11.1). Nurses have professionalized their occupation over the past 100 years. It should be noted that women in subordinate arbitrary set groups, such as, historically, the serving class and Irish in England, Irish immigrants in the northeastern United States, and African Americans in the southern United States, perform a disproportional amount of this work. One exception to this pattern is that when immigration laws barred Asian women from entering the United States, and where there were few persons in other subordinate groups, Asian men performed a substantial proportion of domestic service (Amott & Matthaei, 1991, pp. 320–327).

DISCUSSION

Gender inequality can be understood by examining the dynamics of four bases of power: force, resource control, ideological advantage, and asymmetrical obligations. All four bases of power, and roles associated with them, are differentially held by men, which explains why gender inequality can be found in so many domains, such as marriage customs, wages, inheritance laws, use of violence, and ideologies, and in so many societies.

Our focus on power emphasizes *relationships* rather than gender differences, gender roles, economic considerations, or evolutionary processes. Yet our approach is compatible with theories that focus on these aspects of gender and places some of them in a new light. For example, political–psychological factors help account for gender differences in the acquisition of roles and in support for institutional practices that maintain or attenuate social hierarchy (e.g., Pratto, Stallworth, & Sidanius, 1997; Pratto, Stallworth, Sidanius, & Siers, 1997). We attend to social roles because they help to organize relationships, the use of force, obligations, and resource distribution, and are supported by cultural ideologies. Our description of power allows us not only to declare that roles such as soldier and caregiver are associated with gender and prestige but also to describe how such roles pertain to power through force, resource control, and asymmetrical obligations. Furthermore, we emphasize the relation of such roles to institutions that help maintain or attenuate group-based inequality. Our analysis also identifies power imbalances in "economic" and "complementary" gender roles. A number of our points are compatible with expectation states theory: the way gender functions as a status in determining occupational prestige and as a category system in heterosexual relations, and the central role of consensual ideologies in organizing social structure (see Ridgeway & Bourg, Chapter 10, this volume). Many of the data we have presented are compatible with evolutionary theory (see Kenrick, Trost, & Sundie, Chapter 4, this volume). In particular, the greater variability among men's than among women's outcomes, status competition among men, women's participation in restrictions over their bodies and sexuality, and our acknowledgment that child care arrangements are central to social organization and power relationships between men and women are consistent with feminist interpretations of parental investment theory (e.g., Dickemann, 1981; Pratto & Hegarty, 2000). Our focus on the dynamics of power emphasizes the active creation of these patterns in contemporary environments.

Understanding power as relational and dynamic enables us to describe ways that greater equality can be realized. Recent changes in many societies indicate that giving women more control over resources (e.g., by providing appropriate education, reducing job discrimination, increasing pay equity, enacting fair inheritance laws) is a way to increase women's power. Likewise, reducing violence, balancing asymmetrical obligations, and changing cultural ideologies can reduce inequality. However, because power relations are dynamic, there can be active resistance to and backlashes against empowering women (see Ridgeway & Bourg, Chapter 10, this volume). A more detailed discussion of power dynamics can help to identify conditions that can bring about greater equality.

In explicating each basis of power, we explain *fungibility:* the forms of power that can be used to gain power in another form. Table 11.2 provides examples of how each basis of power can influence the other bases. For example, the left-hand column summarizes some of the ways the use of force (enacted in law, the military, or in violence) can bolster

TABLE 11.2. The Fungibility of Each Basis of Power

	Bases of power			
Their impact on other bases of power	Force	Resource control	Social obligations	Ideologies
Force		Resources enable one to buy political influence and legal and police protection, especially for elites.	Obligations to care (e.g., parenting) are viewed as incompatible with forceful roles (e.g., soldier, lawyer).	• Media violence prompts sexist behavior in men. • "Rape myths" blame women rather than men for rape.
Resource control	• Law reserves certain resources (e.g., land, jobs) for men. • Abuse reduces personal resources (health, self-esteem).		• Caregiving obligations may gain one access to resources, but reduce opportunities for resource control. • Recipients are enriched and save the expense of replacing such benefits.	Gender stereotypes entitle men to high-paying jobs.
Social obligations	Abuse reduces women's freedom to exit marriage and employment.	Lack of access to resources drives women into marriage or other relationships and limits their freedom to exit.		Gender stereotypes consign women to having high social obligations.
Ideologies	Law enforces sexist ideologies (e.g., tolerance of rape, occupational segregation).	Men gain (or lose) prestige through control of resources and occupations.	Asymmetric obligations help produce the stereotypes and other ideologies that legitimize such asymmetries (e.g., men as agentic, women as dependent).	

resource control, advantages gained through asymmetrical social obligations, and sexist ideologies. We have shown that forms of power based in force, resource control, and ideologies contribute to each other and to asymmetrical social obligations. Men are not only advantaged in power, then, simply because they are advantaged in each of these arenas, but also because their power in any one arena enables them to gain power in other arenas. Social change toward equality is more likely to be long-lasting if it takes place in more than one arena; otherwise, it is too easy for men to use one form of power to regain yet another.

Power derived from asymmetrical social obligations has a different relationship to the other bases of power. Being advantaged by obligations has resource value and makes one seem more appropriate for forceful roles, and it is consistent with many ideologies advantaging men. However, being disadvantaged in terms of obligations *prevents* one from gaining power in other arenas. This is untrue of the other three bases of power. For example, not using forceful power does not prevent one from controlling resources or from being ideologically advantaged. For this reason, asymmetrical social obligations are pivotal to gender inequality. So long as women are more obliged to others than others are to them, particularly when what they are "owed" by others is not exchangeable (e.g., affection), they will be disadvantaged in power. Hence, caregiving arrangements are critical in determining gender equality or inequality.

Our dynamic explication of power has also shown that no understanding of gender inequality is complete without understanding its dynamic relation to arbitrary set inequality. There are two reasons for this. First, for each basis of power, variability among men and women is systematically related to arbitrary set group distinctions. Specifically, forceful power wielded by the criminal justice system, disproportionately held by dominant-group men, disproportionately targets and punishes men in subordinate ethnic groups (see Sidanius & Pratto, 1999, Ch. 8). For example, nearly half of U.S. death row inmates are black men (Fins, 2002). Similarly, men in dominant groups (rather than all men) are the ones who really have disproportionate resource control. Ownership of land historically accrued to men in elite groups (e.g., noblemen in feudal systems). Now, elite men are overrepresented among the safest, highest paid, and most prestigious jobs, whereas men in subordinate groups are overrepresented among the unemployed and in poorly paid, male-dominated occupations, such as janitor. Such race differentiation in resource control is reflected in ideologies: Stereotypes differentiate white men from black and Hispanic men along social-standing dimensions, but no parallel differentiation is found for women (Pratto & Espinoza, 2001).

Second, men and women can use arbitrary set dominance to gain power vis-à-vis each other, such that certain forms of gender-related power struggles rely on arbitrary set dominance. For example, gender differentiation in roles and stereotypical traits positions men and women in power relation to each other, usually according to the presumption that heterosexuality is normal. Sexist beliefs and practices are therefore also heterosexist. Stereotypes of lesbians and gay men postulate that they have the traits of the opposite sex (Kite & Deaux, 1987). Because one's gender so often confers one's humanity in the eyes of others, the denial of gender for such persons has been grounds for legal denial of rights (Currah & Minter, 2000). In fact, lesbians and gay men earn less money than do straight people (Badgett, 1998), and forgo many other material and ideological benefits accrued through marriage as well.

Race, ethnicity, and class also play a role in gendered power struggles. For example, resource control, which can be aided by racism and classism among men, makes men more attractive to women as marriage partners (Pratto & Hegarty, 2000). Hence, some men can gain power over women via arbitrary set discrimination. One way that women free themselves from obligations to provide care (e.g., cooking, cleaning, child care) is to hire others to do it. Arbitrary set inequality enables dominant-group women to hire women in subordinate classes and ethnic groups as "household help"; these women often have little choice but to take such low-pay, low-prestige positions (e.g., Collins, 1990, pp. 55–66). Ideologies concerning women's sexuality are often colored by racism, so they legitimize not only the control of women in dominant groups but also the abuse of women and of men in subordinate groups by men in dominant groups (Davis, 1981; Pratto, 1996; White, 1985).

In all of these ways, then, power struggles between men and women depend on arbitrary group inequality. Given that, in complex societies, arbitrary set inequality and gender inequality go hand in hand, it is not surprising that a variety of social practices structure both forms. Indeed, some methods of empowering dominant-group women vis-à-vis men (e.g., hiring domestic help as cheaply as possible, realizing racist or classist feminine beauty ideals) reinforce arbitrary group inequality. But note that other ways of empowering women (e.g., providing living wages and education for household help, spreading nonobjectifying ideologies) can help to reduce arbitrary group inequality as well. The challenge for social change efforts is to identify practices that will increase equality for persons throughout the dynamic system, rather than only for some people or some forms of power. Our theory demonstrates that it is necessary to consider the particular bases of power inequalities in question, what forms of power are fungible with other forms, and the ways that gender intersects with arbitrary set distinctions to devise long-lasting, effective solutions.

ACKNOWLEDGMENTS

We thank Wendy Wood, Jim Sidanius, I-Ching Lee, Nancy Naples, and Melanie Dykas for their thoughtful comments on a previous draft of this chapter.

REFERENCES

Acker, J. (1989). *Doing comparable worth: Gender, class and pay equity.* Philadelphia: Temple University Press.

American Bar Association Commission on Women in the Profession. (2001). *Statistics and data on women in the legal profession.* Retrieved January 19, 2003, from *http://womenlaw.stanford.edu/womenlawyerstats.html*

American Medical Association. (2002). *AMA Women In Medicine data source, 2002 Edition.* Retrieved January 19, 2003, from *http://www.ama-assn.org/ama/pub/category/171.html*

Amott, T. L., & Matthaei, J. A. (1991). *Race, gender, and work.* Boston: South End Press.

Archer, J. (2000). Sex differences in aggression between heterosexual partners: A meta-analytic review. *Psychological Bulletin, 126,* 651–680.

Archer, D., Iritani, B., Kimes, D. D., & Barrios, M. (1983). Faceism: Five studies of sex differences in facial prominence. *Journal of Personality and Social Psychology, 45,* 725–735.

Association de Soutien à Touria. (2003). *Touria is sentenced!* Retrieved September 2, 2003, from *http://touria.tiouli.free.fr/index_english.htm*

Babcock, J., Waltz, J., Jacobson, N., & Gottman, J. (1993). Power and violence: The relation between communication patterns, power discrepancies, and domestic violence. *Journal of Consulting and Clinical Psychology, 61,* 40–50.

Badgett, M. V. L. (1998). *Income inflation: The myth of affluence among gay, lesbian and bisexual Americans.* Retrieved January 22, 2003, from *http://www.ngltf.org/downloads/income.pdf*

Bassuk, E. L. (1993). Social and economic hardships of homeless and other poor women. *American Journal of Orthopsychiatry, 63,* 340–347.

Becker, G. S. (1981). *A treatise on the family.* Cambridge, MA: Harvard University Press.

Bielby, W. T., & Baron, J. N. (1984). A woman's place is with other women. In B. F. Reskin (Ed.), *Sex segregation in the workplace: Trends, explanations, remedies* (pp. 27–55). Washington, DC: National Academy Press.

Bielby, W. T., & Baron, J. N. (1986). Men and women at work: Sex segregation and statistical discrimination. *American Journal of Sociology, 91,* 759–799.

Brown, D. E. (1991). *Human universals.* New York: McGraw-Hill.

Burt, M. (1980). Cultural myths and supports for rape. *Journal of Personality and Social Psychology, 38,* 217–230.

Catalyst. (2002). Catalyst census marks gains in numbers of women corporate officers in America's largest 500 companies. Retrieved April 23, 2003, from *http://www.catalystwomen.org/press_room/press_releases/2002_cote.htm*

Cejka, M. A., & Eagly, A. H. (1999). Gender stereotypic images of occupations correspond to the sex segregation of employment. *Personality and Social Psychology Bulletin, 25,* 413–423.

Collins, P. H. (1990). *Black feminist thought: Knowledge, consciousness, and the politics of empowerment.* New York: Routledge.

Conway, M., Pizzimiglio, M. T., & Mount, L. (1996). Status, communality, and agency: Implications for stereotypes of gender and other groups. *Journal of Personality and Social Psychology, 71,* 25–38.

Currah, P., & Minter, S. (2000). Unprincipled exclusions: The struggle to achieve judicial and legislative equality for transgender people. *William and Mary Journal of Women and the Law, 7,* 37–66.

Daly, M., & Wilson, M. (1988). *Homicide.* New York: Aldine de Gruyter.

Davis, A. Y. (1981). *Women, race, and class.* New York: Vintage.

Davis, D. M. (1990). Portrayals of women in prime-time network television: Some demographic characteristics. *Sex Roles, 23,* 325–332.

Dickemann, M. (1981). Paternal confidence and dowry competition: A biocultural analysis of Purdah. In R. A. Alexander & D. W. Tinkle (Eds.), *Natural selection and social behavior* (pp. 417–438). New York: Chiron Press.

Donnerstein, E. (1980). Aggressive erotica and violence against women. *Journal of Personality and Social Psychology, 39,* 269–277.

Eagly, A. H., & Steffen, V. J. (1984). Gender stereotypes stem from the distribution of women and men into social roles. *Journal of Personality and Social Psychology, 46,* 735–754.

Ebrey, P. (1990). Women, marriage, and the family. In P. S. Roop (Ed.), *Heritage of China: Contemporary perspectives on Chinese civilization* (pp. 197–223). Berkeley: University of California Press.

Engels, F. (1902). *The origin of the family, private property, and the state* (E. Untermann, Trans.). Chicago: E. H. Kerr. (Original work published in 1884)

Federal Bureau of Investigation. (2001). *Crime in the U.S. 2000: Uniform crime reports.* Washington, DC: U.S. Department of Justice. Retrieved January 19, 2003, from *http://www.fbi.gov/ucr/cius_00/contents.pdf*

Fins, D. (2002, Fall). *Death row U.S.A.: A quarterly report of the Criminal Justice Project of the NAACP Legal Defense and Education Fund. Retrieved January 19, 2003, from http://www.deathpenaltyinfo.org/deathrowusarecent.pdf*

Fitzgerald, L. F., Gelfand, M. J., & Drasgow, F. (1995). Measuring sexual harassment: Theoretical and psychometric advances. *Basic and Applied Social Psychology, 17,* 425–445.

Fredrickson, B. L., & Roberts, T. (1997). Objectification theory: Toward understanding women's lived experiences and mental health risks. *Psychology of Women Quarterly, 21,* 173–206.

Fredrickson, B. L., Roberts, T., Noll, S. M., Quinn, D. M., & Twenge, J. M.

(1998). That swimsuit becomes you: Sex differences in self-objectification, restrained eating, and math performance. *Journal of Personality and Social Psychology, 75,* 269–284.

Frieze, I. H., & McHugh, M. C. (1992). Power and influence strategies in violent and nonviolent marriages. *Psychology of Women Quarterly, 16,* 449–465.

Gerstel, N. (2000). The third shift: Gender and work outside the home. *Qualitative Sociology, 3,* 467–483.

Glick, P., Zion, C., & Nelson, C. (1988). What mediates sex discrimination in hiring decisions? *Journal of Personality and Social Psychology, 55,* 178–186.

Gove, W. R., & Shin, H. C. (1989). The psychological well-being of divorced and widowed men and women: An empirical analysis. *Journal of Family Issues, 10,* 122–144.

Grall, T. (2002). *Custodial mothers and fathers and their child support 1999.* Retrieved January 22, 2003, from *http://www.census.gov/prod/2002pubs/p60-217.pdf*

Hanson, T. L., McLanahan, S. S., & Thomsen, E. (1998). Windows on divorce: Before and after. *Social Science Research, 27,* 329–349.

Hornung, C. A., McCullough, B. C., & Sugimoto, T. (1981). Status relationships in marriage: Risk factors in spouse abuse. *Journal of Marriage and the Family, 43,* 675–692.

Human Rights Watch. (2002a). *Women in conflict and refugees.* Retrieved August 27, 2003, from *http://www.hrw.org/wr2k2/women/women.html*

Human Rights Watch. (2001b). *Women's status in the family.* Retrieved August 27, 2003, from *http://www.hrw.org/wr2k2/women/women.html#status*

Independent Sector. (1999). *The demographics of household contributors and volunteers.* Retrieved January 19, 2003, from *http://www.independentsector.org/GandV/s_demo.htm*

Jackman, M. R. (1994). *The velvet glove.* Berkeley: University of California Press.

Jamieson, K. H. (2001, March 14). *Progress or no room at the top?: The role of women in telecommuniations, broadcast, cable and e-companies.* Annenberg Public Policy Center. Retrieved January 22, 2003, from *http://www.appcpenn.org/internet/publicpolicy/progress-report.pdf*

Johnson, M. P. (1995). Patriarchal terror and common couple violence: Two forms of violence against women. *Journal of Marriage and the Family, 57,* 283–294.

Jordan, M. (2002, June 30). In Mexico: An unpunished crime. *Washington Post,* p. A1.

Keegan, J. (1993). *A history of warfare.* New York: Knopf.

Kite, M., & Deaux, K. (1987). Gender belief systems: Homosexuality and the implicit inversion theory. *Psychology of Women Quarterly, 11,* 83–96.

Lauzen, M. M. (2002, June 24). *Executive summary: Statistics on women directors. The Celluloid Ceiling Study.* Retrieved January 19, 2003, from *http://www.5050summit.com/stats2001.html*

Lenski, G. (1984). *Power and privilege: A theory of social stratification.* Chapel Hill: University of North Carolina Press.

Linz, D. G., Donnerstein, E., & Adams, S. M. (1989). Physiological desensitization and judgments about female victims of violence. *Human Communication Research, 15,* 509–522.

Linz, D. G., Donnerstein, E., & Penrod, S. (1988). Effects of long-term exposure to violent and sexually degrading depictions of women. *Journal of Personality and Social Psychology, 55,* 758–768.

Malamuth, N., & Check, J. (1981). The effects of media exposure on acceptance of violence against women: A field experiment. *Journal of Research in Personality, 15,* 436–446.

Marx, K., & Engels, F. (1846). *The German ideology.* New York: International Publishers.

Mullin, C. R., & Linz, D. (1995). Desensitization and resensitization to violence against women: Effects of exposure to sexually violent films on judgments of domestic violence victims. *Journal of Personality and Social Psychology, 69,* 449–459.

O'Connell, E. C., & Korabik, K. (2000). Sexual harassment: The relationship of personal vulnerability, work context, perpetrator status, and type of harassment to outcomes. *Journal of Vocational Behavior, 56,* 299–329.

Peterson, R. R. (1996). A re-evaluation of the economic consequences of divorce. *American Sociological Review, 61,* 528–536.

Pratto, F. (1996). Sexual politics: The gender gap in the bedroom, the cupboard, and the cabinet. In D. M. Buss & N. Malamuth (Eds.), *Sex, power, and conflict: Evolutionary and feminist perspectives* (pp. 179–230). New York: Oxford University Press.

Pratto, F. (1999). The puzzle of continuing group inequality: Piecing together psychological, social, and cultural forces in social dominance theory. In M. P. Zanna (Ed.), *Advances in experimental social psychology* (Vol. 31, pp. 191–263). San Diego: Academic Press.

Pratto, F., & Espinoza, P. (2001). Gender, ethnicity, and power. *Journal of Social Issues, 57,* 763–780.

Pratto, F., & Hegarty, P. (2000). The political psychology of reproductive strategies. *Psychological Science, 11,* 57–62.

Pratto, F., Liu, J., Levin, S., Sidanius, J., Shih, M., Bachrach, H., & Hegarty, P. (2000). Social dominance orientation and the legitimization of inequality across cultures. *Journal of Cross-Cultural Psychology, 31,* 369–409.

Pratto, F., Stallworth, L. M., & Sidanius, J. (1997). The gender gap: Differences in political attitudes and social dominance orientation. *British Journal of Social Psychology, 36,* 49–68.

Pratto, F., Stallworth, L. M., Sidanius, J., & Siers, B. (1997). The gender gap in occupational role attainment: A social dominance approach. *Journal of Personality and Social Psychology, 72,* 37–53.

Pratto, F., & Walker, A. (2000). Dominance in disguise: Power, beneficence, and exploitation in personal relationships. In A. Lee-Chai & J. A. Bargh (Eds.), *The use and abuse of power* (pp. 93–114). Philadelphia: Psychology Press.

Qvist, E. (1998). *Women's access, control, and tenure of land, property and settlement.* Retrieved January 19, 2003, from *http://www.geom.unimelb.edu.au/fig7/Brighton98/Comm7Papers/TS26-Qvist.html*

Reskin, B. F. (1988). Bringing the men back in: Sex differentiation and the devaluation of women's work. *Gender and Society, 2,* 58–81.

Riger, S. (1991). Gender dilemmas in sexual harassment policies and procedures. *American Psychologist, 46,* 497–505.

Rodrigue, G. (1993, May 14). In Bosnia, shocking reality of policy of rape. *San Francisco Examiner,* pp. A1, A20.

Rosaldo, M. Z. (1974). Woman, culture, and society: A theoretical overview. In M. Z. Rosaldo & L. Lamphere (Eds.), *Women, culture, and society* (pp. 17–42). Stanford, CA: Stanford University Press.

Rudman, L. A., & Borgida, E. (1995). The afterglow of construct accessibility: The behavioral consequences of priming men to view women as sexual objects. *Journal of Experimental Social Psychology, 31,* 493–517.

Sacks, K. (1974). Engels revisited: Women, the organization of production, and private property. In M. Z. Rosaldo & L. Lamphere (Eds.), *Women, culture, and society* (pp. 207–222). Stanford, CA: Stanford University Press.

Sagrestano, L. M., Heavey, D. L., & Christianson, A. (1999). Perceived power and physical violence in marital conflict. *Journal of Social Issues, 55,* 65–79.

Sanday, P. (1981). *Female power and male dominance.* New York: Cambridge University Press.

Sanday, P. R. (1974). Female status in the public domain. In M. Z. Rosaldo & L. Lamphere (Eds.), *Women, culture, and society* (pp. 189–206). Stanford, CA: Stanford University Press.

Sanderson, L. P. (1981). *Against the mutilation of women: The struggle to end unnecessary suffering.* London: Ithaca Press.

Schwendinger, J. R., & Schwendinger, H. (1983). *Rape and equality.* Beverly Hills, CA: Sage.

Sidanius, J., & Pratto, F. (1999). *Social dominance: An intergroup theory of social hierarchy and oppression.* New York: Cambridge University Press.

Solomon, S. (2003, February 20). *YRGCARE: Shaping the response to HIV/AIDS in India.* Colloquium given to Center for Health/HIV Intervention and Prevention, University of Connecticut, Storrs.

Sommers-Flanagan, R., Sommers-Flanagan, J., & Davis, B. (1993). What's happening on music television?: A gender role analysis. *Sex Roles, 28,* 745–753.

Spence, J. T., Helmreich, R., & Stapp, J. (1975). Ratings of self and peers on sex role attributes and their relations to self-esteem and conceptions of masculinity and femininity. *Journal of Personality and Social Psychology, 9,* 51–77.

Terpestra, D. E., & Baker, D. D. (1986). Emotional and psychological consequences of sexual harassment: A descriptive study. *Journal of Psychology, 130,* 429–446.

Tessler, R., Rosenheck, R., & Gamache, G. (2001). Gender differences in self-reported reasons for homelessness. *Journal of Social Distress and the Homeless, 10,* 243–254.

Thibaut, J. W., & Kelly, H. H. (1959). *The social psychology of groups.* New York: Wiley.

Tomaskovic-Devey, D. (1993). *Gender and racial inequality at work: The sources and consequences of job segregation.* Ithaca, NY: ILR Press.

United Nations Statistics Division. (2002a). *Physical abuse against women by an intimate partner.* Retrieved January 19, 2003, from *http://unstats.un.org/unsd/demographic/ww2000/table6c.htm*

United Nations Statistics Division. (2002b). *Women's wages relative to men's.* Retrieved January 19, 2003, from *http://unstats.un.org/unsd/demographic/ww2000/table5g.htm*

United Nations Statistics Division. (2002c). *Women in public life.* Retrieved January 19, 2003, from *http://unstats.un.org/unsd/demographic/ww2000/table6a.htm*

U.S. Bureau of the Census. (2002, September). *Number of children, marital status, and work experience in 2001 of people 16 years and over.* Retrieved March 24, 2003, from *http://ferret.bls.census.gov/macro/032002/pov/new09_003.htm*

U.S. Bureau of Labor Statistics. (2001a, August 14). *National census of fatal occupational injuries in 2000.* Washington, DC: Author. Retrieved January 19, 2003, from *http://www.bls.gov/iif/oshwc/cfoi/cfnr0007.pdf*

U.S. Bureau of Labor Statistics. (2001b, December 18). *Workplace injuries and illnesses in 2000.* Washington, DC: Author. Retrieved January 19, 2003, from *http://www.bls.gov/iif/oshwc/osh/os/osnr0013.pdf*

U.S. Bureau of Labor Statistics. (2001c). *Employed persons by detailed occupation, sex, race, and Hispanic origin.* Washington, DC: Author. Retrieved January 19, 2003, from *http://www.bls.gov/cps/cpsaat11.pdf*

U.S. Bureau of Labor Statistics. (2001d). *Median weekly earnings of full time wage and salary workers by detailed occupation and sex.* Washington, DC: Author. Retrieved January 19, 2003, from *http://www.bls.gov/cps/cpsaat39.pdf*

U.S. Department of Defense. (1998). *Active duty military strength, male/female for September, 1998.* Retrieved January 19, 2003, from *http://www.dior.whs.mil/mmid/military/ms5.pdf*

Vianello, M., & Siemienska, R. (1990). *Gender inequality: A comparative study of discrimination and participation.* Newbury Park, CA: Sage.

Weismantle, M. (2001, July). *Reasons people do not work, 1996. Washington, DC: U.S. Bureau of the Census.* Retrieved January 20, 2003, from *http://landview.census.gov/prod/2001pubs/p70-76.pdf*

Weitzman, L. (1985). *Divorce revolution: The unexpected social and economic consequences for women and children in America.* New York: Free Press.

White, D. G. (1985). Jezebel and Mammy: The mythology of female slavery. In D. G. White, *Ar'n't I a woman?* (pp. 27–61). New York: Norton.

White, W. F. (1969). *Rope and faggot: A biography of Judge Lynch.* New York: Arno Press.

Williams, J. E., & Best, D. L. (1990). *Measuring sex stereotypes: A multinational study.* Newbury Park, CA: Sage.

Wirth, L. (2001). *Summary: Breaking through the glass ceiling: Women in management.* International Labor Organization. Retrieved August 27, 2003, from *http://www.ilo.org/public/english/support/publ/pdf/btgc.pdf*

Women's Environment and Development Organization. (2001). *Financing for development gender policy briefing kit.* Retrieved January 19, 2003, from *http://www.wedo.org/ffd/representation.htm*

World Health Organization. (2002a, July 1). *Sexual violence.* Retrieved January 19, 2003, from *http://www.who.int/violence_injury_prevention/main.cfm?p=0000000162*

World Health Organization. (2002b, June). *Fact sheet 241, female genital mutilation.* Retrieved January 19, 2003, from *http://www.who.int/inf-fs/en/fact241.html*

12

Social Role Theory of Sex Differences and Similarities

Implications for the Partner Preferences of Women and Men

ALICE H. EAGLY
WENDY WOOD
MARY C. JOHANNESEN-SCHMIDT

Why do human females and males behave differently in some circumstances and similarly in others? Social role theory provides a comprehensive answer to this question by encompassing several types of causes. Among these causes, social role theorists call special attention to the impact of the distribution of men and women into social roles within societies (Eagly, 1987; Eagly, Wood, & Diekman, 2000). The more ultimate causes responsible for these sex differences in roles are the inherent, physical sex differences that cause certain activities to be accomplished more efficiently by one sex or the other, depending on a society's circumstances and culture (Wood & Eagly, 2002). The benefits of each sex efficiently performing certain tasks emerge because women and men are allied in societies and engage in a division of labor. As this chapter explains, sex is therefore an important organizing feature in all known societies, yet many of the specific behaviors typical of men and women vary greatly from society to society.

The social roles of women and men cause sex differences in behavior through the mediation of social and psychological processes. One such process is the formation of gender roles, by which people are expected to have characteristics that equip them for the activities typical of their sex. For example, in industrialized societies, husbands are more likely than wives to be the main family provider and head of the household, and in workplaces, men are more likely than women to hold positions of authority. Given these sex differences in typical family and occupational roles, gender roles include the expectation that men possess directive leadership qualities (Eagly & Karau, 2002). Gender roles, along with the specific roles occupied by men and women (e.g., occupational and marital roles), then guide social behavior. This guidance is in turn mediated by various developmental and socialization processes, as well as by processes involved in social interaction (e.g., expectancy confirmation) and self-regulation. In addition, biological processes, including hormonal changes, orient men and women to certain social roles and facilitate role performance. In brief, social role theory presents a set of interconnected causes that range from more proximal, or immediate, to more distal, or ultimate (see Figure 12.1). This chapter reviews this theory and then applies it to illuminate a specific area of sex-differentiated behavior, namely, the preferences that men and women have for mates.

ORIGINS OF DIVISION OF LABOR AND GENDER HIERARCHY

The question of why men and women are differently positioned in the social structure is profoundly important for understanding sex differences in behavior. The best answer to this question emerges from the study of sex-typed social roles in a wide range of societies. Wood and Eagly (2002) reviewed this cross-cultural evidence, produced primarily by anthropologists, to provide a framework for a theory of the origins of sex differences in behavior. Their review distinguished between sex differences that are universally evident across cultures and those that emerge less consistently. Universal sex differences indicate essential features of humans that may derive from innate attributes inherent in the human species or from cultural conventions that emerge similarly across societies (e.g., women carrying infants in a sling or papoose). Sex differences that are not consistent across cultures reflect more variable aspects of human functioning that are dependent on societies' external environments.

One cross-cultural universal is that societies have a division of labor between the sexes. Murdock and Provost's (1973) classic analysis of 185

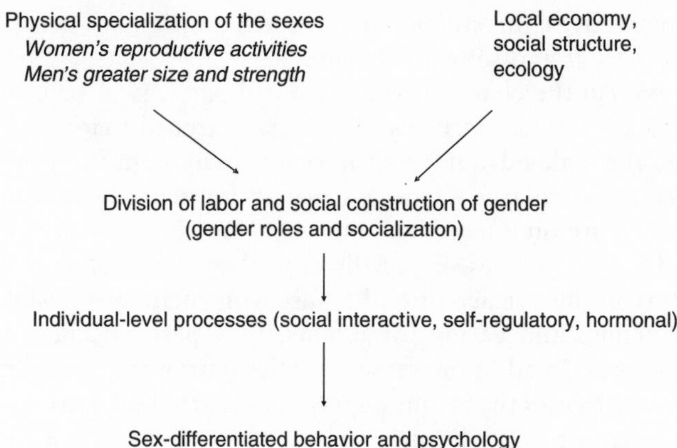

FIGURE 12.1. Social role theory of sex differences and similarities.

nonindustrial societies revealed that, within societies, the majority of productive activities were carried out solely or typically by men or women, and not by both sexes jointly. Even in industrialized societies, women are more likely than men to assume domestic roles of homemaker and primary caretaker of children, whereas men are more likely than women to assume roles in the paid economy and the domestic role of primary family provider (Shelton & John, 1996). Although the majority of women are employed in the paid workforce in many industrialized societies, the sexes tend to be concentrated in different paid occupations, with more men than women in most occupations that yield high levels of income and power (e.g., U.S. Bureau of Labor Statistics, 2001).

Despite this universal pattern of a division of labor, Murdock & Provost (1973) found considerable flexibility across societies in the specific tasks allocated to men or women; that is, the majority of tasks were not uniquely performed by men or women across societies. In some societies, men performed tasks such as planting and tending crops, milking, or preparing skins; in other societies, women performed these tasks. Yet a minority of activities were consistently associated with one sex across societies. For example, only men smelted ores and worked metals, and women cooked and prepared foods from plant sources.

Another universal pattern across societies concerns status and power. Although the existence of some egalitarian societies illustrates that sex differences in status and power do not occur in all societies, all the gender hierarchies that exist favor men (Whyte, 1978). Gender hierarchies take different specific forms across societies: In some societies, women possess fewer resources than men; in others, less value is placed on women's lives; in still others, greater restrictions are placed on women's marital and sexual behavior.

To explain the characteristic sex-typed patterns of behavior in human societies, Wood and Eagly (2002) have argued that the division of labor and the male-advantaged gender hierarchy stem from physical sex differences, particularly women's capacity for reproduction and men's size and strength, in interaction with the demands of socioeconomic systems and local ecologies. Especially critical to the division of labor are women's reproductive activities. Because women are responsible for gestating, nursing, and caring for infants, they perform child care roles across societies. In addition, these activities limit women's ability to perform other activities that require speed, uninterrupted periods of activity and training, or long-distance travel away from home. Therefore, women's reproductive activities lead them generally to eschew tasks such as hunting large animals, plowing, and conducting warfare, in favor of activities more compatible with child care. Yet reproductive activities have less impact on women's roles in societies with low birthrates, less reliance on lactation for feeding infants, and more nonmaternal care of young children. These conditions have become more common in postindustrial societies than in societies that, for example, rely on agriculture for subsistence.

Another determinant of the social roles of men and women is men's larger size and greater strength and speed. Because of these physical differences, the average man is more likely than the average woman to be able to perform with efficiency tasks that demand brief bursts of force and upper-body strength. In foraging, horticultural, and agricultural societies, these tasks include hunting large animals, plowing, and conducting warfare. However, some anthropologists have questioned whether men's size and strength are critical to societies' division of labor given the strength-intensive nature of some of the tasks usually performed by women, which include fetching water, carrying children, and doing laundry (Mukhopadhyay & Higgins, 1988). Regardless of the overall impact of men's size and strength, this aspect of physical differences has a much weaker effect on role performance in postindustrial and other societies in which few occupational roles demand these attributes.

The question of why some societies have a gender hierarchy and others do not also can be answered by considering the sexes' physical attributes in conjunction with societal and ecological conditions (Wood & Eagly, 2002). One underlying principle is that men have more status and power than women in societies in which their greater upper-body strength and speed enable them to perform certain physically demanding activities, such as warfare, that can lead to decision-making power, authority, and access to resources. Another underlying principle is that men have more status and power than women in societies in which women's reproductive activities impair their ability to perform the activities that yield status and power. Typically, this lowering of women's status occurs when their reproductive responsibilities limit their participation in roles that require intensive specialized training, skills acquisition, and task performance outside of the household (e.g., scribe, warrior). Then women have only limited participation in the activities that produce influence outside of the household and yield resources to be traded in the broader economy. Consistent with this argument, relatively egalitarian relations between the sexes are often found in decentralized societies that lack more complex technologies, especially in very simple economies in which people subsist by foraging (Hayden, Deal, Cannon, & Casey, 1986; Salzman, 1999; Sanday, 1981). Such societies generally lack the specialized roles that give some subgroups power over others and, in particular, give men power over women. In contrast, in more socioeconomically complex societies that have specialized roles, men's power and status are enhanced by the relations that develop between the physical attributes of women and men, and the exploitation of technological and economic developments (e.g., the plow, ownership of private property).

In summary, sex-typed social roles involving gender hierarchy and a division of labor emerge from a set of socioeconomic and ecological factors that interact with the physical sex differences inherent in female reproductive activity and male size and strength (Wood & Eagly, 2002). These biosocial interactions provide the "big picture" set of causes that accounts for sex differences in roles across human societies. Although physical sex differences have more limited consequences for role performance in postindustrial societies, even these societies retain some degree of male–female division of labor and aspects of patriarchy. As we explain in the remainder of the chapter, these sex-typed social roles in turn produce sex differences in social behavior, including people's preferences for their long-term partners.

SOCIAL CONSTRUCTION OF GENDER THROUGH GENDER ROLES

Gender roles consist of shared expectations about behavior that apply to people on the basis of their socially identified sex (Eagly, 1987). This definition derives from the general concept of *social role*, which refers to the shared expectations that apply to people who occupy a certain social position or are members of a particular social category (e.g., Biddle, 1979). At an individual level, roles exist in people's minds as *schemas*, or abstract knowledge structures about groups of people. Because they are to a great extent consensual, role schemas exist at the societal level as shared ideologies communicated among society members. As we detail in the next section of this chapter, these gender roles are the products of sex-typed social roles.

Gender roles are diffuse because they apply to the general social categories of male and female. These roles, like other diffuse roles based on age, race, and social class, are broadly relevant across situations. In contrast, more specific roles based on factors such as family relationships (e.g., mother, son) and occupation (e.g., bank teller, firefighter) are mainly relevant to behavior in a particular group or context. Gender roles can work with specific roles to structure interaction (Ridgeway, 2001). In particular, because gender roles are relevant in the workplace, people have somewhat different expectations for women and men employed in the same work role (Eagly & Karau, 2002). For example, male managers, more than female managers, are expected to be self-confident, assertive, firm, and analytical (Heilman, Block, Martell, & Simon, 1989).

Evidence that gender roles exist comes mainly from research on gender stereotypes, which has consistently found that people have differing beliefs about the typical characteristics of men and women (e.g., Diekman & Eagly, 2000; Newport, 2001). The majority of these beliefs about the sexes pertain to *communal* and *agentic* attributes. Communal characteristics, which are typical of women, reflect a concern with the welfare of others and involve affection, kindness, interpersonal sensitivity, and nurturance. In contrast, agentic characteristics, which are typical of men, involve assertion, control, and confidence. Gender roles also encompass beliefs about many other aspects of men and women, including their physical characteristics, cognitive abilities, skills, and emotional dispositions (Deaux & Lewis, 1984).

Gender roles represent the characteristics that are descriptively normative for the sexes, that is, the qualities that differentiate men from women. These *descriptive norms* (also called *descriptive stereotypes*) are guides to the behaviors that are likely to be effective in a given situation (Cialdini & Trost, 1998). Especially when a situation is ambiguous or confusing, people can follow these guides by acting in ways that are typical for their sex. For example, teenagers who are just beginning to date may act in sex-stereotypical ways when they are uncertain what to do next. However, gender role beliefs are not limited to descriptions of male and female behavior; they also include *injunctive norms* (also called *prescriptive stereotypes*), which specify the desirable, admirable behaviors for each sex (Cialdini & Trost, 1998). Injunctive norms indicate which behaviors are likely to elicit approval from others and to yield personal feelings of pride or shame. In general, people desire and approve of communal qualities in women and agentic qualities in men, as demonstrated in research on (1) the differing beliefs that people hold about ideal women and men (e.g., Spence & Helmreich, 1978; Williams & Best, 1990b), (2) the differing beliefs that women and men hold about their ideal selves (Wood, Christensen, Hebl, & Rothgerber, 1997), and (3) the attitudes and prescriptive beliefs that people hold about the roles and responsibilities of women and men (e.g., Glick & Fiske, 1996; Spence & Helmreich, 1978). For example, to the extent that dating partners follow injunctive norms for male and female behavior, women may act nurturant and warm on dates and men may act dominant and chivalrous. Thus, men are more likely to hold doors open for women in a dating situation than in other everyday contexts (Yoder, Hogue, Newman, Metz, & LaVigne, 2002).

The injunctive and descriptive aspects of gender role norms are likely to be closely linked. Hall and Carter (1999b) showed that behaviors are judged appropriate for one sex to the extent that they are believed to be performed more by that sex. In general, people seem to think that women and men ought to differ especially in those behaviors associated with larger sex differences. Furthermore, the typical attributes of a group can be especially desirable in certain situations, such as when the attributes differentiate between an ingroup and an outgroup (Christensen, Rothgerber, Wood, & Matz, 2002). Thus, in contexts that highlight distinctions between the sexes, people may experience pride in possessing and displaying typical, sex-typed attributes.

Despite some individual differences in beliefs about typical and appropriate male and female behavior (e.g., Spence & Buckner, 2000), these beliefs appear to be widely shared by men and women, students and older adults, and people who differ in social class and income (Diekman & Eagly, 2000; Hall & Carter, 1999a). It seems that virtually everyone cognitively represents stereotypical beliefs about the sexes (e.g., Zenmore, Fiske, & Kim, 2000). Although stereotypes can be automatically activated and serve as baseline judgments of men and women, they are nonetheless moderated in their impact by various contextual, informational, and motivational factors (Blair, 2002; Zenmore et al., 2000). These consensual beliefs about groups are likely to develop and to be shared through social interaction when group members regularly cooperate with one another in the tasks of daily living, as do men and women (Ridgeway, 2001).

Gender roles form an important part of the culture of every society (see Best & Thomas, Chapter 13, this volume). In an analysis of gender stereotypes among university students in 25 nations, Williams and Best (1990a) found considerable cross-cultural similarity in the beliefs people held about the communal and agentic characteristics of women and men. However, the tendency for people to perceive men as more active and stronger than women was less pronounced in more economically developed nations, in which literacy and the percentage of women attending universities were high. Thus, in countries in which the sexes have greater social and political equality, gender stereotypes and roles may become less traditional.

In summary, gender roles represent the typical and desirable behavior of the sexes within a society. As we explain in the next section, these gender role beliefs emerge from the social roles of men and women.

RELATION OF GENDER ROLES TO THE SOCIAL POSITION OF WOMEN AND MEN

Gender roles emerge from the typical social roles of the sexes because perceivers infer that people's actions tend to correspond to their inner dispositions (Eagly & Steffen, 1984). This cognitive process constitutes a basic principle of social psychology labeled *correspondent inference*, or *correspondence bias* (Gilbert, 1998). To demonstrate this principle, research has shown that people fail to give much weight to the constraints of social roles in inferring role players' dispositions (e.g., Ross, Amabile, & Steinmetz, 1977). Thus, the communal, nurturing behaviors required by women's domestic and child care roles and by many female-dominated occupational roles favor inferences that women possess communal traits. Similarly, the assertive, task-oriented activities required by many male-dominated occupations produce expectations that men are agentic.

Given the greater power and status more typical of men's than women's roles in patriarchal societies, gender roles also encompass expectations about traits of dominance and submission (e.g., Conway, Pizzamiglio, & Mount, 1996; Eagly, 1983; Wood & Karten, 1986). People in more powerful roles behave in a more dominant style than do people in less powerful roles. Thus, men are believed to be more dominant, controlling, and assertive, and women are believed to be more subordinate and cooperative, compliant to social influence, and less overtly aggressive.

The principle of correspondence bias suggests that gender stereotypes can develop in the absence of any true dispositional differences between the sexes. To test this idea experimentally, Hoffman and Hurst (1990) informed participants that members of two occupational groups, city workers and child raisers, were comparable in their communal and agentic traits. Nonetheless, participants ascribed role-consistent traits to both occupational groups, specifically, agentic traits to city workers and communal traits to child raisers. These findings show that instructions to consider the groups equivalent in their traits were not sufficient to overcome the correspondent inference from roles to underlying dispositions.

In summary, beliefs about the actual and ideal attributes of the sexes emerge because people assume correspondence between each sex's personal attributes and its typical role behaviors in a society. Although these beliefs emerge in large part from individuals' observations of behaviors, their communication contributes to their consensual character. These stereotypical beliefs have their roots in (1) the division of labor in the sexes' performance of family and occupational roles, and (2) the gender hierarchy by which men are more likely than women to occupy roles of higher power and status. Through a variety of proximal mechanisms discussed in the next section, the resulting gender role expectations influence behavior in many domains, including mate preferences.

GENDER ROLES' INFLUENCE ON BEHAVIOR

How do gender roles influence behavior? In terms of the broader, distal causes for sex differences, men's physical attributes and women's reproductive activities frame the effects of gender role beliefs. These attributes and activities establish the perceived costs and benefits of behaviors for each sex within particular societal structures and ecologies. In terms of more proximal, immediate causes, gender roles have an effect because they convey the costs and benefits of behaviors for men and women. Because communal behaviors often appear to have greater utility for women and agentic behaviors for men, both sexes then engage in sex-typed behaviors that in turn foster their preferences for and performance of sex-typical family and occupational roles. This personal participation in sex-typical roles that ensues throughout the life cycle is critical to the socialization and maintenance of sex differences. Insofar as they occupy different specific roles, women and men behave differently, learn different skill sets, and orient themselves toward different life goals. Moreover, based on their experience in specific sex-typed roles, women and men develop general behavioral tendencies that extend beyond these roles. These tendencies emerge as men and women confirm others' gender-stereotypic expectancies, regulate their own behavior based on gender-stereotypic self-concepts, and experience hormonal changes that accompany role performance.

People conform to gender-appropriate behavior in part because others expect them to do so. Other people can deliver penalties for deviation from gender roles and rewards for role-congruent behaviors. Research on sex-stereotypical expectations has yielded some of the clearest demonstrations of such behavioral confirmation (see Deaux & LaFrance, 1998; Geis, 1993), even though the link between expectancies and behavior is contingent on various conditions (Olson, Roese, & Zanna, 1996). The sanctions against role-inconsistent behavior may be overt (e.g., losing a job) or subtle (e.g., being ignored, disapproving looks). People communicate these expectations through verbal and nonverbal behaviors, although they are not necessarily aware of these processes because such communication can operate at a relatively implicit or automatic level (Blair, 2002; Dijksterhuis & Bargh, 2001). It is important to recognize, too, that there are likely to be circumstances in which the benefits of gender nonconformity outweigh its possible social costs; therefore, people act in ways that counter gender stereotypes.

Much evidence indicates that people react negatively to deviations from gender roles. For example, in a meta-analytic review of 61 studies of evaluations of male and female leaders, Eagly, Makhijani, and Klonsky (1992) showed that women who adopt a male-stereotypical, assertive, and directive leadership style are evaluated more negatively than men who adopt this style. Also, in small-group interaction, women tend to lose likability and influence when they behave in a dominant or extremely competent manner (see Carli, 2001). Additional evidence indicates that men may be penalized for behaving passively, unassertively, and negatively (e.g., Anderson, John, Keltner, & Kring, 2001; Costrich, Feinstein, Kidder, Marecek, & Pascale, 1975).

Evidence that people are rewarded for acting in ways that are congruent with gender role expectations derives from studies of socialization practices across nonindustrial societies. Parents use both rewards and punishments to inculcate nurturance in girls, and achievement and self-reliance in boys, although the strength of these socialization pressures also varies with societal attributes (e.g., Barry, Bacon, & Child, 1957). Socialization research in North America and other Western nations has produced less evidence of parents' delivery of differential rewards and punishments for boys and girls, with the important exception of parents' encouragement of gender-typed activities and interests—for example, toys, games, and chores (Lytton & Romney, 1991). Nonetheless, sex-typed expectations are also communicated through more subtle processes, such as the modeling of behaviors (see Bussey & Bandura, Chapter 5, this volume).

Differential rewards for gender-consistent behaviors are also evident in adult social interaction. For example, in a study of college organizations, Cotes and Feldman (1996) found that in female groups, women were better liked to the extent that they could display happiness, an emotion useful in relations characterized by support and understanding. In contrast, in male groups, men were better liked to the extent that they effectively displayed anger, an emotion useful in competitive interactions within a hierarchy. Finally, evidence of approval of sex-appropriate attributes comes from the research on preferences for long-term partners, which we discuss in the final section of this chapter. As we explain, preferences for sex-typed mates vary with both the attributes valued in men and women within a society and individual society members' gender role ideologies.

Gender roles can produce sex differences in behavior not only through behavioral confirmation of expectancies but also by affecting people's self-concepts. The idea that gender roles influence people's perceptions of themselves is supported by research findings that self-concepts, on average, tend to be gender-stereotypical (e.g., Spence & Buckner, 2000; Spence & Helmreich, 1978). Specifically, women's identities are oriented toward interdependence, in the sense that representations of others are treated as part of the self (e.g., Cross & Madson, 1997). Thus, women's self-concepts tend to be relational and to include others who are important to them, especially in close, dyadic relationships. Although some researchers have argued that men's self-concepts are oriented toward independence and separation from others (e.g., Cross & Madson, 1997), instead, it appears that men have an interdependent self-concept that focuses on hierarchical relationships within larger groups (Baumeister & Sommer, 1997; Gabriel & Gardner, 1999; Gardner & Gabriel, Chapter 8, this volume). Men's construal of themselves in terms of competition for power and status in larger collectives is compatible with the social role theory principle that the male gender role follows in part from men's greater access to status and power.

Self-concepts guide the behavior of men and women through a variety of cognitive and motivational mechanisms (Hannover, 2000; Bussey & Bandura, Chapter 5, this volume). In one such process, gender role norms are internalized and adopted as personal standards against which people judge their own behavior. Men and women tend to evaluate themselves favorably to the extent that they conform to these standards, and unfavorably to the extent that they deviate from them. In a demonstration of such processes, Wood et al. (1997) investigated normative beliefs that men are powerful, dominant, and self-assertive, and that women are caring, intimate with others, and emotionally expressive. Participants who had internalized gender role norms felt good about themselves when their behavior was consistent with these norms; that is, dominant experiences for men and communal experiences for women had the effect of shifting participants' actual self-concepts closer to their standards about how they wished to behave and believed they should behave. Alternatively, when people fail to live up to these sex-typed normative standards, they may experience depression and lowered self-esteem (e.g., Crocker & Wolfe, 2001). Thus, gender roles can affect behavior when people incorporate them into their self-concepts and use them as personal standards against which to evaluate their own behavior.

Consideration of self-construals helps to explain individual differences in the extent to which people engage in behavior consistent with the gender roles of their culture. Although many people think of themselves in conventional masculine or feminine terms, many other people are not highly gender-identified. People influenced by culturally atypical environments may not internalize conventional gender role norms and may thus have self-concepts that are not typical of their gender. In support of this idea, only about half of Wood et al.'s (1997) student participants reported that their desired behaviors were congruent with the sex-appropriate standard. Furthermore, research relating self-report personality measures of masculinity and femininity to behavior has demonstrated that people vary in the degree to which their self-concepts are sex-typed, and that nontypical people are less likely to show traditionally sex-typed behavior (Taylor & Hall, 1982). In addition, the differing self-concepts of men and women may become cognitively accessible only in some social contexts, with some situations evoking a stronger awareness of oneself as male or female (Deaux & Major, 1987).

Biological processes, especially hormonal changes, provide another mechanism through which gender role norms influence behavior. A direct link between hormonal processes and the demands of social roles has been demonstrated by studies showing that testosterone levels in males rise in anticipation of athletic and other competition, and in response to insults, presumably to energize and direct their physical and cognitive performance (e.g., Booth, Shelley, Mazur, Tharp, & Kittok, 1989; Cohen, Nisbett, Bowdle, & Schwarz, 1996). Hormonal changes, particularly increases in cortisol, also occur with mothers' initiation of their parental role at childbirth and evidently stimulate nurturing behavior (Corter & Fleming, 1995; Fleming, Ruble, Krieger, & Wong, 1997). Although some of these hormonal effects are likely sex-specific, other hormonal changes are common to both sexes. Especially compelling evidence that hormonal mechanisms can mediate the effects of roles on behavior was provided by the finding that fathers anticipating childbirth experienced hormonal changes parallel to the changes that occurred in mothers (i.e., involving estradiol, cortisol, and prolactin) and, in addition, experienced a drop in testosterone (Berg & Wynne-Edwards, 2001; Storey, Walsh, Quinton, & Wynne-Edwards, 2000). To facilitate the role performance of women and men, such biological processes work in concert with psychological processes involving sex-typed social expectations and self-concepts.

Gender roles are not the only influence on behavior; they coexist with specific roles based on factors such as family relationships (e.g., father, daughter) and occupation (e.g., secretary, electrician). In workplace settings, for example, a manager has a role defined by occupation and, simultaneously, a gender role of being a man or woman. Expectations for specific roles and those for more diffuse gender roles are typically combined to give greater weight to expectations that are relevant to the task at hand (Hembroff, 1982). Because specific roles have more direct implications for behavior in many settings, they may often be more important than gender roles. This conclusion was foreshadowed by experimental demonstrations that stereotypical sex differences can be eliminated by providing information that specifically counters gender-based expectations (e.g., Wood & Karten, 1986). In employment settings, occupational roles no doubt have primary influence on how men and women accomplish the tasks required by their jobs. However, gender roles may "spill over" to influence discretionary behaviors, such as the style in which an occupational role is carried out (e.g., in leadership roles, women tend to be more democratic than men; Eagly & Johnson, 1990). Thus, gender roles influence behavior, even if they assume secondary status in settings in which specific roles are of primary importance.

Although a general review of research on sex differences and similarities is beyond the scope of this chapter, much evidence suggests that actual differences are, in general, gender-stereotypical, just as social role theory predicts. Furthermore, people are relatively accurate in their beliefs about men's and women's behavior. This accuracy is not surprising given that these beliefs emerge from the social roles of men and women and in turn foster role-appropriate sex differences. Hall and Carter (1999a) provided evidence of this accuracy in their research on perceptions of sex differences and similarities in 77 traits, abilities, and behaviors. They reported that student judges' mean estimates of these differences and similarities correlated .70 with the actual research findings (as meta-analytically summarized). The judges understood which differences tended to be larger and which smaller; they also understood the direction of the difference, meaning whether males or females were more likely to possess the attribute or perform the behavior.

Despite the evidence of accuracy in gender-stereotypical beliefs, some systematic biases in judgments lessen the accuracy of perceptions of men and women (e.g., Boldry, Wood, & Kashy, 2001; Diekman, Eagly, & Kulesa, 2002). Furthermore, accurate perceptions of men and women in general do not imply accuracy in perceptions of an individual man or woman. Instead, when categorized into groups, people tend to be perceived as similar to one another; therefore, predictions of individual behavior from group membership tend to be overly homogeneous. Even given these limitations, however, people's ideas about men and women generally are congruent with behavioral evidence of sex differences.

As a final point in our presentation of social role theory, we note that we have oversimplified our presentation of the distal and proximal causes of sex differences, especially in Figure 12.1, by confining our treatment mainly to a forward causal direction. Yet causation is more complex, and the various causes in the model influence one another in reciprocal fashion. Although our diagram depicts the forward causation from the physical specialization of the sexes and socioeconomic factors to the division of labor and the social construction of gender, and then to individual-level mediating processes that influence patterns of behavior, these causal arrows can be reversed. In particular, to the extent that people exhibit gender-stereotypical behavior, these behavioral differences act back to strengthen gender roles and stereotypes and to channel men and women into different social roles. Thus, the causal sequence of social role theory allows for both forward and backward causal flow. Moreover, to the extent that any causes of sex differences not mentioned in this chapter (e.g., inherited differences in cognitive tendencies or temperament) have some influence, they also act on gender roles and role distributions.

SEX DIFFERENCES AND SIMILARITIES IN PARTNER PREFERENCES

Social role theory explains why men and women desire somewhat different attributes in a long-term partner. To illustrate the utility of this theory, we summarize our research on this topic in the remainder of this chapter. From a social role perspective, the psychology of mate selection reflects people's efforts to maximize their positive outcomes and to minimize their negative ones in an environment in which these outcomes are constrained by both societal gender roles and the more specific expectations associated with marital roles (see also Pratto, 1996). The criteria that women and men use to select mates reflect the divergent responsibilities and obligations inherent in their current and anticipated social roles. An important aspect of these roles in many Western cultures has been (and still is, to some extent) a family system based on a male provider and a female homemaker. Within this division of labor, women typically maximize their outcomes by seeking a mate who is likely to be successful in the wage-earning role—in short, a good provider. In turn, men typically maximize their outcomes by seeking a mate who is likely to be successful in the domestic role—in short, a skilled homemaker and child caretaker.

This marital system also underlies women's preferences for older husbands and men's preferences for younger wives. With this combination, it is easier for marriage partners to assign to men the relatively powerful position that is normative for this form of marriage. Also, younger women tend to lack independent resources and are therefore more likely to regard their marital role as attractive. In complementary fashion, older men are more likely to have acquired the resources that make them good candidates to be providers. Older men and younger women thus fit the culturally expected pattern of breadwinner and homemaker. In summary, mate preferences are influenced by the division of labor and marital system in a society and in turn become embedded in gender roles and the broader cultural ideology of societies.

To test social role theory's predictions about mate selection, we conducted several studies that relate variation in the social roles of men and women to the characteristics that people desire in mates. This variation in social roles occurs both across societies (because some societies have a stronger division of labor than do others) and within societies (because people occupy homemaker or employee roles). In addition, variation in people's beliefs about social roles emerges across individuals within a society because people differ in the degree to which they endorse traditional gender ideology. The research that we present relates each of these forms of role variation to sex differences in mate selection preferences.

A Cross-Cultural Test

To examine cross-cultural variation in mate preferences of women and men, we reanalyzed data from a well-known study of mate selection (Buss, 1989; Buss et al., 1990). The participants were young adults of 37 diverse, primarily urbanized, cash-economy cultures, with 54% from European and North American cultures. These participants responded to questionnaire measures of the characteristics they desired in mates. In these data, certain sex differences in mate preferences were apparent across cultures. Specifically, men, more than women, preferred mates who were skilled homemakers and cooks, physically attractive, and younger than themselves; whereas women, more than men, preferred mates who were good providers and older than themselves (see also Kenrick & Keefe, 1992).

From a social role perspective, sex differences in mate preferences become smaller as the traditional division of labor weakens in industrial and postindustrial societies. As societies become more egalitarian, men and women become more similarly positioned in the social structure and, therefore, more similar psychologically in many ways, including in their preferences for long-term partners. To test these predictions, Eagly and Wood (1999) related the mate preferences reported by each culture's women and men to the degree of gender equality in the culture (as reported by the United Nations Development Programme, 1995).

Most relevant to this hypothesis is the *Gender Empowerment Measure* (GEM), which represents the extent to which women participate equally with men in economic, political, and decision-making roles. This index increases as (1) women's share of administrative and managerial jobs and of professional and technical jobs approaches equality with men's share; (2) women's share of parliamentary seats rises; and (3) women's income approaches parity with that of men. Another relevant United Nations index, the *Gender-Related Development Index* (GDI), assesses a society's ability to provide its citizens with greater life expectancy, education and literacy, and income in general, and imposes a penalty when women have lower outcomes on these measures than men.

As predicted, women's preferences for older mates and mates with resources, and men's preferences for younger mates and mates with housekeeping and cooking skills were most pronounced in patriarchal societies; these sex differences became less pronounced as the traditional division of labor weakened and societies became more egalitarian (see Tables 12.1 and 12.2). Providing additional evidence that the preferences of men and women were a common response to a sex-typed division of labor, the sex differences in mate preferences tended to coexist within societies. Specifically, in societies in which women expressed especially strong preferences for mates with resources and older mates, men also expressed especially strong preferences for mates with domestic skills and younger mates.

Additional evidence that mate preferences reflect social roles comes from Kasser and Sharma's (1999) separate reexamination of the 37 cultures study. They found that women, but not men, were more likely to prefer a good provider to the extent that women in the culture had limited reproductive freedom and educational opportunity. These findings lend additional support to the social role prediction that mate selection preferences reflect societal gender and marital roles.

Experimental Test of Playing Homemaker or Employee Role

To supplement the evidence that mate preferences vary across cultures with the roles of men and women, Johannesen-Schmidt (2003) carried out a role-playing experiment to explore the relation between specific marital roles and mate preferences. In this research, student participants

TABLE 12.1. Correlations of Mean Rankings and Ratings of Mate Selection Criteria with United Nations Indexes of Gender Equality for Buss et al.'s (1990) 37 Cultures Sample

	Ranked criteria		Rated criteria	
Mate selection criterion and raters	Gender Empowerment Measure ($n = 33$)	Gender-Related Development Index ($n = 34$)	Gender Empowerment Measure ($n = 35$)	Gender-Related Development Index ($n = 36$)
Good earning capacity (financial prospect)				
Sex difference	–.43*	–.33†	–.29†	–.23
Women	–.29	–.18	–.49**	–.42**
Men	.24	.27	–.40*	–.36*
Good housekeeper (and cook)				
Sex difference	–.62***	–.54**	–.61***	–.54**
Women	.04	–.01	.11	–.07
Men	–.46**	–.42*	–.60***	–.61***

Note. The criteria were described slightly differently in the ranking and the rating tasks. The ranking term is given first, with the rating term following in parentheses. Higher values on the gender equality indexes indicate greater equality. For the preferences of women or men, higher values of the mean rankings and ratings of mate selection criteria indicate greater desirability in a mate; therefore, a positive correlation indicates an increase in the desirability of a criterion as gender equality increased, and a negative correlation indicates a decrease. Sex differences in these preferences were calculated as female-minus-male means for good earning capacity and male-minus-female means for good housekeeper. A positive correlation thus indicates an increase in the sex difference as gender equality increased, and a negative correlation indicates a decrease in the sex difference.

†$p < .10$; *$p < .05$; **$p < .01$; ***$p < .001$.

from a U.S. university imagined that they had the role of primary breadwinner or primary homemaker and reported on their preferences for mates. Individuals assigned to the breadwinner role placed greater emphasis on finding a younger mate with good domestic skills than did those assigned to the domestic role; individuals assigned to the domestic role placed greater emphasis on finding an older mate with good provider skills than did individuals assigned to the breadwinner role. These findings suggest that people seek mates with attributes that complement their marital role.

Although all sex differences in preferences were not eliminated by the role variation, the assigned roles had a similar impact on male and

TABLE 12.2. Correlations of Mean Preferred Age Difference between Self and Spouse with United Nations Indexes of Gender Equality for Buss et al.'s (1990) 37 Cultures Sample

	Gender Empowerment Measure (n = 35)	Gender-Related Developmental Index (n = 36)
Sex difference	–.73***	–.70***
Women	–.64***	–.57***
Men	.70***	.70***

Note. Higher values on the gender equality indexes indicate greater equality. Positive ages indicate preference for an older spouse, and negative ages indicate preference for a younger spouse. Therefore, for the preferences of women, a negative correlation indicates a decrease in the tendency to prefer an older spouse as gender equality increased, whereas for the preferences of men, a positive correlation indicates a decrease in the tendency to prefer a younger spouse. Because the sex difference in preferred age was calculated as female minus male mean preferred spousal age in relation to self, a negative correlation indicates a decrease in the sex difference in preferred age as gender equality increased. From Eagly and Wood (1999). Copyright 1999 by the American Psychological Association. Reprinted by permission.

***$p < .001$.

female participants. Thus, this study provides important evidence that expected roles in society are related to preferred mate characteristics.

Tests of Within-Society Individual Differences

Another way to test social role predictions is to examine within a society the mate preferences of people who differ in their personal endorsement of the traditional male–female division of labor. Illustrating this approach, Johannesen-Schmidt and Eagly (2002) explored whether individual differences in gender ideology are associated with mate selection preferences. Because change toward nontraditional gender arrangements has mainly taken the form of women entering the paid labor force rather than men performing a larger proportion of domestic labor (Bianchi, Milkie, Sayer, & Robinson, 2000), it is attitudes toward change in women's roles that are crucial. People who approve of traditional roles for women or disapprove of nontraditional roles for women should be especially likely to make traditionally sex-differentiated choices of mates.

Glick and Fiske's (1996) Ambivalent Sexism Inventory (ASI) provides appropriate measures of individual differences to test these predictions because it assesses endorsement of the traditional female role. The ASI includes scales of (1) benevolent sexism, defined as approval of women in traditional roles; and (2) hostile sexism, defined as disapproval of women in nontraditional roles. Despite men's generally greater sexism (Glick & Fiske, 1996), these measures should relate to mate preferences within both sexes. To the extent that men or women favor the traditional female role by manifesting benevolent or hostile sexism, they should show stronger mate preferences that support this division of labor.

To test these predictions within a sample of university students, Johannesen-Schmidt and Eagly (2002) correlated participants' endorsement of traditional female roles on the ASI and the characteristics they preferred in a spouse. In general, people with traditional expectations about women also had sex-typed preferences that enhance the classic division of labor between husbands and wives. For example, for age preferences, the more men supported the traditional female role, the younger the age they preferred in a spouse; the more women supported the traditional female role, the older the age they preferred in a spouse (albeit significant only for the benevolent sexism measure). In summary, the three studies we have presented provide strong converging evidence that partner preferences, like many other social attributes and behaviors, are associated with the social roles of men and women.

Evolutionary Psychology as a Theory of Mate Selection

Social role theory is surely not the only theory of sex differences in mate selection. In particular, evolutionary psychologists have contended that these differences reflect the unique adaptive problems experienced by men and women as they evolved (e.g. Buss, 1989; Kenrick, Trost, & Sundie, Chapter 4, this volume). Thus, the sexes developed different strategies to ensure their survival and to maximize reproductive success. Buss et al. (1990) interpreted the results of the 37 cultures study as providing evidence that sex differences in preferred mate characteristics are universal and, therefore, reflect evolved tendencies that are general to the human species. However, the systematic cross-cultural variation in the magnitude of sex differences raises questions about this interpretation (Eagly & Wood, 1999; Kasser & Sharma, 1999).

Although evolutionary psychologists, in principle, acknowledge the possibility of cultural variation, they have claimed that mate preferences are unrelated to individuals' economic resources and other such role-related factors within a given society (e.g., Kenrick & Keefe, 1992; Townsend, 1989). For example, in a well-known study, Wiederman and Allgeier (1992) found that women in our society who themselves anticipated a high income still valued financial resources in their mates. This finding provides a poor test of role variables because achieving a high-paying occupation does not neutralize the impact of broader gender role expectations. Consistent with these broader norms, most women regard themselves as secondary wage earners (Ferree, 1991) and anticipate being partially dependent on their husband's income during a portion of their lifespan (e.g., while raising a family; Herzog, Bachman, & Johnston, 1983). Furthermore, women who themselves have a higher income are likely to select partners from their own higher level socioeconomic group (e.g., Kalmijn, 1994; Mare, 1991). In general, tests of social role theory predictions should assess the influences of specific role requirements (e.g., actual or anticipated marital roles) and more diffuse role expectations (e.g., gender roles and expectations based on social class and education).

Changes in Gender Roles and Sex Differences over Time

The view that gender roles are rooted in the division of labor and gender hierarchy implies that when these features of social structure change, expectations about men and women change accordingly. Indeed, the employment of women has increased rapidly in the United States and many other nations in recent decades. This change in the occupational structure may reflect declines in the birthrate and increased compatibility of employment and family roles, along with the increasing rarity of occupations that favor male size and strength. Their greatly increased education has qualified women for jobs with more status and income than the jobs they typically held in the past. Even though men's tendency to increase their responsibility for child care and other domestic work is modest (Bianchi et al., 2000), these changes in the division of labor have resulted in decreasing acceptance of the traditional gender roles and a redefinition of the patterns of behavior most appropriate to women and men.

Because women's roles have changed to become more like those of men, some convergence should occur in the behavior of men and women and take the form of changes in women's attributes in masculine domains. Consistent with this idea, analyses of sex differences across time periods in recent decades show some convergence of the attributes of women and men in traditionally masculine domains such as risk-taking and assertiveness (see review by Eagly & Diekman, in press). These changes presumably reflect women's increasing labor force participation and lessening concentration on child care and other domestic activities.

These shifts in women's roles have also affected both sexes' preferences for mates (Buss, Shackelford, Kirkpatrick, & Larsen, 2001). Specifically, in the United States, from 1939 to 1996, men's preference for a good housekeeper and cook decreased and their preference for partners with good financial prospects and similar level of education increased. In turn, women's preference for a mate with ambition and industriousness decreased. These sex-typed changes reflect societal revisions of marital roles as wives come to share more breadwinning responsibility with their husbands.

Not only does scientific evidence suggest some convergence of the sexes but also people believe that men and women are becoming more similar. Thus, social perceivers tend to believe women and men have converged in their personality, cognitive, and physical characteristics during the past 50 years, and will continue to converge for the next 50 years (Diekman & Eagly, 2000). This perceived convergence occurs because women increasingly possess qualities typically associated with men. Perceivers function like implicit role theorists by assuming that because the roles of women and men have become more similar, their attributes have become more similar. This demise of many sex differences with increasing gender equality is a prediction of social role theory that will be more adequately tested to the extent that societies produce conditions of equality or near-equality between women and men.

CONCLUSIONS

This chapter has outlined the basic assumptions of the social role theory of sex differences and similarities. Tests of the model with preferences for long-term partners revealed that, as anticipated, sex differences depend on role differences. Specifically, women tend to prefer an older partner with resources, and men tend to prefer a younger partner with homemaking skills, to the extent that they hold or endorse traditional roles. Furthermore, we have argued that these (and other) relations between social roles and behavior are mediated by proximal causes, including confirmation of others' sex-typed expectancies, self-regulation, and hormonal influences. At a societal level, the concentration of women and men in different roles is a consistent feature of human societies because the sexes cooperate in a division of labor. Moreover, in many societies, the roles of men and women manifest patriarchal relationships whereby men have more power and authority than women. Patriarchy and the division of labor in turn emerge because women's reproductive activities and men's size and strength facilitate performance of certain activities. In more socioeconomically complex societies, activities compatible with women's child care duties tend not to accord especially high levels of status or power. However, in postindustrial societies, with their low birthrates, women have greatly increased their access to roles that yield higher levels of power and authority.

ACKNOWLEDGMENTS

Preparation of this chapter was supported by awards from the National Science Foundation (Grant No. SBR-9729449) to Alice H. Eagly and from the National Institute of Mental Health (Grant No. 1R01MH619000-01) to Wendy Wood. We thank Jeff Pasch, Felicia Pratto, and Carmen Tanner for comments on a draft of the chapter.

REFERENCES

Anderson, C., John, O. P., Keltner, D., & Kring, A. M. (2001). Who attains social status?: Effects of personality and physical attractiveness in social groups. *Journal of Personality and Social Psychology, 81*, 116–132.

Barry, H., III, Bacon, M. K., & Child, I. L. (1957). A cross-cultural survey of some sex differences in socialization. *Journal of Abnormal and Social Psychology, 55*, 327–332.

Baumeister, R. F., & Sommer, K. L. (1997). What do men want? Gender differences and two spheres of belongingness: Comment on Cross and Madson (1997). *Psychological Bulletin, 122*, 38–44.

Berg, S. J., & Wynne-Edwards, K. E. (2001). Changes in testosterone, cortisol, and estradiol levels in men becoming fathers. *Mayo Clinic Proceedings, 76*, 582–592.

Bianchi, S. M., Milkie, M. A., Sayer, L. C., & Robinson, J. P. (2000). Is anyone doing the housework?: Trends in the gender division of household labor. *Social Forces, 79*, 191–228.

Biddle, B. J. (1979). *Role theory: Expectancies, identities, and behaviors.* New York: Academic Press.

Blair, I. V. (2002). The malleability of automatic stereotypes and prejudice. *Personality and Social Psychology Review, 6*, 242–261.

Boldry, J., Wood, W., & Kashy, D. A. (2001). Gender stereotypes and the evaluation of men and women in military training. *Journal of Social Issues, 57*, 689–705.

Booth, A., Shelley, G., Mazur, A., Tharp, G., & Kittok, R. (1989). Testosterone, and winning and losing in human competition. *Hormones and Behavior, 23*, 556–571.

Buss, D. M. (1989). Sex differences in human mate preferences: Evolutionary hypotheses tested in 37 cultures. *Behavioral and Brain Sciences, 12*, 1–14.

Buss, D. M., Abbott, M., Angleitner, A., Biaggio, A., Blanco-Villasenor, A., Bruchon Schweitzer, M., et al. (1990). International preferences in selecting mates: A study of 37 cultures. *Journal of Cross-Cultural Psychology, 21*, 5–47.

Buss, D. M., Shackelford, T. K., Kirkpatrick, L. A., & Larsen, R. J. (2001). A half century of mate preferences: The cultural evolution of values. *Journal of Marriage and the Family, 63*, 491–503.

Carli, L. L. (2001). Gender and social influence. *Journal of Social Issues, 57,* 725–741.

Christensen, P. N., Rothgerber, H., Wood, W., & Matz, D. C. (2002). [Social norms and the self: A motivational approach to normative behavior]. Unpublished manuscript, San Diego State University, CA.

Cialdini, R. B., & Trost, M. R. (1998). Social influence: Social norms, conformity, and compliance. In D. T. Gilbert, S. T. Fiske, & G. Lindzey (Eds.), *The handbook of social psychology* (4th ed., Vol. 2, pp. 151–192). Boston: McGraw-Hill.

Cohen, D., Nisbett, R. E., Bowdle, B. F., & Schwarz, N. (1996). Insult, aggression, and the southern culture of honor: An "experimental ethnography." *Journal of Personality and Social Psychology, 70,* 945–960.

Conway, M., Pizzamiglio, M. T., & Mount, L. (1996). Status, communality, and agency: Implications for stereotypes of gender and other groups. *Journal of Personality and Social Psychology, 71,* 25–38.

Corter, C. M., & Fleming, A. S. (1995). Psychobiology of maternal behavior in human beings. In M. H. Bornstein (Ed.), *Handbook of parenting* (Vol. 2, pp. 87–116). Mahwah, NJ: Erlbaum.

Costrich, N., Feinstein, J., Kidder, L., Marecek, J., & Pascale, L. (1975). When stereotypes hurt: Three studies of penalties for sex-role reversals. *Journal of Experimental Social Psychology, 11,* 520–530.

Cotes, E. J., & Feldman, R. S. (1996). Gender differences in nonverbal correlates of social status. *Personality and Social Psychology Bulletin, 22,* 1014–1022.

Crocker, J., & Wolfe, C. T. (2001). Contingencies of self-worth. *Psychological Review, 108,* 593–623.

Cross, S. E., & Madson, L. (1997). Models of the self: Self-construals and gender. *Psychological Bulletin, 122,* 5–37.

Deaux, K., & LaFrance, M. (1998). Gender. In D. T. Gilbert, S. T. Fiske, & G. Lindzey (Eds.), *The handbook of social psychology* (4th ed., Vol. 1, pp. 788–827). Boston: McGraw-Hill.

Deaux, K., & Lewis, L. L. (1984). Structure of gender stereotypes: Interrelationships among components and gender label. *Journal of Personality and Social Psychology, 46,* 991–1004.

Deaux, K., & Major, B. (1987). Putting gender into context: An interactive model of gender related behavior. *Psychological Review, 94,* 369–389.

Diekman, A. B., & Eagly, A. H. (2000). Stereotypes as dynamic constructs: Women and men of the past, present, and future. *Personality and Social Psychology Bulletin, 26,* 1171–1188.

Diekman, A. B., Eagly, A. H., & Kulesa, P. (2002). Accuracy and bias in stereotypes about the social and political attitudes of women and men. *Journal of Experimental Social Psychology, 38,* 268–282.

Dijksterhuis, A., & Bargh, J. (2001). The perception–behavior expressway: Automatic effects of social perception on social behavior. In M. P. Zanna (Ed.), *Advances in experimental social psychology* (Vol. 33, pp. 1–40). San Diego: Academic Press.

Eagly, A. H. (1983). Gender and social influence: A social psychological analysis. *American Psychologist, 38*, 971-981.

Eagly, A. H. (1987). *Sex differences in social behavior: A social-role interpretation.* Hillsdale, NJ: Erlbaum.

Eagly, A. H., & Diekman, A. B. (in press). The common-sense psychology of changing social groups. In J. Jost, M. Banaji, & D. Prentice (Eds.), *The ying and yang of social psychology: Perspectivism at work.* Washington, DC: American Psychological Association Books.

Eagly, A. H., & Johnson, B. T. (1990). Gender and leadership style: A meta-analysis. *Psychological Bulletin, 108*, 233–256.

Eagly, A. H., & Karau, S. J. (2002). Role congruity theory of prejudice toward female leaders. *Psychological Review, 109*, 573–598.

Eagly, A. H., Makhijani, M. G., & Klonsky, B. G. (1992). Gender and the evaluation of leaders: A meta-analysis. *Psychological Bulletin, 111*, 3–22.

Eagly, A. H., & Steffen, V. J. (1984). Gender stereotypes stem from the distribution of women and men into social roles. *Journal of Personality and Social Psychology, 46*, 735–754.

Eagly, A. H., & Wood, W. (1999). The origins of sex differences in human behavior: Evolved dispositions versus social roles. *American Psychologist, 54*, 408–423.

Eagly, A. H., Wood, W., & Diekman, A. (2000). Social role theory of sex differences and similarities: A current appraisal. In T. Eckes & H. M. Trautner (Eds.), *The developmental social psychology of gender* (pp. 123–174). Mahwah, NJ: Erlbaum.

Ferree, M. M. (1991). The gender division of labor in two-earner marriages: Dimensions of variability and change. *Journal of Family Issues, 12*, 158–180.

Fleming, A. S., Ruble, D., Krieger, H., & Wong, P. Y. (1997). Hormonal and experiential correlates of maternal responsiveness during pregnancy and the puerperium in human mothers. *Hormones and Behavior, 31*, 145–158.

Gabriel, S., & Gardner, W. L. (1999). Are there "his" and "hers" types of interdependence?: The implications of gender differences in collective versus relational interdependence for affect, behavior, and cognition. *Journal of Personality and Social Psychology, 77*, 642–655.

Geis, F. L. (1993). Self-fulfilling prophecies: A social psychological view of gender. In A. E. Beall & R. J. Sternberg (Eds.), *The psychology of gender* (pp. 9–54). New York: Guilford Press.

Gilbert, D. T. (1998). Ordinary personology. In D. T. Gilbert, S. T. Fiske, & G. Lindzey (Eds.), *The handbook of social psychology* (4th ed., Vol. 2, pp. 89–150). Boston: McGraw-Hill.

Glick, P., & Fiske, S. T. (1996). The Ambivalent Sexism Inventory: Differentiating hostile and benevolent sexism. *Journal of Personality and Social Psychology, 3*, 491–512.

Hall, J. A., & Carter, J. D. (1999a). Gender-stereotype accuracy as an individual difference. *Journal of Personality and Social Psychology, 77*, 350–359.

Hall, J. A., & Carter, J. D. (1999b). [Unpublished data]. Northeastern University, Boston, MA.

Hannover, B. (2000). Development of the self in gendered contexts. In T. Eckes & H. M. Trautner (Eds.), *The developmental social psychology of gender* (pp. 177–206). Mahwah, NJ: Erlbaum.

Hayden, B., Deal, M., Cannon, A., & Casey, J. (1986). Ecological determinants of women's status among hunter/gatherers. *Human Evolution, 1*, 449–473.

Heilman, M. E., Block, C. J., Martell, R. F., & Simon, M. C. (1989). Has anything changed?: Current characterizations of men, women, and managers. *Journal of Applied Psychology, 74*, 935–942.

Hembroff, L. A. (1982). Resolving status inconsistency: An expectation states theory and test. *Social Forces, 61*, 183–205.

Herzog, A. R., Bachman, J. G., & Johnston, L. D. (1983). Paid work, child care, and housework: A national survey of high school seniors' preferences for sharing responsibilities between husband and wife. *Sex Roles, 9*, 109–135.

Hoffman, C., & Hurst, N. (1990). Gender stereotypes: Perception or rationalization? *Journal of Personality and Social Psychology, 58*, 197–208.

Johannesen-Schmidt, M. C. (2003). *Social role theory and sex differences in preferred mate characteristics: Correlational and experimental approaches.* Doctoral dissertation, Northwestern University, Evanston, IL.

Johannesen-Schmidt, M. C., & Eagly, A. H. (2002). Another look at sex differences in preferred mate characteristics: The effects of endorsing the traditional female gender role. *Psychology of Women Quarterly, 26*, 322–328.

Kalmijn, M. (1994). Assortative mating by culture and economic occupational status. *American Journal of Sociology, 100*, 422–452.

Kasser, T., & Sharma, Y. S. (1999). Reproductive freedom, educational equality, and females' preferences for resource-acquisition characteristics in mates. *Psychological Science, 10*, 374–377.

Kenrick, D. T., & Keefe, R. C. (1992). Age preferences in mates reflect sex differences in human reproductive strategies. *Behavioral and Brain Sciences, 15*, 75–133.

Lytton, H., & Romney, D. M. (1991). Parents' differential socialization of boys and girls: A meta-analysis. *Psychological Bulletin, 109*, 267–296.

Mare, R. D. (1991). Five decades of educational assortative mating. *American Sociological Review, 56*, 15–32.

Mukhopadhyay, C. C., & Higgins, P. J. (1988). Anthropological studies of women's status revisited: 1977–1987. *Annual Review of Anthropology, 17*, 461–495.

Murdock, G. P., & Provost, C. (1973). Factors in the division of labor by sex: A cross-cultural analysis. *Ethnology, 12*, 203–225.

Newport, F. (2001, February 21). *Americans see women as emotional and affectionate, men as more aggressive.* Gallup Poll News Service. Retrieved August 18, 2001, from *http://www.gallup.com/poll/releases/pr010221.asp*

Olson, J. M., Roese, N. J., & Zanna, M. P. (1996). Expectancies. In E. T. Higgins & A. W. Kruglanski (Eds.), *Social psychology: Handbook of basic principles* (pp. 211–238). New York: Guilford Press.

Pratto, F. (1996). Sexual politics: The gender gap in the bedroom, the cupboard, and the cabinet. In D. M. Buss & N. Malamuth (Eds.), *Sex, power, and conflict: Evolutionary and feminist perspectives* (pp. 179–230). New York: Oxford University Press.

Ridgeway, C. L. (2001). Gender, status, and leadership. *Journal of Social Issues, 57*, 637–656.

Ross, L., Amabile, T. M., & Steinmetz, J. L. (1977). Social roles, social control, and biases in social–perception processes. *Journal of Personality and Social Psychology, 35*, 485–494.

Salzman, P. C. (1999). Is inequality universal? *Current Anthropology, 40*, 31–44.

Sanday, P. R. (1981). *Female power and male dominance: On the origins of sexual inequality.* New York: Cambridge University Press.

Shelton, B. A., & John, D. (1996). The division of household labor. *Annual Review of Sociology, 22*, 299–322.

Spence, J. T., & Buckner, C. E. (2000). Instrumental and expressive traits, trait stereotypes, and sexist attitudes. *Psychology of Women Quarterly, 24*, 44–62.

Spence, J. T., & Helmreich, R. (1978). *Masculinity and femininity: Their psychological dimensions, correlates, and antecedents.* Austin: University of Texas Press.

Storey, A. E., Walsh, C. J., Quinton, R. L., & Wynne-Edwards, K. E. (2000). Hormonal correlates of paternal responsiveness in new and expectant fathers. *Evolution and Human Behavior, 21*, 79–95.

Taylor, M. C., & Hall, J. A. (1982). Psychological androgyny: Theories, methods, and conclusions. *Psychological Bulletin, 92*, 347–366.

Townsend, J. M. (1989). Mate selection criteria: A pilot study. *Ethology and Sociobiology, 10*, 241–253.

United Nations Development Programme. (1995). *Human development report, 1995.* New York: Oxford University Press.

U. S. Bureau of Labor Statistics. (2002). *Median weekly earnings of full-time wage and salary workers by detailed occupation: Current Population Survey* (Table 39). Retrieved on September 4, 2003 from *http://www.bls.gov/cps/cpsaat39.pdf*

Whyte, M. K. (1978). *The status of women in preindustrial societies.* Princeton, NJ: Princeton University Press.

Wiederman, M. W., & Allgeier, E. R. (1992). Gender differences in mate selection criteria: Sociobiological or socioeconomic explanation? *Ethology and Sociobiology, 13*, 115–124.

Williams, J. E., & Best, D. L. (1990a). *Measuring sex stereotypes: A multination study* (rev. ed.). Newbury Park, CA: Sage.

Williams, J. E., & Best, D. L. (1990b). *Sex and psyche: Gender and self viewed cross culturally.* Newbury Park, CA: Sage.

Wood, W., Christensen, P. N., Hebl, M. R., & Rothgerber, H. (1997). Conformity to sex-typed norms, affect, and the self-concept. *Journal of Personality and Social Psychology, 73*, 523–535.

Wood, W., & Eagly, A. H. (2002). A cross-cultural analysis of the behavior of women and men: Implications for the origins of sex differences. *Psychological Bulletin, 128*, 699–727.

Wood, W., & Karten, S. J. (1986). Sex differences in interaction style as a product of perceived sex differences in competence. *Journal of Personality and Social Psychology, 50*, 341–347.

Yoder, J. D., Hogue, M., Newman, R., Metz, L., & LaVigne, T. (2002). Exploring moderators of gender differences: Contextual differences in door-holding behavior. *Journal of Applied Social Psychology, 32*, 1682–1686.

Zenmore, S. E., Fiske, S. T., & Kim, H.-J. (2000). Gender stereotypes and the dynamics of social interaction. In T. Eckes & H. M. Trautner (Eds.), *The developmental social psychology of gender* (pp. 207–241). Mahwah, NJ: Erlbaum.

13

Cultural Diversity and Cross-Cultural Perspectives

DEBORAH L. BEST
JENNIFER J. THOMAS

"Is it a boy or a girl?" In practically every culture, this is the first question asked following the announcement of the birth of a healthy child, and the response to this question affects almost every aspect of that child's subsequent life. In some societies, differences between females and males are emphasized, whereas in others, there is less interest in such diversity. Highlighting sex differences leads to the expectation that gender is a critical determinant of human behavior. However, it is important to remember that anatomically and physiologically, human males and females are more similar than different. Consequently, with the exception of childbearing, the sexes are mostly interchangeable with regard to social roles and behaviors. It may be surprising to see how little difference gender makes when considered against the background of broad variability in psychological characteristics across cultural groups.

In this chapter, we briefly discuss the methods and value of cross-cultural research in regard to questions of gender, followed by a review of adult gender issues concerning the individual and interpersonal relationships. Subsequently, gender role development and related cultural factors are considered. One caveat to bear in mind is that, unlike the other chapters in this volume, cross-cultural psychology does not advance any specific theory but offers a comparative approach that emphasizes the importance of the sociocultural context. Cross-cultural psychology seeks to understand the "interface between culture and psychology through careful research . . . it is conceptually, philosophically, and methodologically pluralistic . . . [with a] focus on culture as an important dynamic ingredient in both theory and application" (Adamopoulos & Lonner, 2001, p. 19). Virtually no theory or model of gender is inconsistent with this orientation, but with only a few exceptions (e.g., Munroe, Shimmin, & Munroe, 1984), gender theories have not been examined cross-culturally. Researchers have simply assumed that their theories are universally applicable.

CROSS-CULTURAL RESEARCH

Despite ample research and theory concerning gender and sex differences, the majority of the literature is based on Western, primarily U.S. samples. Such studies represent only a small segment of the world's population and fail to consider the entire range of variation in human behavior. Cross-cultural research helps to correct this imbalance by examining gender-related behaviors within the context of numerous cultural variations.

Cross-cultural psychology examines the degree to which psychological processes and behaviors are relatively invariant across cultures, universal, or tend to vary systematically with cultural influences. Some cross-cultural psychologists are more interested in pancultural generalities, but others search for significant differences that can be linked to cultural factors. Cross-cultural psychology becomes critical when investigating the robustness or generalizability of a psychological theory or empirical finding in cultural settings that differ from the one in which it was originally derived.

The standard protocol in cross-cultural psychology is the transfer, test, and discovery procedure that involves (1) selecting a psychological principle or model that has worked well in one culture, (2) "testing" its generalizability in one or more other cultures, and (3) discovering factors in the other cultures that are not present in the originating culture (Adamopoulos & Lonner, 2001). This orthodox model of cross-cultural research assumes that persons in various cultures have experienced different cultural influences that may be conceptualized as different "experimental treatments," or quasi-independent variables (Campbell & Stanley, 1963).

At first glance, cross-cultural psychology may seem qualitatively different from other psychological research. However, closer examination suggests that the methodological considerations and problems of equivalence (e.g., participants, procedures, materials) differ not in kind but in degree. For example, a psychologist comparing sex stereotypes in Great Britain and France would certainly face the problem of language equivalence between the English and French versions of a questionnaire administered to participants. Likewise, if the researcher were comparing European American and African American participants, in principle, the same question of language appropriateness would apply. Although both groups of U.S. participants "speak English," connotations of various words may differ between groups. Hence, cross-cultural psychologists may face the same problems as do researchers working in a single culture, but they must do so more directly.

When conceptualizing important methodological problems, cross-cultural psychologists often distinguish between *emic* concerns, those related to intracultural validity, and *etic* concerns, or intercultural validity. Logically, emic concerns should always precede etic concerns; that is, researchers should first ensure that their procedures are appropriate within each of the cultures being studied. Only after emic concerns are addressed can one consider etic concerns and ask whether the methods will permit valid comparisons between cultural groups. An etic method that is sensitive to emic concerns, called a *derived etic*, is considered appropriate for comparisons between groups. However, when a method originally developed in one cultural setting is simply used in another, without consideration for its appropriateness in the new setting, it is labeled *pseudoetic*, or *imposed etic*, and is methodologically inappropriate.

The emic–etic issue is illustrated by researchers that have translated masculinity–femininity scales developed in the United States into other languages, and administered and scored them using American scoring systems (e.g., Basow, 1984; Spence & Helmreich, 1978). Sometimes such research has shown substantial cross-cultural generality in the meaning of masculinity and femininity. Studies with the California Personality Inventory Fe (now F/M) scale have shown that when American scoring systems are used in other countries, men's self-descriptions usually are more masculine and women's self-descriptions are more feminine (Gough, 1966). In contrast, Kaschak and Sharratt (1983) reported a dramatic failure of the translated items in their efforts to develop a sex role inventory with Costa Rican university students. Using Spanish translations of 200 items, including the Personal Attributes Questionnaire (PAQ; Spence & Helmreich, 1978) and the Bem Sex Role Inventory (BSRI; Bem, 1974), they found that only two of the 55 PAQ items and half of the 60 BSRI items discriminated between men and women. Thus, many items representing masculinity–femininity in the United States do not do so in Costa Rica. Similar failures have occurred with BSRI items used in South India, Malaysia (Ward & Sethi, 1986), and Mexico (Lara-Cantu & Navarro-Arias, 1987). Clearly, evaluating masculinity–femininity across cultures requires careful attention to culture-specific (emic) definitions of the concepts.

As noted earlier, cross-cultural psychology examines both similarities and differences in behavior across cultural groups, but the relative ease of interpretation differs. Many methodological problems encountered in cross-cultural psychology (e.g., poor selection of participants, poor translation of materials) are likely to lead to spurious evidence of behavioral differences rather than spurious evidence of similarities. Consequently, similarities are often taken at face value, because they are assumed to have occurred in spite of existing methodological problems. This is particularly true when examining similarities in *patterns* of findings across cultural groups rather than when dealing with a single score. In contrast, differences in behaviors of various cultural groups are interpreted more cautiously and are not considered true cultural differences, unless they are related systematically to independently measured cultural variables. Thus, ideal cross-cultural studies involve a large sample of groups, perhaps 10 or more, so that observed differences can be correlated with cultural measures (e.g., indices of socioeconomic development). In studies with fewer cultural groups, it may be hard to identify which of the dimensions (e.g., individualism–collectivism) or cultural practices (e.g., child-rearing behaviors) that vary between groups contribute to the differences found on the particular measure of interest (e.g., sex role behavior).

Although interpreting cross-cultural findings may be easier with a larger number of countries, studies involving two or three countries also have merit. Their value depends on how the countries were selected relative to the variable of interest. Consider a study of three countries chosen for their known differences on a theoretically relevant cultural variable that predicts a particular pattern of group differences. If the observed differences conform to the predicted pattern, the theory is supported. However, if the three countries were chosen simply because they were convenient opportunities, with no predicted pattern of differences, then whatever differences are found most likely can be attributed only to "chance factors," including whatever methodological problems there may be in the study.

In light of these considerations, several large-scale, cross-cultural studies of gender at the adult level are reviewed. Studies of masculine work-related values, gender stereotypes, and the self-perceptions of women and men are considered first, followed by a discussion of two areas relevant to the relations between men and women: sex role ideology and mate preferences.

GENDER AT THE ADULT LEVEL

Gender-Related Values, Stereotypes, and Self-Perceptions

Masculine Work-Related Values

Using attitude survey data gathered between 1968 and 1972 by IBM, a large, multinational high-technology business, on more than 116,000 of its employees, Hofstede (1980) compared work-related values in 40 countries (primarily European, Asian, and South American countries). One scale that Hofstede derived via factor analysis concerned the extent to which the values of assertiveness, money, and things prevail in a society rather than the values of nurturance, quality of life, and people. Hofstede named the scale Masculinity (MAS), because male employees assigned greater importance to the first set of values, and female employees assigned greater importance to the second set.

For each of his 40 countries, Hofstede computed a MAS index derived from country factor scores. The five most masculine countries were Japan, Austria, Venezuela, Italy, and Switzerland, and the five most feminine countries were Sweden, Norway, the Netherlands, Denmark, and Finland. Using country indices from other sources (e.g., economic, geographic indicators), Hofstede (1980) looked at correlations with MAS scores across countries and found numerous interesting relationships. For example, highly masculine countries were closer to the equator and had stronger support for independent decision making, stronger achievement motivation, and higher job stress, and work was more central in people's lives.

Although the MAS dimension is obviously a meaningful one, perhaps it should have been designated Materialism. Calling the scale Masculinity led to expectations that MAS scores would be associated with cross-country variations in other gender-related concepts. However, Best and Williams (1998) found no relationship between cross-country variations in their sex stereotypes or masculinity–femininity scores (discussed later) and Hofstede's MAS scores. Similarly, Ward's (1995) Attitude Toward Rape scores were unrelated to MAS scores.

Gender Stereotypes

In contrast to Hofstede's country-level analyses based on factor scores for each country, Williams and Best (1982/1990a, 1990b) examined means derived from scores of individual participants in their cross-cultural gender studies. They defined gender stereotypes as the psychological traits believed to be more characteristic of one gender than the other. Williams and Best (1982/1990a) presented the 300 person-descriptive adjectives (e.g., absentminded, active, adventurous, affectionate, aggressive) from the Adjective Checklist (ACL; Gough & Heilbrun, 1980) to approximately 100 university students in each of 27 countries and asked them to indicate whether, in their culture, each adjective was more frequently associated with men, more frequently associated with women, or not differentially associated by gender.

Item frequencies for each of the 300 adjectives were tallied separately for men and women in each country, and these frequencies were correlated across countries. The correlation between female and male participants' frequencies across countries showed general agreement on the adjectives most often associated with men and with women. Male and female stereotypes differed most in the Netherlands, Finland, Norway, and Germany, and least in Scotland, Bolivia, and Venezuela. Stereotypes of women and men differed more in Protestant than in Catholic countries, in more developed countries, and in countries relatively high in Hofstede's Individualism work-related value. In an examination of agreement between countries, correlations between pairs of countries ranged from .35 for Pakistan versus Venezuela to .94 for Australia versus England. The mean common variance across all countries was 42%, indicating substantial pancultural agreement about stereotypical characteristics.

Given the large number of items involved, the high-agreement male- and female-stereotypical items in each country, designated the focused sex–trait stereotypes, were summarized by three theoretically derived scoring systems. Only the affective meaning scoring system based on Osgood's three factors of connotative or affective meaning are discussed here, because it has substantial cross-cultural generality (Osgood, May, & Miron, 1975; Osgood, Suci, & Tannenbaum, 1957). In a large number of studies examining the connotative meaning of words and other classes of stimuli, Osgood and his associates found that the principal component of affective meaning, or "feelings" toward concepts, was an evaluation factor (good–bad) usually accompanied by two secondary factors, potency (strong–weak) and activity (active–passive). Using an approximation of Osgood's system, Williams and Best (Best, Williams, & Briggs, 1980) had university students rate each of the 300 ACL items for favorability, strength, and activity along a 5-point scale. They used these mean ratings to calculate the mean favorability, strength, and activity of the items that other university students identified as focused stereotypical traits.

In all countries, the focused male sex–trait stereotypical items were stronger and more active than the female stereotypical items. Interestingly, there was no pancultural effect for favorability; the male stereotype was more positive in some countries (e.g., Japan, South Africa, Nigeria), and the female stereotype, in others (e.g., Italy, Peru, Australia). Strength and activity differences between male and female stereotypes were greater in socioeconomically less developed countries, in countries with low literacy rates, and with small percentages of women attending university. Economic and educational advancement reduced, but did not eliminate, the tendency to view men as stronger and more active than women.

A finding of cross-cultural similarity in the psychological characteristics differentially associated with men and women leads to the conclusion that gender stereotypes follow a general pancultural model, with cultural factors producing minor variations. Williams and Best (1982/1990a) proposed that biological differences set the stage (e.g., women bear children, men have greater physical strength) and led to a division of labor (discussed later in the chapter), with women mainly being responsible for child care and other domestic activities, and men primarily responsible for hunting (providing) and protection. Gender stereotypes that evolve as a rationale for this division of labor are assumed on the basis that each sex has or can develop characteristics congruent with the assigned role. Once established, stereotypes become socialization models that encourage boys to become masculine, adventurous and independent, and girls to become feminine, nurturant and affiliative. Consistent with the ecocultural framework (Berry, Poortinga, Segall, & Dasen, 1992) that recognizes biological and cultural influences at both the population and individual levels, this model demonstrates how widely different cultures come to associate one set of characteristics with men and another with women, with only minor variations around these central themes.

Masculinity–Femininity of Self-Concepts

Man-like or woman-like are the essential meanings of the paired concepts of masculinity–femininity (M-F). A person can be masculine or feminine in a number of ways, including physical appearance, dress, mannerisms, or tone of voice. Here, the definition is restricted to self-concepts and the degree to which they incorporate traits that are differentially associated with women or men in one's own culture.

Williams and Best (1990b) employed culture-specific measures of masculinity–femininity in a study with approximately 100 university students in 14 (primarily Asian and European countries) of the 30 countries in the stereotype study. Each participant described him- or herself and his or her ideal self using the 300 ACL adjectives, and these descriptions were scored relative to the local gender stereotypes (e.g., a culture-specific measure such as Venezuelan self-descriptions was scored relative to Venezuelan male and female stereotypes rather than to stereotypes derived in the United States or to some generalized stereotype of women and men; Williams & Best, 1982/1990a). Not unexpectedly, men in all countries described themselves as more masculine than women. Conversely, for the ideal self, *both* gender groups wished to be "more masculine" than they thought they were.

Although some cultural variation in self-concepts was found, there were no substantial associations with cultural comparison variables, such as economic–social development. Across cultural groups, relative to each culture's definition of femininity and masculinity, there was no evidence that women in some societies were more feminine than women in others, or that men in some societies were more masculine than men in others.

In contrast, when self-concepts were examined in terms of affective meaning scores, substantial differences in self and ideal self-concepts existed across countries, and these correlated with cultural comparison variables. Self-descriptions faintly "echoed" some of the stereotypical characteristics, such that in most countries, men's self-concepts were stronger and more active than those of women. However, these differences did not occur in all countries, which suggests that stereotypical characteristics are not necessarily incorporated into men's and women's self-concepts. Men's and women's self-concepts were more similar in more developed countries, where women were employed outside the home and attended university, and where sex role ideology was relatively modern.

An interesting paradox occurs in these findings. When analyzing scores based on culture-specific definitions of masculinity–femininity, a methodologically superior measure, there is less evidence of cross-cultural variation and more evidence of pancultural similarity in masculinity–femininity. Surprisingly, with use of the affective meaning scores based on ratings by persons in the United States, which may be culturally biased, a number of robust relationships with cultural comparison variables exist. This paradox is not easily resolved.

Relations between Men and Women

Sex Role Ideology

Stereotypes about the differential characteristics of women and men are sometimes used to justify prescriptive beliefs about how they should relate to one another. Sex role ideology concerns an individual's beliefs about those proper role relationships, ranging along a continuum from traditional to modern. Traditional ideologies contend that men are more "important" than women, and that it is appropriate for men to control and dominate women (Larsen & Long, 1988; Williams & Best, 1990b). In contrast, modern ideologies are more egalitarian, and consider women and men to be equals; dominance of one sex over the other is rejected.

Sex roles have been studied extensively in contemporary India, where traditional and modern ideologies are juxtaposed. Compared with American students, Indian university students hold more traditional views, but women in both cultures are more liberal than men (Agarwal & Lester, 1992; Rao & Rao, 1985). Indian women with nontraditional attitudes tend to come from nuclear families, have educated mothers, and are involved in professional or career-oriented disciplines (Ghadially & Kazi, 1979). Similarly, educational level and professional managerial jobs are strong predictors of sex role attitudes for both Japanese and American women (Suzuki, 1991).

In many sex role ideology studies, Americans, the reference group, are usually found to be rather liberal, suggesting they may be unusual in this respect. However, Williams and Best (1990b) did not find this to be true in their 14-country sex role ideology study with university students. In the self-concept study described earlier, participants completed the Kalin Sex Role Ideology (SRI) measure (Kalin & Tilby, 1978), a 30-item scale that measures role relationships between men and women (e.g., "A woman should have exactly the same freedom of action as a man"). Cooperating researchers evaluated item appropriateness for their culture and deleted inappropriate items. European countries (the Netherlands, Germany, Finland, England, Italy) had the most modern ideologies, the United States was in the middle of the distribution, and the most traditional ideologies were found in Africa and Asia (Nigeria, Pakistan, India, Japan, Malaysia). Generally, women had more modern, egalitarian views than did men, but not in all countries (e.g., Malaysia, Pakistan). However, a high correspondence existed between men's and women's scores in a given country, and overall, the effect of culture was greater than the effect of gender. Sex role ideology tended to be more modern in more developed, urbanized countries, in more Christian countries, and in countries in the higher latitudes.

Mate Preferences

Another area relevant to male–female relations deals with mate preferences. Buss and associates (1989, 1990) examined mate preferences in

37 samples, totaling over 10,000 respondents from 33 countries. Although social scientists often assume that mate preferences are highly culture-bound and arbitrary, the Buss et al. findings are to the contrary.

Using two similar lists of potential-mate characteristics, Buss asked participants to indicate their preferences by rating or ranking the items. Most striking was the remarkable agreement in mate-characteristic preferences between men and women. Both sexes ranked "kind and understanding" first, "intelligent" second, "exciting personality" third, "healthy" fourth, and "religious" last. Despite the overall similarity, women generally valued good earning capacity in a potential mate slightly more than did men, whereas men generally valued physical appearance slightly more than did women. In a reanalysis of Buss et al.'s (1990) data, Eagly and Wood (1999) also found that men valued a good cook and housekeeper more than did women.

In the Buss et al. (1990) data, cultural differences were found for virtually every item, and variation on some items was quite large. The greatest cultural effect occurred for chastity, with Northern Europeans considering it irrelevant, whereas Chinese, Indians, and Iranians greatly emphasized it. More men than women valued chastity in a prospective mate.

GENDER DEVELOPMENT

Seeing the relationship between gender and culture at the adult level, it is natural to ask: How do conceptions of gender develop? What roles are played by biological and cultural factors? In the following sections, cross-cultural studies of gender roles and stereotypes are discussed, followed by a review of gender role behaviors and of cultural factors that influence their development.

Gender Roles and Stereotypes

Gender roles and behaviors develop within the context of cultural stereotypes about male–female differences. In the United States, as early as age 2, children stereotype objects as masculine or feminine (Thompson, 1975; Weinraub et al., 1984), and by age 3–4, children correctly use stereotypical labels with toys, activities, and occupations (Edelbrook & Sugawara, 1978; Guttentag & Longfellow, 1977).

In Africa, similar gender stereotyping of toys occurs among girls playing with dolls and boys constructing vehicles and weapons (Bloch & Adler, 1994). By age 4–5, Sri Lankan village children display gender differences in play, similar to those found with British children (Prosser, Hutt, Hutt, Mahindadasa, & Goonetilleke, 1986). Cultural factors determine the content of children's play (e.g., sword fights vs. fashioning cars of wire), but most forms of play (e.g., constructive, role-playing, imaginative, and rule-based games) are found across cultures (Edwards, 2000). Interestingly, role playing, which was common in most communities, is more prevalent among girls than among boys (Edwards, 2000), supporting Sutton-Smith's (1974) hypothesis that role playing allows children, especially girls, to prepare for adult roles.

Development of Sex–Trait Stereotypes

For children in the United States, sex–trait stereotypes are learned somewhat later than is stereotypical knowledge of toys and occupations (Best et al., 1977; Reis & Wright, 1982; Williams & Best, 1982/1990). With the use of the Sex Stereotype Measure (SSM) to assess children's knowledge of adult-defined stereotypes, European American children show a consistent pattern of increasing knowledge from kindergarten through high school, similar to a typical learning curve. Stereotypical knowledge increases dramatically in the early elementary school years and plateaus in the middle school years. African American children's scores also increase with age but do not reach the level of scores of European American children, which reflects subcultural variation. Stereotypes become more differentiated with age (Biernat, 1991) and often incorporate gender-incongruent information (e.g., expressive attributes in males, instrumental attributes in females; Hannover, 2000).

Cross-Cultural Findings

Williams and Best (1982/1990) administered the SSM II to 5-, 8-, and 11-year-olds in 25 countries. Across all countries, the percentage of stereotyped responses rose from around 60% at age 5 to around 70% at age 8. Traits such as strong, aggressive, cruel, coarse, and adventurous were consistently associated with men by all age groups, whereas weak, appreciative, softhearted, gentle, and meek were traits consistently associated with women.

Relative to the other countries studied, stereotype scores were unusually high in Pakistan and relatively high in New Zealand and England. Scores were atypically low in Brazil, Taiwan, Germany, and France. Although countries varied in learning rates, there was a general developmental pattern of stereotype acquisition beginning prior to age 5, accelerating during the early school years, and becoming complete during adolescence.

Girls and boys learned the stereotypes at the same rate, but male traits were learned somewhat earlier than female traits. In 17 of the 25 countries, children knew more male stereotype items than female items. Germany was the only country in which female stereotype items were better known than the male ones. Interestingly, female stereotype items were learned earlier than male items in Latin/Catholic cultures (Brazil, Chile, Portugal, Venezuela), where the adult-defined female stereotype is more positive than that of the male.

Compared with children in non-Muslim countries, 5-year-olds in predominantly Muslim countries associated traits with the two sexes in a more highly differentiated manner, and they learned the stereotypes, particularly male items, at an earlier age. Initially, children in Christian countries were slower in learning stereotypes, perhaps reflecting the less-differentiated adult stereotypes, particularly in Catholic countries.

Albert and Porter (1986) found that stereotyping increased with age for 4- to 6-year-olds in the United States and South Africa. South African children stereotyped the male role more than did American children, but there were no differences for the female role. South African children from liberal Christian and Jewish backgrounds stereotyped less than did children from more conservative religious groups, but religion had no effects in the United States.

In a study of 11- to 18-year-olds, Intons-Peterson (1988) found that Swedish adolescents attributed more instrumental qualities to women than did American adolescents. Male and female stereotypes were more similar in Sweden than in the United States, perhaps reflecting the egalitarian Swedish culture. Surprisingly, there were gender differences in ideal occupations for Swedish but not for American adolescents. Swedish girls aspired to service occupations (e.g., flight attendant, hospital worker, nanny), and Swedish boys, to business occupations. In the United States, doctor, dentist, attorney, and business executive were top occupational choices for both sex groups.

Gibbons, Stiles, and Shkodriani (1991) studied attitudes toward gender and family roles among adolescents from 46 different countries, who attended schools in the Netherlands. Students from less affluent, more collectivistic countries had more traditional attitudes than students from wealthier, individualistic countries, and boys were more traditional than girls.

In summary, similarities found across diverse cultures, particularly with different measures, suggest that sex stereotypes are universal. Culture modifies both the rate of learning and minor aspects of content. Indeed, cross-cultural consistency in stereotypes suggests a uniform cross-cultural pattern of differences in the behaviors of males and females.

Differences in Male and Female Gender Role Behaviors

The classic Six Culture Study (Edwards & Whiting, 1974; Minturn & Lambert, 1964; Whiting, 1963; Whiting & Edwards, 1973) begun in 1954 by teams of social scientists from Harvard, Yale, and Cornell, and its sequel, the Children of Different Worlds (Whiting & Edwards, 1988), represent the first systematic cross-cultural data sets collected by standard methods in multiple cultures. The data focused on child and family life observed over 20 years in communities undergoing immense economic, political, and cultural changes. Mothers and their 3- to 11-year-old children were observed in India, Kenya, Mexico, Okinawa, the Philippines, and the United States. Gender differences in behaviors are reviewed.

Nurturance

Between ages 5 and 12, gender differences in nurturance were more consistent in behavior directed toward infants and toddlers than toward mothers and older children (Edwards & Whiting, 1980). Because infants elicit nurturant behavior and girls spend more time with infants than do boys, girls displayed more nurturant behaviors than boys.

Consistent with these findings, using the Human Relations Area Files data, Barry, Bacon, and Child (1957, 1967) found that, compared with boys, girls were socialized to be more nurturant (82% of cultures), obedient (35% of cultures), and responsible (61% of cultures). However, boys were socialized to be more achievement oriented (87% of cultures) and self-reliant (85% of cultures) than girls. In 108 preindustrial cultures (Welch, Page, & Martin, 1981), boys had more pressure to conform to their roles, and girls had greater role variability.

Aggression

Cross-culturally, prepubertal boys consistently showed higher levels of aggression, competitiveness, dominance-seeking, and rough-and-tumble play than girls (Ember, 1981; Freedman & DeBoer, 1979; Rohner, 1976; Strube, 1981). Data from the Six Culture Study and additional African samples (Whiting & Edwards, 1988) indicated sex differences in aggression and dominance, but contrary to earlier findings, aggression did not decrease with age, and it was more physical among the oldest boys. In playground observations in Ethiopia, Switzerland, and the United States (Omark, Omark, & Edelman, 1975), boys were more aggressive than girls, and similar patterns were found in four African !Kung Bushmen villages and in London (Blurton Jones & Konner, 1973). Observers in four nonindustrial cultures found more frequent aggression in boys than girls (Munroe, Hulefeld, Rodgers, Tomeo, & Yamazaki, 2000). Although both girls and boys to some degree segregated themselves by sex, aggregating with same-sex peers was more closely related to boys' episodes of aggression.

Mothers in the Six Culture Study reacted similarly to boys' and girls' aggression, but in Okinawa and the United States, some differential aggression training substantiated fathers' roles in socializing boys' aggression (Minturn & Lambert, 1964). In western European countries, acceptance of verbal aggression was similar for boys and girls, but boys were more accepting of physical violence (Ramirez, 1993), and girls were more emotionally and verbally aggressive (Burbank, 1987).

Proximity to Adults and Activity

Observations of 5- to 7-year-olds at play in eight cultures (Australian Aboriginal, Balinese, Ceylonese, Japanese, Kikuyu, Navajo, Punjabi, and Taiwanese) showed boys running in larger groups, covering more physical space, and engaging in more physical, unpredictable activities, and girls engaging in more conversations and repetitive games (Freedman, 1976). Girls were usually found closer to home (Draper, 1975; Munroe & Munroe, 1971; Whiting & Edwards, 1973). Boys interacted more with other boys, and girls interacted more with adults (Blurton Jones & Konner, 1973; Omark et al., 1975; Whiting & Edwards, 1973). Both task assignment (Whiting & Edwards, 1973) and behavioral preferences may have contributed to these gender differences (Draper, 1975). Children's drawings in nine cultures, which may reflect differential preferences, showed boys drawing more vehicles, monsters, and violence scenes, and girls drawing more flowers (Freedman, 1976).

Self-Esteem

In spite of similar gender role attributions, girls seemed less satisfied with being girls than were boys with being boys (Burns & Homel, 1986), and boys perceived themselves to be more competent than did girls in scholastic and athletic abilities, in physical appearance, and in general self-worth (van Dongen-Melman, Koot, & Verhulst, 1993). Surprisingly, girls' dissatisfaction was not consistently manifested in lower self-esteem (Calhoun & Sethi, 1987). Adolescent girls in Nepal, the Philippines, and Australia had lower opinions of their physical and mathematical abilities than did boys, but girls in Australia and Nigeria felt more competent in reading (Watkins & Akande, 1992; Watkins, Lam, & Regmi, 1991). Nigerian boys believed themselves to be more intelligent than did Nigerian girls (Olowu, 1985). A recent meta-analysis of global self-esteem questionnaire data found that gender differences peaked during adolescence, but the difference was not large (Kling, Hyde, Showers, & Buswell, 1999).

In summary, differences between girls and boys in nurturance, aggression, and mobility are robust and found consistently across cultures, but self-esteem differences are less systematic. Although theories of sex role development differ, most recognize the role of gender information readily available in the child's culture.

THE ROLE OF CULTURE: SOCIALIZATION AND CULTURAL PRACTICES

Socialization of Boys and Girls

Culture shapes the social behaviors of children by determining the company they keep and the activities that engage their time. Parents' behaviors communicate the importance of gender by reactions to their children's behavior, by the behaviors they model, and by family activities. Peers, teachers, and other socialization agents help shape sex-appropriate behaviors, toy and playmate choices, and activities. Caretaking, task assignment, and the educational environment are among the cultural influences that socialize children's gender role behaviors. Socialization experiences can minimize, maximize, or even eliminate gender differences in social behaviors.

Parents

Baby X studies (e.g., the sex of the infant is not known to study participants) in the United States have shown that parents and young adults treat infants differently depending on whether they think they are interacting with a girl or a boy (Karraker, Vogel, & Lake, 1995; Rubin, Provezano, & Luria, 1974; Seavey, Katz, & Zalk, 1975; Sidorowicz & Lunney, 1980; Sweeney & Bradbard, 1989). Boys are described as big and strong, and are bounced and handled more physically than are girls, who are described as pretty and sweet, and are handled gently. Parental expectations are not peculiar to the United States (Greenfield, Brazelton, & Childs, 1989) and may affect how children are treated.

Gender differences in behavior are often attributed to differences in socialization. Barry and colleagues (1957) examined socialization practices in over 100 societies and found that, generally, boys are reared to achieve, and to be self-reliant and independent, and girls are reared to be nurturant, responsible, and obedient. However, Hendrix and Johnson (1985) reanalyzed these data and found that the instrumental–expressive dichotomy popularly used to describe socialization differences were not polar opposites but were instead orthogonal, unrelated dimensions, with similar emphases in the training of boys and girls. Both instrumental and expressive behaviors were emphasized in the training of girls and boys, and achievement was stressed more for boys. In a more recent study of parental socialization practices in Germany and the United States (Barber, Chadwick, & Oerter, 1992), the only sex difference found across a number of behaviors was that adolescent girls in both cultures reported more physical affection from their fathers than did boys.

In a meta-analysis of 158 North American socialization studies (Lytton & Romney, 1991), the only significant effect was the encouragement of sex-typed behaviors. In 17 additional studies from other Western countries, boys received significantly more physical punishment than girls, but differential treatment decreased with age.

Socialization studies suggest that there may be subtle differences in how parents treat boys and girls. However, these differences are only occasionally significant, perhaps reflecting the ways that behaviors are measured, or which parent is observed. Fathers are especially important in signaling what behaviors they consider appropriate, particularly for sons, who have fewer male role models, and whose deviations are more undesirable (Jacklin, DiPietro, & Maccoby, 1984; Langlois & Downs, 1980). Even if parents do not differentiate between daughters and sons, the same parental treatment may affect girls and boys differently. Indeed, parents model different behaviors, and children pay more attention to same-sex models and to those that display more sex-typical behaviors (Perry & Bussey, 1979).

Caretaking

Analysis of 186 nonindustrial societies (Weisner & Gallimore, 1977) revealed that female adult relatives and female children are usually the primary caretakers of infants. However, when infants reach early childhood, both-sex peers share caretaking responsibilities. Sibling caretakers play an important socialization role in societies in which 2- to 4-year-olds spend more than 70% of every day in their care. Mothers in such societies engage in productive activities and are not devoted exclusively to mothering (Greenfield, 1981; Minturn & Lambert, 1964). Nonetheless, children in all cultures see mothers as more responsible for children than are fathers.

Moreover, in 20% of 80 cultures surveyed (Katz & Konner, 1981), fathers were rarely, or never, near their infants. Father–infant relationships were close in only 4% of the cultures, but even when close, fathers spent only 14% of their time with their infants and provided only 6% of the actual caregiving. In most societies, father–child interactions are characterized by play (Munroe & Munroe, 1975/1994).

Father absence has been associated with both effeminate (e.g., dependent) and hypermasculine (e.g., aggressive) behaviors (Katz & Konner, 1981; Segall, 1988; Stevenson & Black, 1988; Whiting, 1965). Fathers pay less attention to daughters than to sons, and they promote sex-typed activities more than do mothers (Lytton & Romney, 1991). Mothers are equally involved in caring for sons and daughters, but fathers are more involved with sons (Rohner & Rohner, 1982). Observers in public places in 10 cultures found girls more often in groups with no adult males, and boys frequently in all male groups; these differences increased with age (Mackey, 1981, 1985; Mackey & Day, 1979). Across 22 cultures, when no women are present, men are rarely seen with infants and have a high level of association with older boys (Mackey, 2001).

Task Assignment

Cultural differences in learning environments help shape children's gender roles. In the Six Culture Study (Edwards & Whiting, 1974; Minturn & Lambert, 1964; Whiting & Edwards, 1973), fewer gender differences in behaviors (e.g., aggression, responsibility, dependence, nurturance) were found in the three cultures (the United States, the Philippines, Kenya) in which both girls and boys cared for younger siblings and performed household chores. In contrast, more differences were found when boys and girls were treated dissimilarly, with girls assuming more responsibility for siblings and household tasks (India, Mexico, Okinawa). Indeed, the fewest gender differences were found between American girls and boys, the group assigned the fewest child care or household tasks. Overall, girls spent more of their time in responsible, productive work, and boys spent relatively more time playing (Edwards, 2000).

From the cultures in the Standard Cross-Cultural Sample (Murdock & White, 1969), Bradley (1993) selected ethnographic records from 91 nonindustrial societies that are considered by anthropologists to be representative of world cultures. They found that children younger than age 6 perform little work, whereas children older than 10 perform work similar to that of same-sex adults. Both girls and boys do women's work (e.g., fetching water) more frequently than men's work (e.g., hunting), and children usually do chores that adults consider demeaning or unskilled.

Peers

Peers play an important socialization role throughout childhood and adolescence. In some cultures, boys and girls are separated by the end of infancy (Whiting & Edwards, 1988), but in others, children play freely within mixed-gender and -age groups (Rogoff, 1990). Gender segregation is the overriding rule of social interaction during middle childhood (ages 6–10; Edwards, 2000). Peer influences increase with age, structuring the transition from childhood to adulthood (Edwards, 1992).

Maccoby (1988, 1998) contends that peers may be more important than parents in the socialization of gender roles and identifies three gender-linked phenomena in children's social development: gender segregation, differentiation of interaction styles, and group asymmetry. In the United States and cross-culturally (Whiting & Edwards, 1988), children as early as age 3 have a powerful tendency to seek out same-sex mates and to avoid other-sex children, and this tendency strengthens throughout grade school (Edwards, 1992; Edwards & Whiting, 1993). In their segregated groups, boys strive for dominance, engage in rough-and-tumble play, take risks, "grandstand," and are reluctant to reveal weaknesses to each other. In contrast, girls self-disclose more, try to maintain positive social relationships, and avoid open conflict. Compared with girls' groups, boys' groups are more cohesive, exclusionary, and separate from adult culture. Segregated groups lead to different activities and toy choices that in turn may lead to differences in intellectual and emotional development (Block, 1983).

Culturally prescribed adolescent initiation rites also lead to gender segregation by separating initiates from their families, socializing them to culturally appropriate sexual behaviors, creating peer-group loyalty, and solidifying political ties. Collective rituals are more common for boys than for girls and are frequently found in societies that emphasize adult gender differences (Edwards, 1992). Western education has led to changes in initiation rites, but vestiges of them still remain.

Education

Educational settings and expectations influence children's gender role development. Japanese and American fifth-grade teachers pay more attention to boys than to girls, particularly negative attention, but the greater attention is not a result of boys' off-task or bad behavior (Hamilton, Blumenfeld, Akoh, & Miura, 1991).

Parents' beliefs about academic performance also affect children's achievement. In Zambia, education is considered more important for boys than for girls (Serpell, 1993). In China, Japan, and the United

States, mothers expect boys to be better at mathematics and girls to be better at reading (Lummis & Stevenson, 1990) even though the sexes perform equally well in some aspects of both disciplines.

Interestingly, over the second half of the 20th century, women's level of education increased and has surpassed that of men in the United States and in several other Western countries (United Nations Development Programme, 1995). This shift is important, considering that, in some countries, women are not permitted to participate in formal education (United Nations Development Programme, 1995).

Cultural Practices That Influence Behaviors of Males and Females

In the previous section, we examined proximal socialization activities that influence gender role learning, but there are also broader, more distal cultural practices that provide an important context for gender-related behavior, including women's status and political influence, gender division of labor and economic factors, and religious beliefs and values.

Status and Political Influence

At least to some degree, every society assigns traits and tasks according to gender (Munroe & Munroe, 1975/1994), and in no society is the status of women superior to that of men, whereas the reverse is common (Hoyenga & Hoyenga, 1993; Population Crisis Committee, 1988; Whyte, 1978). Women's status is multidimensional (e.g., power, autonomy, prestige, economic impact, ideology; Mukhopadhyay & Higgins, 1988) and is related to reproductive roles, physical differences, and complexity of the society (Berry, 1976; Ember, 1981).

Across cultures, men are more involved in political activities and possess greater power than do women (Ember, 1981; Ross, 1985, 1986). The long-standing stereotyped dichotomy of public/male versus private/female suggests that men are in the public eye, active in business, politics, and culture, whereas women stay at home, caring for home and family (Peterson & Runyan, 1993). However, recent cross-cultural studies indicate that this dichotomy is crumbling, with women working outside the home and in public life, and men more involved with their families (Vianello et al., 1990). Adolescents' images of women reflect the changing conditions and attitudes toward women around the world (Gibbons et al., 1991, 1993).

Even though attitudes are changing, sexism and gender inequality still exist, and women are clearly a disadvantaged group. Examining sexist attitudes of more than 15,000 men and women in 19 nations, Glick and Fiske (2001) found cross-culturally prevalent ideologies of chivalry (benevolent sexism) and antipathy (hostile sexism) that predict gender inequality.

Gender Division of Labor

Ethnographic analysis of jobs and tasks in 224 societies indicated that men were involved with hunting, metal work, weapon making, and travel farther from home, and women were responsible for cooking, carrying water, caring for clothing, and making household goods (D'Andrade, 1966; Murdock & Prevost, 1973). Women's subsistence activities were consistent with child-rearing demands (Brown, 1970; Segal, 1983), and women hunted in societies in which this activity did not compete with child care (Goodman, Griffin, Estioko-Griffin, & Grove, 1985). Men had major child-rearing responsibilities in only 10% of 80 cultures examined (Katz & Konner, 1981). However, both sexes seem to be flexible enough to adapt to a wide range of socioeconomic roles (Wood & Eagly, 2002).

Decreases in infant mortality and technological advances have made it easier for women to participate in the labor force outside the home (Huber, 1986). However, compared to men, women remain economically disadvantaged and are paid less than their male counterparts (Ottaway & Bhatnagar, 1988). Even in societies in which women are active in the labor force, a commensurate reduction in their household duties has not taken place (Population Crisis Committee, 1988).

Indeed, the difficulty of eliminating gender divisions in labor is illustrated by the Israeli *kibbutz*, established in the 1920s, a deliberate attempt to develop egalitarian societies (Rosner, 1967; Spiro, 1956, 1995). Initially, there was no sexual division of labor. Both women and men worked in the fields, drove tractors, and worked in the kitchen and in the laundry. However, with time and increases in the birthrate, women found they could not undertake many of the physical tasks that men were capable of doing. Women soon found themselves in the roles they had tried to escape—cooking, cleaning, laundering, teaching, caring for children. Surprisingly, the *kibbutz* efforts toward an equitable division of labor had little effect on children's sex roles or their self-attributions (Carlsson & Barnes, 1986).

The persistence of traditional roles in the *kibbutz* is consistent with the "role overload" women experience when moving into the labor force. Although women may work outside the home, there has been no commensurate reduction in their household duties (Population Crisis

Committee, 1988). In the United States, Switzerland, Sweden, Canada, Italy, Poland, and Romania, the overwhelming majority of household work is performed by women, regardless of the extent of their occupational demands (Calasanti & Bailey, 1991; Charles & Höpflinger, 1992; Guberman, Maheu, & Maillé, 1992; Vianello et al., 1990; Wright, Shire, Hwang, Dolan, & Baxter, 1992).

Economic Factors

Economic factors appear to influence gender-related cultural practices. In his examination of 386 cultures, Heath (1958) found that bride price was a form of compensation for the loss of a daughter's economic contributions to her family, was frequently greater when her contribution was substantial. A dowry accompanied the bride when her economic contributions to her family were relatively small. Economic factors may affect males' reproductive success more than that of females, particularly when men may have more than one wife and must pay a bride price for them (Cronk, 1993). In families with high socioeconomic status, whose sons can pay for wives, parents favor males, but parents with low status favor females, because they can be married off to wealthier, higher status neighbors.

Socioeconomic conditions may also affect sex-biased parental investment in children. Among the Mukogodo of Kenya, who are at the bottom of the regional hierarchy of wealth and prestige, the male–female birth ratio is about equal, but the 1986 census recorded 98 girls and 66 boys less than 4 years of age. Although there is no evidence of male infanticide, boys' higher death rate is most likely due to favoritism toward girls. Compared with sons, daughters are breast-fed longer, are well-fed, and visit the doctor more often. Because men in the Mukogodo area can have as many wives as they can afford, women are in short supply, and they all find husbands.

In sharp contrast, in most other traditional parts of the world (e.g., India, China, Turkey, Korea) cultural practices favor boys, who are highly valued by their families, and whose births lead to great rejoicing (Kagitçibasi, 1982). Bride burning (Ghadially & Kumar, 1988), wife beating (Flavia, 1988), and female infanticide (Krishnaswamy, 1988) are cultural practices that demonstrate the low regard for females in some traditional Indian cultures. In the United States (Oakley, 1979; Pooler, 1991) and in non-Western countries (Arnold et al., 1975), preference for boys continues to be strong even though many of the economic circumstances and religious traditions that created male preferences no longer apply in contemporary society.

Religious Beliefs and Values

Religious beliefs about gender roles and family honor influence perceptions of women (Williams & Best, 1982/1990a), women's work outside the home (Rapoport, Lomski-Feder, & Masalha, 1989), and role models that children see. Some religious communities prescribe proper roles and behaviors for males and females, and children are brought up in a manner that is consistent with these views.

BIOLOGICAL AND CULTURAL INFLUENCES ON GENDER DEVELOPMENT

When similar gender differences in behavior are found across cultural groups, it is sometimes considered to be evidence for the role of genes and hormones, implying genetic or biological determinism. Biological determinism assumes that any biological influence or bias always leads to an irreversible sex difference, making biology both the necessary and sufficient cause of those sex differences. Biology is neither. The long-standing nature–nurture controversy in developmental psychology demonstrates that biology does not cause behavior, and that such a notion is quite naive.

Sex chromosomes and hormones do not cause behaviors; they simply change the probability of occurrence of certain behaviors (Hoyenga & Hoyenga, 1993; Stewart, 1988). Epigenesis (development) is probabilistic, and a particular phenotype may come from either a gene or a given developmental environment, or both (Cairns, Gariépy, & Hood, 1990; Gottlieb, 1997). The gene–behavior pathway is bidirectional, with influences in both directions (Gottlieb, 1983). Just as people inherit genes, they may "inherit" environments and cultures by living close to family. Both genes and environment determine sexual dimorphism (Hampson, 1965; Hoyenga & Hoyenga, 1993), and gender is an added factor that affects their interaction. Gender assignment at birth influences later gender identity, roles, stereotypes, ideology, and other cultural–environmental aspects of gender.

CONCLUSIONS

Although biological factors impose predispositions and restrictions on development, sociocultural factors are crucial determinants of development (Best & Williams, 1993; Munroe & Munroe, 1975/1994). Culture has profound effects on behavior, prescribing how babies are delivered, how children are dressed and socialized, what tasks children are taught, what is considered intelligent behavior, and what roles adult men and women adopt. Children's behaviors, even those considered biologically determined, are governed by culture (Super & Harkness, 1982). Pancultural gender differences or universals are sometimes explained by similarities in socialization practices, whereas cultural differences are attributed to differences in socialization. Cultural practices shape children to fit differing life circumstances, and gender plays an important part in those practices.

Children grow up within other people's scripts, which guide their actions long before they themselves can understand or carry out culturally appropriate actions. For cross-cultural researchers, one of the crucial tasks is to identify the mechanism responsible for developmental change. This means that broadly defined cultural variables must be "unpackaged" to identify the processes that lead to the development of specific gender-related behaviors. Gender must be examined in relation to cultural processes (e.g., practices, beliefs, myths, rituals, social systems) and the broader cultural context, including the history and economics of a society. Not only are the parent and child changing across time but also those changes take place in a cultural system that is itself changing.

Cultural mechanisms responsible for developmental change must account for both within-culture variation of individuals and between-culture variation across cultural groups. Variations between cultural groups are certainly greater than variations within a single, homogeneous culture; as a consequence, cross-cultural studies provide an excellent "testing ground" for theoretical concepts and predictions. Predictions that are supported and replicated across very different populations are certainly robust and are likely to result in richer, more complete explanations of gender-related behavior. Indeed, the cross-cultural approach is not inconsistent with any of the views of gender described in this volume. In itself, it is not a theory but an amalgam of comparative orientations and methodologies that stress the formative role of the sociocultural context; consequently, it may provide a valuable means for understanding other viewpoints.

REFERENCES

Adamopoulos, J., & Lonner, W. J. (2001). Culture and psychology at a crossroad: Historical perspective and theoretical analysis. In D. Matsumoto (Ed.), *The handbook of culture and psychology* (pp. 11–34). New York: Oxford University Press.

Agarwal, K. S., & Lester, D. (1992). A study of perception of women by Indian and American students. In S. Iwawaki, Y. Kashima, & K. Leung (Eds.), *In-*

novations in cross-cultural psychology (pp. 123–134). Amsterdam: Swets & Zeitlinger.

Albert, A. A., & Porter, J. R. (1986). Children's gender role stereotypes: A comparison of the United States and South Africa. *Journal of Cross-Cultural Psychology, 17*, 45–65.

Arnold, F., Bulatao, R., Buripakdi, C., Chung, B. J., Fawcett, J. T., Iritani, et al. (1975). *The value of children: Introduction and comparative analysis* (Vol. 1). Honolulu: East–West Center Population Institute.

Barber, B. K., Chadwick, B. A., & Oerter, R. (1992). Parental behaviors and adolescent self-esteem in the United States and Germany. *Journal of Marriage and the Family, 54*, 128–141.

Barry, H., III, Bacon, M. K., & Child, I. L. (1957). A cross-cultural survey of some sex differences in socialization. *Journal of Abnormal and Social Psychology, 55*, 327–332.

Barry, H., III, Bacon, M. K., & Child, I. L. (1967). Definitions, ratings and bibliographic sources of child-training practices of 110 cultures. In C. S. Ford (Ed.), *Cross-cultural approaches* (pp. 293–331). New Haven, CT: Human Relations Area Files Press.

Basow, S. A. (1984). Cultural variations in sex typing. *Sex Roles, 10*, 577–585.

Bem, S. L. (1974). The measurement of psychological androgyny. *Journal of Consulting and Clinical Psychology, 42*, 155–162.

Berry, J. W. (1976). Sex differences in behavior and cultural complexity. *Indian Journal of Psychology, 51*, 89–97.

Berry, J. W., Poortinga, Y. H., Segall, M. H., & Dasen, P. R. (1992). *Cross-cultural psychology: Research and applications*. New York: Cambridge University Press.

Best, D. L., & Williams, J. E. (1993). Cross-cultural viewpoint. In A. E. Beall & R. J. Sternberg (Eds.), *The psychology of gender* (pp. 215–248). New York: Guilford Press.

Best, D. L., & Williams, J. E. (1998). Masculinity and femininity in the self and ideal self descriptions of university students in 14 countries. In G. Hofstede (Ed.), *Masculinity and femininity: The taboo dimensions of national cultures* (pp. 106–116). Thousand Oaks, CA: Sage.

Best, D. L., Williams, J. E., & Briggs, S. R. (1980). A further analysis of the affective meanings associated with male and female sex-trait stereotypes. *Sex Roles, 6*, 735–746.

Best, D. L., Williams, J. E., Cloud, J. M., Davis, S. W., Robertson, L. S., Edwards, J. R., et al. (1977). Development of sex–trait stereotypes among young children in the United States, England, and Ireland. *Child Development, 48*, 1375–1384.

Biernat, M. (1991). Gender stereotypes and the relationship between masculinity and femininity: A developmental analysis. *Journal of Personality and Social Psychology, 61*, 351–365.

Bloch, M. N., & Adler, S. M. (1994). African children's and the emergence of the sexual division of labor. In J. L. Roopnarine, J. E. Johnson, & F. H. Hooper

(Eds.), *Children's play in diverse cultures* (pp. 148–178). Albany: State University of New York Press.

Block, J. H. (1983). Differential premises arising from differential socialization of the sexes: Some conjectures. *Child Development, 54*, 1335–1354.

Blurton Jones, N. B., & Konner, M. (1973). Sex differences in behavior of London and Bushman children. In R. P. Michael & J. H. Crook (Eds.), *Comparative ecology and behavior of primates* (pp. 690–749). London: Academic Press.

Bradley, C. (1993). Women's power, children's labor. *Cross-Cultural Research, 27*, 70–96.

Brown, J. K. (1970). A note on the division of labor by sex. *American Anthropologist, 72*, 1073–1078.

Burbank, V. K. (1987). Female aggression in cross-cultural perspective. *Behavior Science Research, 21*(1–4), 70–100.

Burns, A., & Homel, R. (1986). Sex role satisfaction among Australian children: Some sex, age, and cultural group comparisons. *Psychology of Women Quarterly, 10*, 285–296.

Buss, D. M. (1989). Sex differences in human mate preferences: Evolutionary hypotheses tested in 37 cultures. *Behavioral and Brain Sciences, 12*, 1–49.

Buss, D. M., Abbott, M., Angleitner, A., Biaggio, A., Bianco-Villasenor, A., Bruchon Schweitzer, M., et al. (1990). International preferences in selecting mates. *Journal of Cross-Cultural Psychology, 21*, 5–47.

Cairns, R. B., Gariépy, J. L., & Hood, K. E. (1990). Development, microevolution, and social behavior. *Psychological Review, 97*, 49–65.

Calhoun, G., Jr., & Sethi, R. (1987). The self-esteem of pupils from India, the United States, and the Philippines. *Journal of Psychology, 121*, 199–202.

Campbell, D. T., & Stanley, J. C. (1963). *Experimental and quasi-experimental designs for research*. Chicago: Rand McNally.

Carlsson, M., & Barnes, M. (1986). Conception and self-attribution of sex-role behavior: A cross-cultural comparison between Swedish and kibbutz-raised Israeli children. *Scandinavian Journal of Psychology, 27*, 258–265.

Cronk, L. (1993). Parental favoritism toward daughters. *American Scientist, 81*, 272–279.

D'Andrade, R. (1966). Cultural meaning systems. In R. A. Shweder & R. A. LeVine (Eds.), *Culture theory: Essays on mind, self and emotion* (pp. 88–122). New York: Cambridge University Press.

Draper, P. (1975). Cultural pressure on sex differences. *American Ethnologist, 2*(4), 602–616.

Eagly, A. H., & Wood, W. (1999). The origins of sex differences in human behavior: Evolved dispositions versus social roles. *American Psychologist, 54*, 75–133.

Edelbrock, C., & Sugawara, A. I. (1978). Acquisition of sex-typed preferences in preschool-aged children. *Developmental Psychology, 14*, 614–623.

Edwards, C. P. (1992). Cross-cultural perspectives on family–peer relations. In R. D. Parke & G. W. Ladd (Eds.), *Family–peer relationships: Modes of linkages* (pp. 285–315). Mahwah, NJ: Erlbaum.

Edwards, C. P. (2000). Children's play in cross-cultural perspective: A new look at the Six Cultures Study. *Cross-Cultural Research*, *34*, 318–338.

Edwards, C. P., & Whiting, B. B. (1974). Women and dependency. *Politics and Society*, *4*, 343–355.

Edwards, C. P., & Whiting, B. B. (1980). Differential socialization of girls and boys in light of cross-cultural research. *New Directions for Child Development*, *8*, 45–57.

Edwards, C. P., & Whiting, B. B. (1993). "Mother, older sibling, and me": The overlapping roles of caretakers and companions in the social world of 2–3 year olds in Ngeca, Kenya. In K. MacDonald (Ed.), *Parent–child: Descriptions and implications* (pp. 305–329). Albany: State University of New York Press.

Ember, C. R. (1981). A cross-cultural perspective on sex differences. In R. H. Munroe, R. L. Munroe, & B. B. Whiting (Eds.), *Handbook of cross-cultural human development* (pp. 531–580). New York: Garland.

Flavia. (1988). Violence in the family: Wife beating. In R. Ghadially (Ed.), *Women in society: A reader* (pp. 151–166). New Delhi: Sage.

Freedman, D. G. (1976). Infancy, biology, and culture. In L. P. Lipsitt (Ed.), *Developmental psychobiology: The significance of infancy* (pp. 35–55). New York: Wiley.

Freedman, D. G., & DeBoer, M. M. (1979). Biological and cultural differences in early child development. *Annual Review of Anthropology*, *8*, 579–600.

Ghadially, R., & Kazi, K. A. (1979). Attitudes toward sex roles. *Indian Journal of Social Work*, *40*, 65–71.

Ghadially, R., & Kumar, P. (1988). Stress, strain, and coping styles of female professionals. *Indian Journal of Applied Psychology*, *26*(1), 1–8.

Gibbons, J. L., Lynn, M., Stiles, D. A., de Berducido, E. J., Richter, R., Walker, K., et al. (1993). Guatemalan, Filipino, and U.S. adolescents' images of women as office workers and homemakers. *Psychology of Women Quarterly*, *17*, 373–388.

Gibbons, J. L., Stiles, D. A., & Shkodriani, G. M. (1991). Adolescents' attitudes toward family and gender roles: An international comparison. *Sex Roles*, *25*, 625–643.

Glick, P., & Fiske, S. T. (2001). An ambivalent alliance: Hostile and benevolent sexism as complementary justifications for gender inequality. *American Psychologist*, *56*, 109–118.

Goodman, M. J., Griffin, P. B., Estioko-Griffin, A. A., & Grove, J. S. (1985). The compatibility of hunting and mothering among the Agta hunter–gatherers of the Philippines. *Sex Roles*, *12*, 1199–1209.

Gottlieb, G. (1983). The psychobiological approach to development. In P. H. Mussen (Series Ed.), M. M. Haith & J. J. Campos (Vol. Eds.), *Handbook of child psychology: Vol. 2. Infancy and Infancy and developmental psychobiology* (pp. 1–26). New York: Wiley.

Gottlieb, G. (1997). *Synthesizing nature–nurture: Prenatal roots of instinctive behavior.* Mahwah, NJ: Erlbaum.

Gough, H. G. (1966). A cross-cultural analysis of the CPI femininity scale. *Journal of Consulting Psychology, 30*, 136–141.

Gough, H. G., & Heilbrun, A. B., Jr. (1980). *The Adjective Check List manual.* Palo Alto, CA: Consulting Psychologists Press.

Greenfield, P. M. (1981). Child care in cross-cultural perspectives: Implications for the future organization of child care in the United States. *Psychology of Women Quarterly, 6*, 41–54.

Greenfield, P. M., Brazelton, T. B., & Childs, C. P. (1989). From birth to maturity in Zinacantan: Ontogenesis in cultural context. In V. Bricker & G. Gosen (Eds.), *Ethnographic encounters in southern Mesoamerica: Celebratory essays in honor of Evon Z. Vogt* (pp. 177–216). Albany: Institute of Mesoamerican Studies, State University of New York.

Guttentag, M., & Longfellow, C. (1977). Children's social attributions: Development and change. In C. B. Keasey (Ed.), *Nebraska Symposium on Motivation* (pp. 305–341). Lincoln: University of Nebraska Press.

Hamilton, V. L., Blumenfeld, P. C., Akoh, H., & Miura, K. (1991). Group and gender in Japanese and American elementary classrooms. *Journal of Cross-Cultural Psychology, 22*, 317–346.

Hampson, J. L. (1965). Determinants of psychosexual orientation. In F. A. Beach (Ed.), *Sex and behavior* (pp. 108–132). New York: Wiley.

Hanover, B. (2000). Development of the self in gendered contexts. In T. Eckes & H. M. Trautner (Eds.), *The developmental social psychology of gender* (pp. 177–206). Mahwah, NJ: Erlbaum.

Heath, D. B. (1958). Sexual division of labor and cross-cultural research. *Social Forces, 37*, 77–79.

Hendrix, L., & Johnson, G. D. (1985). Instrumental and expressive socialization: A false dichotomy. *Sex Roles, 13*, 581–595.

Hofstede, G. (1980). *Culture's consequences: International differences in work-related values.* Beverly Hills, CA: Sage.

Hoyenga, K. B., & Hoyenga, K. T. (1993). *Gender-related differences: Origins and outcomes.* Boston: Allyn & Bacon.

Huber, J. (1986). Trends in gender stratification, 1970–1985. *Sociological Forum, 1*, 476–495.

Intons-Peterson, M. J. (1988). *Gender concepts of Swedish and American youth.* Hillsdale, NJ: Erlbaum.

Jacklin, C. N., DiPietro, J. A., & Maccoby, E. E. (1984). Sex typing behavior and sex typing pressure in child/parent interaction. *Archives of Sexual Behavior, 13*, 413–425.

Kagitçibasi, Ç. (1982). Old-age security value of children: Cross-national socioeconomic evidence. *Journal of Cross-Cultural Psychology, 13*, 29–42.

Kalin, R., & Tilby, P. (1978). Development and validation of a sex-role ideology scale. *Psychological Reports, 42*, 731–738.

Karraker, K. H., Vogel, D. A., & Lake, M. A. (1995). Parents' gender-stereotyped perceptions of newborns: The eye of the beholder revisited. *Sex Roles, 33*, 687–701.

Kaschak, E., & Sharratt, S. (1983). A Latin American sex role inventory. *Cross-Cultural Psychology Bulletin*, *18*, 3–6.

Katz, M. M., & Konner, M. J. (1981). The role of the father: An anthropological perspective. In M. E. Lamb (Ed.), *The role of the father in child development* (2nd ed., pp. 155–185). New York: Wiley.

Kling, K. C., Hyde, J. S., Showers, C. J., & Buswell, B. N. (1999). Gender differences in self-esteem: A meta-analysis. *Psychological Bulletin*, *125*, 470–500.

Krishnaswamy, S. (1988). Female infanticide in contemporary India: A case study of Kallars of Tamilnadu. In R. Ghadially (Ed.), *Women in Indian society: A reader* (pp. 186–195). New Delhi: Sage.

Langlois, J. H., & Downs, C. (1980). Mothers, fathers and peers as socialization agents of sex-typed behavior in young children. *Child Development*, *51*, 1217–1247.

Lara-Cantu, M. A., & Navarro-Arias, R. (1987). Self-descriptions of Mexican college students in response to the Bem Sex Role Inventory and other sex role items. *Journal of Cross-Cultural Psychology*, *18*, 331–344.

Larsen, K. S., & Long, E. (1988). Attitudes toward sex-roles: Traditional or egalitarian? *Sex Roles*, *19*, 1–12.

Lummis, M., & Stevenson, H. W. (1990). Gender differences in beliefs and achievement: A cross-cultural study. *Developmental Psychology*, *26*, 254–263.

Lytton, H., & Romney, D. M. (1991). Parents' differential socialization of boys and girls: A meta-analysis. *Psychological Bulletin*, *109*, 267–296.

Maccoby, E. E. (1988). Gender as a social category. *Developmental Psychology*, *24*, 755–765.

Maccoby, E. E. (1998). *The two sexes: Growing up apart, coming together.* Cambridge, MA: Belnap Press.

Mackey, W. C. (1981). A cross-cultural analysis of adult-child proxemics in relation to the Plowman–Protector Complex: A preliminary study. *Behavior Science Research*, *3/4*, 187–223.

Mackey, W. C. (1985). *Fathering behaviors: The dynamics of the man–child bond.* New York: Plenum Press.

Mackey W. C. (2001). Support for the existence of an independent man-to-child affiliative bond: Fatherhood as a biocultural invention. *Psychology of Men and Masculinity*, 2, 51–66.

Mackey, W. C., & Day, R. (1979). Some indicators of fathering behaviors in the United States: A cross-cultural examination of adult male–child interaction. *Journal of Marriage and the Family*, *41*, 287–299.

Minturn, L., & Lambert, W. W. (1964). *Mothers of six cultures: Antecedents of child rearing.* New York: Wiley.

Mukhopadhyay, C. C., & Higgins, P. J. (1998). Anthropological studies of women's status revisited: 1977–1987. *Annual Review of Anthropology*, *17*, 461–495.

Munroe, R. L., Hulefeld, R., Rodgers, J. M., Tomeo, D. L., & Yamazaki, S. K. (2000). Aggression among children in four cultures. *Cross-Cultural Research*, *34*, 3–25.

Munroe, R. L., & Munroe, R. H. (1971). Effect of environmental experiences on spatial ability in an East African society. *Journal of Social Psychology, 83,* 3–10.

Munroe, R. L., & Munroe, R. H. (1994). *Cross-cultural human development* (rev. ed.). Prospect Heights, IL: Waveland Press. (Original work published 1975)

Munroe, R. H., Shimmin, H. S., & Munroe, R. L. (1984). Gender understanding and sex role preference in four cultures. *Developmental Psychology, 20,* 673–682.

Murdock, G. P., & Prevost, C. (1973). Factors in the division of labor by sex: A cross-cultural analysis. *Ethnology, 12,* 203–225.

Murdock, G. P., & White, D. R. (1969). Standard cross-cultural sample. *Ethnology, 8,* 329–369.

Oakley, A. (1979). *Becoming a mother.* Oxford, UK: Martin Robertson.

Olowu, A. A. (1985). Gender as a determinant of some Nigerian adolescents' self-concepts. *Journal of Adolescence, 8,* 347–355.

Omark, D. R., Omark, M., & Edelman, M. (1975). Formation of dominance hierarchies in young children: Action and perspective. In T. Williams (Ed.), *Psychological anthropology* (pp. 289–315). The Hague: Mouton.

Osgood, C. E., May, W. H., & Miron, M. S. (1975). *Cross-cultural universals of affective meaning.* Urbana: University of Illinois Press.

Osgood, C. E., Suci, G. J., & Tannenbaum, P. H. (1957). *The measurement of meaning.* Urbana: University of Illinois Press.

Ottaway, R. N., & Bhatnagar, D. (1988). Personality and biographical differences between male and female managers in the United States and India. *Applied Psychology: An International Review, 37,* 201–212.

Perry, D. G., & Bussey, K. (1979). The social learning theory of sex differences: Imitation is alive and well. *Journal of Personality and Social Psychology, 37,* 1699–1712.

Peterson, V. S., & Runyan, A. S. (1993). *Global gender issues.* Boulder, CO: Westview Press.

Pooler, W. S. (1991). Sex of child preferences among college students. *Sex Roles, 25,* 569–576.

Population Crisis Committee. (1988, June). *Country rankings of the status of women: Poor, powerless, and pregnant* (Issue Brief No. 20). Washington, DC: Author.

Prosser, G. V., Hutt, C., Hutt, S. J., Mahindadasa, K. J., & Goonetilleke, M. D. J. (1986). Children's play in Sri Lanka: A cross-cultural study. *British Journal of Developmental Psychology, 4,* 179–186.

Ramirez, J. M. (1993). Acceptability of aggression in four Spanish regions and a comparison with other European countries. *Aggressive Behavior, 19,* 185–197.

Rao, V. V. P., & Rao, V. N. (1985). Sex-role attitudes across two cultures: United States and India. *Sex Roles, 13,* 607–624.

Rapoport, T., Lomski-Feder, E., & Masalha, M. (1989). Female subordination in the Arab–Israeli community: The adolescent perspective of "social veil." *Sex Roles, 20,* 255–269.

Williams, J. E., & Best, D. L. (1990a). *Measuring sex stereotypes: A multination study* (rev. ed.). Newbury Park, CA: Sage. (Original work published 1982)

Williams, J. E., & Best, D. L. (1990b). *Sex and psyche: Gender and self viewed cross-culturally.* Newbury Park, CA: Sage.

Wood, W., & Eagly, A. H. (2002). A cross-cultural analysis of the behavior of women and men: Implications for the origins of sex differences. *Psychological Bulletin, 128*, 699–727.

Wright, E. O., Shire, K., Hwang, S. L., Dolan, M., & Baxter, J. (1992). The non-effects of class on the gender division of labor in the home: A comparative study of Sweden and the United States. *Gender and Society*, 6, 252–282.

14

Sex Changes

A Current Perspective on the Psychology of Gender

MARIANNE LAFRANCE
ELIZABETH LEVY PALUCK
VICTORIA BRESCOLL

As this volume attests, the psychology of gender comprises a rich array of topics pursued by top-notch researchers drawing on the latest theories and using the most sophisticated methodologies. The psychological study of gender has clearly come of age. No longer the concern of a handful of researchers, the psychology of gender embraces researchers from across the domain of psychology. No longer regarded as an upstart or an area of questionable legitimacy, the study of the psychology of gender is now accepted as a serious scholarly pursuit. No longer viewed as stridently political, the psychology of gender has entered the scientific mainstream. But all this expansion, acceptance, and growing coherence should not be taken to mean that all the issues prompting the rise of the field have now been settled.

In what follows, we discuss several issues that were instigated by the chapters in this volume. These issues, however, are not unique to these chapters but, we believe, have applicability across the domain of the psychology of gender. Specifically, we draw attention to four issues. First, we look at the changes in content of the psychology of gender, specifically, with reference to observing the increased presence of theory, the greater prevalence of biology, and the diminution of feminist politics. Second, we take a close look at terminology in order to determine whether word choice provides information about the tacit belief systems that continue to link *sex* with biological processes and *gender* with sociocultural processes. Third, we note the persistence of between-sex comparisons, which continue to be the central focus in general for psychologists interested in gender. Finally, we reiterate the point that because gender processes necessarily operate in conjunction with other social categories (e.g., race, class, and age), investigators should attend more to these and other situation and group interactions.

THE PSYCHOLOGY OF GENDER: PAST AND PRESENT

The psychology of gender today subsumes a diverse collection of topics, questions, methods, and political underpinnings. Everything from hormonal and genetic influences on sex differences to societal conditions affecting gender inequality is included. This second edition of *The Psychology of Gender* mirrors this far-ranging collection of topics. For example, Hampson and Moffat (Chapter 3) ask how reproductive hormones affect sex differences in behavior, and answer the question by drawing on evidence from both animal and human studies. Ridgeway and Bourg (Chapter 10) examine the ways that gender-linked status beliefs create power inequities between men and women, and investigate these links with social psychological experiments.

Perspectives and Trends

As the field of the psychology of gender has expanded, so too have the attempts to characterize how it has developed (e.g., Banaji, 1993; Crawford & Marecek, 1989; Deaux, 1984; Deaux & LaFrance, 1998; Unger, 1998, 2001; West & Zimmerman, 1987). Most researchers agree that the earliest tack taken by psychologists in the study of gender focused on the ways that men and women differ or are similar to each other. At least early on, this approach sometimes led to seeing women as a problem, and somewhat later it led to seeing women as special (Crawford & Marecek, 1989). The "woman as problem" focus documented the ways in which women appeared to be deficient relative to men. For example, researchers in achievement motivation sought to understand why women have a "fear of success" (Horner, 1972). Gilligan's (1984) description of women's unique ethic of care exemplifies the "woman as special" focus, in which women's noteworthy characteristics were given special attention. Regardless of how women were seen relative to men, the common thread was an emphasis on sex comparisons.

The second major perspective emerged in the 1970s, when psychologists began to conceptualize gender as multidimensional rather than binary. Masculinity and femininity were conceptualized as two independent sets of psychological traits rather than as opposite ends of a single scale (Bem, 1974). Studies in this area distinguished sex-typed people (e.g., self-described masculine males and feminine females) from more androgynous people (e.g., males and females who identified themselves as both masculine and feminine). The aim was to demonstrate that androgyny might be a way out of the problems associated with bipolar measurements of masculinity and femininity then in use. For conceptual and methodological reasons, androgyny has not lived up to its initial promise. For example, the measurement of masculinity and femininity was found to be somewhat unreliable because of shifting ideas of what constituted typical male and female characteristics. Moreover, androgynous individuals were not consistently found to be healthier psychologically than sex-typed individuals (see Hoffman & Borders, 2001). Bell (Chapter 7) touches on similar issues when she considers individuals who are uncomfortable with their sex.

The research on androgyny nonetheless showed that masculinity and femininity were differentially valued and that the evaluations varied with the contexts in which they took place. Attention thus turned to seeing sex as a stimulus variable. In other words, researchers began to investigate people's stereotypes of males and females as social categories. Reflecting this substantial shift in focus (Deaux, 1984), the "psychology of women," as it was typically known, was renamed the "psychology of gender" as researchers began to concentrate on how gender is perceived and enacted (Crawford & Marecek, 1989). In this volume, gender as social category is reflected by Ridgeway and Bourg's (Chapter 10) study of people's different expectations for men and women. It also shows up in Pomerantz, Ng, and Wang's (Chapter 6) discussion of how parents' gender-based expectations influence their treatment of sons and daughters.

Most recently, some psychologists have begun to challenge the prevailing assumptions, methods, and values of the positivist take on the psychology of gender. Maracek, Crawford, and Popp (Chapter 9) provide a vigorous endorsement of this social constructivist perspective on the understanding of gender. A constructivist stance has gathered adherents on both sides of the Atlantic, yet it appears to have more support in Europe and the United Kingdom than in the United States.

Although we have described these four perspectives as though the later ones have subsumed or replaced the earlier ones, a truer description is that all four perspectives continue to have their adherents, not only in this volume but in the psychology of gender as a whole.

What's New in This Volume?

Twenty years ago, Deaux (1984) urged researchers to develop better theories to explain the processes and mechanisms underlying the psychology of gender. If this volume is any indication, psychologists have heeded her advice. Several chapters present theoretically derived research programs. Social role theory (Eagly, Wood, & Johannesen-Schmidt, Chapter 12), parent × child interaction theory (Pomerantz et al., Chapter 6), evolutionary psychological theory (Kenrick, Trost, & Sundie, Chapter 4), social cognitive theory (Bussey & Bandura, Chapter 5), and expectation states theory (Ridgeway & Bourg, Chapter 10) all constitute well-developed, empirically supported models of gender-related behavior.

Besides the greater salience of theory, this volume also places greater emphasis on biology than the previous edition (Beall & Sternberg, 1993). Three chapters stress biological processes (Hampson & Moffat, Chapter 3; Hines, Chapter 2; Kenrick et al., Chapter 4), whereas three others incorporate biological components into their models (e.g., Bussey & Bandura, Chapter 5; Eagly et al., Chapter 12; Pomerantz et al., Chapter 6). Previously, some gender psychologists were reluctant to incorporate biological aspects. The concern (to use the familiar refrain) was that biology signaled destiny, that is, the biological processes would be used to explain inequality between the sexes. Indeed, there is legitimacy in this concern, because biological explanations for psychological sex differences have been used to bolster unequal treatment of women (Bleier, 1984; Fausto-Sterling, 1985; Hubbard, 1989).

So why is biology more prevalent in this second edition, and in the psychology of gender generally? Partly it is because researchers now recognize that gender-correlated biological processes are flexible, and not fixed elements that explain the origins of sex differences (Rogers, 1999). Biological processes are now viewed as both effects and causes of gender-related behavior. For example, research shows that testosterone levels vary as a function of situation. Specifically, sports fans' testosterone levels increase when their team wins and decreases when their team loses (Bernhardt, Dabbs, Fielden, & Lutter, 1998).

In addition to the increased presence of theory and the greater inclusion of biology, this edition also provides more room for the concepts of power and status. The previous volume barely acknowledged the role of power, whereas several chapters are devoted to its explication in this second edition. Chapters on expectation states theory (Ridgeway &

Bourg, Chapter 10), social role theory (Eagly et al., Chapter 12), social constructivism (Marecek et al., Chapter 9), and a gendered power perspective (Pratto & Walker, Chapter 11) all address why men have more social, economic, and political power than women do. A recurrent theme is that equalization of power between men and women would have the effect of substantially reducing sex differences.

Politics in the Psychology of Gender

Politics has been present since the beginning of a psychology of gender. In the first edition of this volume, Beall and Sternberg (1993) observed that "few fields of study have such political overtones as the study of gender" (p. xix). Although political views affect all research programs, they are seldom explicitly acknowledged as such. The exception has been the psychology of gender, in which many psychologists have acknowledged their debt to feminist politics. Feminist politics, specifically a concern with dismantling sexist practices, generated the field that has come to be known as the psychology of gender. One might even argue that the psychology of women and gender would not exist as a distinct area were it not for feminism. The field began by challenging the notion that women are inherently inferior. Subsequently, responding to calls from feminists, psychologists took up social problems such as rape, domestic violence, and sexual harassment (Koss et al., 1994).

For many psychologists, the concern with gender centers on social issues. The American Psychological Association's involvement in the *Price Waterhouse v. Hopkins* sex discrimination case illustrates how a research basis can be used to influence important legal and policy issues (Fiske, Bersoff, Borgida, Deaux, & Heilman, 1991). When the Supreme Court heard this case, psychologists testified on the role of stereotypes and gender expectations. Hopkins eventually prevailed, in part because of input from psychological research. Research on rape by gender psychologists has also contributed to public policy. For example, Koss's congressional testimony on the factors affecting the incidence of and reactions to rape contributed to the passing of the Violence Against Women Act (Award for Distinguished Contribution, 2000).

This volume devotes rather little explicit attention to politics and social policy implications, although the social constructivist and gendered power perspectives are clear exceptions. The emphasis throughout this volume is on documenting new developments in basic theory and research. The authors have responded by describing the current state of knowledge in several topics. It might be the case, as Unger (1998) has argued, that a greater focus on theory building sometimes results in a decreased application of research to practical issues. Since the best policy and intervention recommendations come from a solid understanding of the processes and mechanisms involved, we look forward to subsequent descriptions of how research findings on topics such as those represented here might be put to use. Application may yet re-emerge as an important element in the field as its scientific credentials are acknowledged.

GENDER TERMS

In the history of the psychology of gender, terminology has been an area of disagreement among social scientists (Nicholson, 1994). Although some perceive language disputes as distracting, issues of wording are important to a complete psychology of gender. Terminology is important because inconsistently used or under-defined labels hamper the development of a coherent and cumulative body of work. Social constructivists go further by arguing that linguistic terms significantly construct and constrain what we know or think we know. Consequently, if language changes, so too does our understanding of the phenomena we study. For example, when people read about a "sex difference," they typically assume that it is more rooted in biology than one described as a "gender difference" (Pryzgoda & Chrisler, 2000).

The field known today as the psychology of gender began with no mention of gender—only sex. Sex was generally understood to mean identities rooted in bodily differences that were believed to significantly affect traits, abilities, and interests regarded as "masculine" or "feminine." The terms *gender* and *gender identity* were invented to describe individuals' outward manifestations of and attitudes toward their status as males or females (Hooker, 1993; Money, 1955; Stoller, 1964; Unger, 2001). Terms like *gender-typical* and *sex-identified* were coined to acknowledge variation in what the psychological attributes attributed to being male or female. The distinction between *sexual harassment* and *gender harassment* made in Chapter 11 of this volume points to two different kinds of hazards for working women. The former term stresses the kind of harassment that comes from sexual coercion, while the latter focuses on hostile working conditions imposed on people because they are deemed to be the wrong sex in a particular environment. All this expansion of terminology has the effect of alerting researchers to possible ideological and social structural underpinnings for the differences between males and females. In particular, it has allowed psychologists interested in changing male–female inequality to think about differences as part of a dynamic, socioculturally based gender system rather than simply a biologically based sex system.

New terms such as *gender role*, *sex-typical*, *sex-typed*, *gender performance*, *gender identity*, *sex category*, *sexual preference*, *biologically assigned sex*, and *sex-identifier* have also come to be used because of the need to recognize and investigate the increasingly complex domain subsumed by the psychology of gender (see West & Zimmerman, 1987). Terminology describing the concept of sexual orientation, specifically, lesbian, gay, bisexual, and transgendered people (LGBT), opened up new areas of research and theory on the relationships between and among sex, gender, and sexuality. Consider the term *transgendered*, which does not refer to lesbian, gay, or bisexual individuals, but rather to people whose appearance and/or sexual behavior runs contrary to their identification as male or female. For example, it can include cross-dressers as well as individuals who self-describe as "butch" or "fem."

In short, terms have developed in order to deal with the nonequivalence among sex, gender, and sexual orientation. The expanded vocabulary has in turn prompted questions about methodology and statistical analyses. For example, on what bases should we measure sex, gender, and sexuality? Eagly et al. (Chapter 12, this volume) use the concept "socially identified sex," which indicates that assessment of someone's "sex" usually draws on social appearances rather than some biological or physical criterion. Theoretical models, in turn, are articulating how sex, gender, and sexuality interrelate, as it is now clear that sex does not necessarily provide information about gender or sexuality.

This volume shows this diversity of new terminology, but—as in the field more generally—identical terms sometimes reflect different meanings, and different terms sometimes reflect similar usage. For example, some authors use *sex* and *gender* interchangeably to convey that they regard the association of sex with nature and gender with nurture as not yet determined. Others, while not explicitly saying so, appear to link *sex* differences with biological correlates and *gender* differences with sociocultural ones.

The *Publication Manual of the American Psychological Association* (2002) does not specify when authors are to use the term *sex* instead of *gender* and vice versa, but instructs investigators to "avoid ambiguity in sex identity or sex role by choosing nouns, pronouns, and adjectives that specifically describe participants" (p. 66). In the *Encyclopedia of Psychology*, Eagly (2000) argued that the labels *sex differences* and *gender differences* should both be considered correct, given that little consensus exists regarding distinctions between them.

We have examined terminological practices in this volume to see whether the various chapter authors have adopted a common language with respect to sex and gender. Because the volume is titled *The Psychology of Gender*, it is not surprising that the majority of chapters include the word *gender* in their titles. Does this mean that the authors deal primarily with sociocultural rather than biological mechanisms, as might be understood by readers not well initiated into the nuances of the field's terminology (Pryzgoda & Chrisler, 2000)? Clearly it does not. What does seem to be the case is that authors who stress biological variables tend to use *sex* more often than *gender*, while authors who stress social variables and explanations tend to employ *gender* more often than *sex*.

In our examination of this book's chapters, we counted four categories of terms. *Sex* terms and *gender* terms constituted two categories. For example, *sex-typed* was included in the *sex* category, and the adjective *gendered* was counted in the *gender* category. The third category, namely *sexual* terms, included words such as *sexual* and *sexuality*, and the fourth category comprised terms describing sexual orientation (e.g., *bisexual*, *lesbian*, *gay*, *heterosexual*, and *homosexual*). The *sexual* and *sexual orientation* language categories appear relatively infrequently in the book, so our analysis will focus primarily on the first two groups of terms.

Not surprisingly, the chapter on evolutionary theory (Kenrick et al., Chapter 4) and the two chapters describing hormonal processes (Hines, Chapter 2; Hampson & Moffat, Chapter 3) employ the greatest proportion of *sex* terms (60–80% of all terms used in our categories). In contrast, chapters with a more social contextual emphasis use proportionally more *gender* terms. The chapter on gender development by Bussey and Bandura (Chapter 5) uses gender terms most often, followed in turn by Gardner and Gabriel (Chapter 8), Bell (Chapter 7), Ridgeway and Bourg (Chapter 10), Best and Thomas (Chapter 13), and Pratto and Walker (Chapter 11) (59–89% of all terms in our categories). Interestingly, the chapters by Eagly et al. and Pomerantz et al. (Chapters 12 and 6, respectively), both of which explicitly incorporate both biological and social processes into their explanations, use equivalent proportions of *sex* terms (47% and 45%, respectively) and *gender* terms (52% and 50%, respectively). For example, in the Eagly et al. chapter (Chapter 12), comparisons between males and females are described as *sex* differences and the social environmental processes that moderate these are described in *gender* terms. Although most researchers in the psychology of gender now eschew the simple equation of *sex* with biology and *gender* with social context, readers of the literature still need to be alert to subtle associations implied by *sex* and *gender* terms. At least for the moment, we have no single term that clearly conveys the idea that both biology and social context are simultaneously implicated whenever gender matters are discussed.

We also took note of whether the authors of these chapters conceptualized sex and/or gender as binary and mutually exclusive. For example, in two chapters that used more *sex* category than *gender* category terms, namely, Chapter 4 on evolutionary theory and Chapter 3 on reproductive hormones, the authors also use the term *opposite sex*. This term clearly entails a view of sex as a dichotomous and mutually exclusive category. But to show that the use of sex does not always imply a dichotomous classification, Hines (Chapter 2) also uses *sex* frequently but introduces the idea of *intersexed* individuals, which by definition avoids implications of mutual exclusivity. Interestingly, most of the chapters that use a greater proportion of *gender* terms also construe gender as binary, despite the priority they give to social contextual influences. The exception is Chapter 7, which discusses current psychoanalytic theories of gender and in which Bell proposes a "multiplicity of genders."

As noted above, sexual orientation appears rarely in this volume, appearing to substantiate Kitzinger's (1994) claim that sexual orientation research constitutes a peripheral area within gender psychology (Kitzinger, 1994). For example, Kenrick et al. (Chapter 4) describe sex behavior in exclusively heterosexual terms, and some other word choices appear to reinforce a marginal status for non-heterosexual people. Hines (Chapter 2) uses the term *homosexual* against the advice of the American Psychological Association's publication manual, which recommends "gay men, lesbians, and bisexuals" as the more precise, less stigmatizing terms. Pratto and Walker (Chapter 11) follow the manual's recommended practice. Bell (Chapter 7) and Marecek et al. (Chapter 9) use the more political term, *queer*, which questions a simple heterosexual–homosexual dichotomy. The social constructivist chapter (Chapter 9), the one most preoccupied with terminology, uses the term *spectrum person* to convey the range, rather than the dichotomy, of sexual orientation.

As is probably evident by now, terminology is central to the understanding of the psychology of gender. This volume shows how the language has grown to keep pace with the ever-evolving set of constructs in the field. It also occasionally reveals an ambiguity in the use of some terms, which is similarly true of the field as a whole. Investigators and readers alike need to be attentive to the selection of terms because of their implied or indeterminate meanings.

EMPHASIZING SEX COMPARISONS

As noted earlier, the psychology of gender was once nearly synonymous with sex comparisons. In its most elementary form, this approach focuses on whether, and to what degree, the sexes differ or are similar in any number of psychological attributes such as hormonal responses, physical capabilities, cognitive faculties, personality traits, social inclinations, styles of communication, and so forth. Although there has been concerted movement away from simple sex comparisons, this volume shows that sex comparisons still tend to dominate the psychology of gender.

The focus on sex comparisons is so entrenched in the fabric of psychology that the subject area "human sex differences" generates over 50,000 citations just for work published since 1974. For many, this focus makes good sense and constitutes a much needed balancing of psychology's early subject matter, which for too long equated psychology as a whole with the psychology of men. A similar rebalancing is now under way in medicine. A recent report from the Institute of Medicine (2001), *Exploring the Biological Contributions to Human Health: Does Sex Matter?*, answered the question in the affirmative. Sex matters, specifically sex differences matter. According to the authors of this report, sex is a basic human variable. Because "every cell has a sex" and "the scientific importance of sex differences throughout the life span abounds," the authors state emphatically that effort should be directed at "understanding sex differences and determinants at the biological level" (p. 20). They recommend that sex be included in the design and analysis of "studies in all areas and at all levels of bio-medical and health related research" (2001, p. 20). From one viewpoint, this call to incorporate sex comparisons is laudable, because diseases and their treatments do sometimes vary depending on a person's sex. Nonetheless, the breadth of such a focus could inadvertently generate a whole new set of problems that we describe in more detail in the section entitled Problems with Sex Comparisons.

This volume also devotes considerable coverage to sex comparisons, although many chapters add important moderating factors to the mix. The kinds of comparisons can be roughly grouped into those that concentrate on showing that men and women have "different bodies," or that they encounter "different worlds," or that they are located in a social system that structurally affords men and women "different power and status."

Several chapters focus on the sexes having "different bodies," but the particular physical features being described vary greatly. Hines (Chapter 2) examines the influences of gonadal hormones on human brain development and behaviors such as childhood play preference and cognitive abilities. Hampson and Moffat (Chapter 3) review evidence pertaining to the idea that estrogen and androgen modulate cognitive functions in women and men, respectively. For Kenrick et al. (Chapter 4) a "different bodies" perspective takes the form of presenting the idea that the sexes possess different genetic endowments. Specifically, they argue that sex differences in aggressiveness, within-sex competition, and sexual behavior are the result of gradual changes in male and female genetics acquired over generations.

Authors of several other chapters emphasize the idea that males and females tend to encounter "different worlds." Chapters by Bussey and Bandura (Chapter 5) and by Pomerantz et al. (Chapter 6) contend that gender differentiation is the result of societal gender typing via the actions of parents, teachers, and peers, although the latter chapter shows how actions by children interact with those by parents to produce sex differences. Bell (Chapter 7) draws from a psychoanalytic perspective to show how people develop a gendered self in response to input from family members and other early caregivers. Eagly et al. (Chapter 12) explicitly contend that sex differences are the result of having different bodies and encountering different worlds. Different worlds show up in both distal environmental factors (e.g., sex-typed socialization) and proximal factors (occupational demands and self-regulatory processes) that impinge on the fact that males and females have different reproductive organs.

In both the "different bodies" and "different worlds" perspectives, the focus is on how individuals come with a gendered-self or develop one. Two chapters, Pratto and Walker (Chapter 11) and Ridgeway and Bourg (Chapter 10), begin with the observation that women and men are asigned to unequal *positions of power*. The "different positions-of-power" perspective stresses the idea that people have different expectations for males and females simply on the basis of sex determination. Such expectations result in different opportunities, evaluations, and behavior.

Problems with Sex Comparisons

The conspicuous weight given to sex comparisons in this volume is familiar to any psychologist who studies gender. Although many of the chapters approach sex comparisons in a more sophisticated way than has previously been the case in psychological approaches to gender, it is nonetheless useful to articulate some of the concerns that sex comparion approaches have spawned in general (Bem, 1993; Deaux & LaFrance, 1998; Kitzinger, 1994). First, critics argue that a focus on sex differences within the psychology of gender can obscure the much larger reality of overlap between the sexes.

Second, perspectives that emphasize sex comparisons sometimes overlook the dissimilarities within each sex. One consequence of this is the neglect of other individual differences that may matter a good deal more in predicting behavior (e.g., age, race, culture, social class, health, experience, and education). For example, a recent cross-cultural investigation of beliefs about love and romantic relationships found cultural differences matter a good deal more than do gender differences (Sprecher & Toro-Morn, 2002). In addition, studies that include other dimensions, along with sex, are commendable in that they allow us to evaluate the importance of sex differences and not just their existence. Statistical techniques such as meta-analyses aim to do just this.

Third, critics charge that concentrating on sex differences can produce gender polarization, which tends to force any psychological attribute into mutually exclusive male and female forms, with the result that the sexes are implicitly, if not explicitly, conceived as "opposites." As noted previously, two chapters in this volume employ the phrase *opposite sex*. Gardner and Gabriel (Chapter 8) make a distinction between two types of social interdependence and report that women rely more on relational aspects of the social self, whereas men evidence more group-based aspects of the social self. Although these are described as relative differences, it is rather easy to conclude, given the relative dearth of information about variability within and between the sexes, that males and females are consistently and largely different in their relational orientation. Our concern is that once the sexes are seen as dissimilar, the probability goes down that there will be interested in searching for within-sex variation and/or variability across contexts. Chapters by Eagly et al. (Chapter 12) on social role theory and Pratto and Walker (Chapter 11) on the bases of gendered power are useful counterexamples. Both deal explicitly with the effect of situational factors in moderating the size of sex differences in psychological behavior.

Despite the concerns we have described, several factors conspire to make sex differences a continued focus for psychologists interested in gender. Psychologists sometimes take their lead from cumulative wisdom about the extent to which women and men are born different or become so. In response, at least one psychologist has proposed relinquishing the study of sex differences altogether (Baumeister, 1988), although his interest has subsequently turned to how the sexes differ in sexual behavior (Baumeister, 2000; Baumeister, Catanese, & Vohs, 2001). Others counter that it is only by studying the sexes—sometimes finding few, weak, or no differences, and other times finding significant differences—that researchers will be persuaded to understand when and why the sexes differ, and not merely whether they do (Eagly, 1987).

A psychology of gender needs to be alert to complexities rather than polarities, as many chapters in this volume have done. On the methodological side, this entails heeding a number of suggestions: Reporting effect sizes when sex differences are described is essential. Hines (Chapter 2), for example, cites mean effects from others' meta-analyses. It means employing multiple-factor designs and looking for interactions with sex, as Best and Williams have done on the interactions of sex with culture in Chapter 13. Conceptually, it means considering sex as a process, as Pratto and Walker (Chapter 11) have done in their discussion of the interaction of sex with power. It means unpacking the constructs "male" and "female," as several chapters here have done, to determine what about them is predicted to be the cause or the result of other processes. Most crucially, it means *not* reducing the psychology of gender to a search for sex differences. To do so can conceal rather than reveal what is important about the gender and its psychological ramifications.

SEX AND OTHER SOCIAL CATEGORIES

Although the psychology of gender originally developed in response to psychology's male-centered bias, it soon became clear that the psychology of gender has also had its own problems of exclusion. Psychology of gender researchers have, until recently, largely ignored how gender interacts with race (Greene et al., 1997), sexual orientation (Rothblum & Cole, 1988), disability (Fine & Asch, 1988), and social class (Reid, 1993).

As outlined earlier, concentrating on sex differences and ignoring other group differences tends to obfuscate factors that may better explain many psychological phenomena. At the very least, examining differences among groups of women and men may help untangle the relative influence of sociocultural and biological factors on sex differences, because society exposes different groups to different experiences. For instance, white women do not experience sex discrimination in the same way as African American women, given that the former are privileged because of their skin color (MacIntosh, 1987). Similarly, sex discrimination likely takes different forms and has different effects depending on race, age, social class, and sexual orientation (Hurtado, 1992). In this volume, the expectation states approach (Ridgeway & Bourg, Chapter 10) and the gendered power approach (Pratto & Walker, Chapter 11) specifically combine other factors such as race, class, sexual orientation with gender processes. According to Marecek et al. (Chapter 9), the connections among biology, physical appearance, social roles, and sexual orientation may be neither stable nor universal.

Toward a More Inclusive Psychology of Gender

Although no psychologist, to our knowledge, explicitly disagrees with the contention that race, class, sexual orientation, and age matter in understanding the psychology of gender, research in the psychology of gender as a whole, and in this volume, is often conducted with samples of convenience. With the exception of research that requires "special" populations, such as women with congenital adrenal hyperplasia (Hines, Chapter 2) or international populations (Best and Thomas, Chapter 13) or children (Pomerantz et al., Chapter 6), college students are often the samples of choice. The problem is they tend to be more educated and literate, more financially secure, and more likely to speak English, even in countries outside the United States.

Consequently, we still know less about gender-related behavior among people who have low incomes or who are immigrants, middle-aged, or elderly. Even outside the United States, researchers use samples of convenience. See, for example, results described by Best and Thomas (Chapter 13), in which an international comparison used participants who attending college in their respective countries.

Samples of convenience in the study of gender-related behavior are a concern, then, because they are unique in a number of respects and may seem more typical and representative than they are and less in need of explanation (Miller, Taylor, & Buck, 1991). Other samples may seem distinctive or applied just because they are less familiar. In addition, research psychologists as a group may, like other scientists and professors, lack the "standpoint" of personal experience with diversity. At the least, this fact should prompt the exercise of care in interpreting results with nontypical samples. Interpretations of the meaning of gender-related behavior may vary with the group being studied; hence, members of the group in question should be consulted (Harding, 1991).

To address concerns about "standpoint," more diversity within academia at the undergraduate, graduate, and faculty levels is likely to bring different perspectives to psychological research on gender. Although it is not the responsibility of gay and lesbian, disabled, racial minority, and working-class investigators to initiate more research and knowledge on diverse groups, the heightened visibility of these individuals in psychology departments would make their identities and group issues more salient and familiar to psychologists.

CONCLUSIONS

Psychologists have discovered that sex and gender matter, and have made discernible inroads into describing when, how, and why that is the case. The chapters in this volume demonstrate how much the field has grown. It has expanded to include biological processes as well as sociological ones. It has become encompassing with respect to methodology and now actively entertains and tests sophisticated theoretical models.

The growth has been such that psychologists across the discipline are now more likely to incorporate gender issues into their research and applications, and gender psychologists are bringing the theories and methods of other areas to bear on gender questions.

This second edition of the *The Psychology of Gender* shows how varied and influential this field has become. Consequently, one suspects that it will be harder in the next edition to capture in a mere thirteen chapters what this volume has done.

REFERENCES

American Psychological Association. (2001). *Publication Manual of the American Psychological Association* (5th ed.). Washington, DC: Author.

Award for Distinguished Contribution to Research in Public Policy: Mary Koss. (2000). *American Psychologist, 55*, 1330–1332.

Banaji, M. (1993). The psychology of gender: A perspective on perspectives. In A. E. Beall & R. J. Sternberg (Eds.), *The psychology of gender* (pp. 251–273). New York: Guilford Press.

Baumeister, R. F. (1988). Should we stop studying sex differences altogether? *American Psychologist, 43*, 1092–1095.

Baumeister, R. F. (2000). Gender differences in erotic plasticity: The female sex drive as socially flexible and responsive. *Psychological Bulletin, 126*, 347–374.

Baumeister, R. F., Catanese, K. R., & Vohs, K. D. (2001). Is there a gender difference in strength of sex drive? Theoretical views, conceptual distinctions, and a review of relevent evidence. *Personality and Social Psychology Review, 5*, 242–273.

Beall, A. E., & Sternberg, R. J. (Eds.). (1993). *The psychology of gender.* New York: Guilford Press.

Bem, S. L. (1974). The measurement of psychological androgyny. *Journal of Consulting and Clinical Psychology, 42*, 155–162.

Bem, S. L. (1993). *The lenses of gender: Transforming the debate on sexual inequality.* New Haven, CT: Yale University Press.

Bernhardt, P. C., Dabbs, J. M., Fielden, J. A., & Lutter, C. D. (1998). Testosterone changes during vicarious experiences of winning and losing among fans at sporting events. *Physiology and Behavior, 65*, 59–62.

Bleier, R. (1984). *Science and gender: A critique of biology and its theories on women.* New York: Pergamon Press.

Crawford, M., & Marecek, J. (1989). Feminist theory, feminist psychology: A bibliography of epistemology, critical analysis, and applications. *Psychology of Women Quarterly, 13*, 477–491.

Crawford, M., & Unger, R. (1997). *Women and gender: a feminist psychology.* Philadelphia: Temple University Press.

Deaux, K., & LaFrance, M. (1998). Gender. In D. Gilbert, S. T. Fiske, & G. Lindzey (Eds.), *The handbook of social psychology* (4th ed.). New York: McGraw Hill.

Deaux, K. (1984). From individual differences to social categories: Analysis of a decade's research on gender. *American Psychologist, 39,* 105–116.

Eagly, A. H. (1987). Reporting sex differences. *American Psychologist, 42,* 756–757.

Eagly, A. H. (2000). Sex differences and gender differences. In A. Kazdin (Ed.), *Encyclopedia of psychology.* New York: Oxford University Press.

Fausto-Sterling, A. (1985). *Myths of gender: Biological theories about women and men.* New York: Basic Books.

Fine, M., & Asch, A. (1988). *Women with disabilities: Essays in psychology, culture, and politics.* Philadelphia: Temple University Press.

Fiske, S. T., Bersoff, D. N., Borgida, E., Deaux, K., & Heilman, M. (1991). Social science research on trial: Use of sex stereotyping research in *Price Waterhouse v. Hopkins. American Psychologist, 46,* 1049–1060.

Gilligan, C. (1984). *In a different voice: Psychological theory and women's development.* Cambridge, MA: Harvard University Press.

Greene, B., Sanchez-Hucles, J., Banks, M., Civish, G., Contratto, S., Griffith, J., et al. (1997). Diversity: Advancing an inclusive feminist psychology. In J. Worell & N. G. Johnson (Eds.), *Shaping the future of feminist psychology: Education, research, and practice* (pp. 173–202). Washington, DC: American Psychological Association.

Harding, S. (1991).*Who's science? Who's knowledge?* Ithaca, NY: Cornell University Press.

Hoffman, R. M., & Borders, L. D. (2001). Twenty-five years after the Bem Sex-Role Inventory: A reassessment and new issues regarding classification variability. *Measurement and Evaluation in Counseling and Development, 34,* 39–55.

Hooker, E. (1993). Reflections of a 40-year exploration: A scientific view on homosexuality. *American Psychologist, 48,* 450–453.

Horner, M. (1972). Toward an understanding of achievement-related conflicts in women. *Journal of Social Issues, 28,* 157–175.

Hubbard, R. (1989). *Politics of women's biology.* New Brunswick, NJ: Rutgers University Press.

Hurtado, A. (1989). Relating to privilege: Seduction and rejection in the subordination of white women and women of color. *Signs: Journal of Women in Culture and Society, 14,* 833–855.

Institute of Medicine. (2001). *Exploring the biological contributions to human health: Does sex matter?* Washington, DC: National Academy Press.

Kitzinger, C. (Ed.). (1994). Should psychologists study sex differences? *Feminism and Psychology, 4,* 501–546.

Koss, M. P., Goodman, L. A., Browne, A., Fitzgerald, L. F., Keita, G. P., & Russo, N. F. (1994). *No safe haven: Male violence against women at home, at work, and in the community.* Washington, DC: American Psychological Association.

McIntosh, P. (1998). White privilege: Unpacking the invisible knapsack. In M. McGoldrick (Ed.), *Re-visioning family therapy: Race, culture, and gender in clinical practice* (pp. 147–152). New York: Guilford Press.

Miller, D. T., Taylor, B., & Buck, M. L. (1991). Gender gaps: Who needs to be explained? *Journal of Personality and Social Psychology, 61*, 5–12.

Money, J. (1955). Hermaphroditism, gender and precocity in hyperadrenocorticism: Psychologic findings. *Bulletin of the Johns Hopkins Hospital, 96*, 253–264.

Nicholson, L. (1994). Interpreting gender. *Signs: Journal of Women in Culture and Society, 20*, 79–105.

Pryzgoda, J., & Chrisler, J. C. (2000). Definitions of gender and sex: The subtleties of meaning. *Sex Roles: A Journal of Research, 43*, 553–569.

Reid, P. T. (1993). Poor women in psychological research: Shut up and shut out. *Psychology of Women Quarterly, 17*, 133–150.

Rogers, L. (1999). *Sexing the brain.* London: Weidenfeld & Nicolson.

Sprecher, S., & Toro-Morn, M. (2002). A study of men and women from different sides of Earth to determine if men are from Mars and women are from Venus in their beliefs about love and romantic relationships. *Sex Roles: A Journal of Research, 46*, 131–147.

Stoller, R. J. (1964). The hermaphroditic identity of hermaphrodites. *Journal of Nervous and Mental Disease, 139*, 453–457.

Unger, R. (1998). *Resisting gender: Twenty-five years of feminist psychology.* Thousand Oaks, CA: Sage.

Unger, R. (2001). *Handbook of the psychology of women and gender.* New York: Wiley.

West, C., & Zimmerman, D. H. (1987). Doing gender. *Gender and Society, 1*, 125–151.

Author Index

Subject Index